The Psychology of Health Care

The Psychology of Health Care
A Humanistic Perspective

Jane E. Chapman, R.N., Ph.D.

Assistant Clinical Professor of Clinical Psychology
University of Colorado Health Sciences Center
Denver Colorado
Private Practice, Clinical and Consulting Psychology,
Denver, Colorado

Harry H. Chapman, Ph.D.

Police Psychologist,
City and County of Denver, Colorado
Private Practice, Clinical Psychology,
Denver, Colorado

W

Wadsworth Health Sciences
Monterey, California

Wadsworth Health Sciences
A Division of Wadsworth, Inc.

Printed in the United States of America

10   9   8   7   6   5   4   3   2   1

Library of Congress Cataloging in Publication Data

Chapman, Jane E., 1932-
    The psychology of health care.

    Bibliography: p.
    Includes index.
    1. Medical personnel and patient. 2. Medical person-
nel—Psychology. 3 Helping behavior.   I. Chapman,
Harry H., 1933-   . II. Title. [DNLM: 1. Attitude of
health personnel. 2. Quality of health care.
3. Attitude to health. 4. Humanism. 5. Delivery of
health care. W 84.1 C466p]
    R727.3.C46   1983   610.69′6   82-21873
    ISBN 0-534-01291-4

Subject Editor: James Keating
Manuscript Editor: Mary Anne Stewart
Production: Ron Newcomer & Associates, San Francisco, California
Interior Design: Ron Newcomer
Cover Design: Albert Burkhardt
Typesetting: Computer Typesetting Services, Inc.
Production Services Manager: Stacey C. Sawyer

We dedicate this book in special thankfulness to a great institution of learning—The University of Wisconsin. We consider this site to be our cradle of educational civilization because as students there, we were stimulated to think, to challenge, to struggle, and to grow. We were respected as persons in that complex system. It is our belief that, in health-care systems, no less can be given to either the helper or the receiver of intended helping.

Contents

Unit V
Humanistic Advocacy as Burnout Prevention   *193*

Preface

This text is concerned with certain aspects of health care that all students and professionals in the field struggle in common to understand: *their own behavior and that of others*. It is a text to be clinically applied, growing out of what we have perceived to be significant problematic issues that we, our patients, our peers, our many students, and their patients have repeatedly encountered: (1) coping with the frustrations of trying to become a productive, humanistic person in an occupation that is stressful, complex, and demanding of increased technological know-how; (2) troublesome patient behavior that seems to get in the way of helping; and (3) troublesome staff behaviors, as professionals from a variety of disciplines collectively attempt to bring a helping process to bear on the patient's situation.

An attempt to understand these problematic issues and to do something about them led to our study of patients', professionals', and students' views of their health-care experiences. From this study, we have evolved an approach to the helping process in health-care delivery that speaks to the needs of helpers, irrespective of discipline, and patients, irrespective of diagnosis.

Our approach to both understanding and carrying out the helping process is put forth in this text as an *advocacy model of humanistic helping*. This model provides helpers, whether beginners or advanced learners, with (1) a framework for evaluating the present health-care delivery system and (2) a method by which to identify more clearly helping roles and behaviors as they apply both to helpers and to their patients. Such a model stresses that *technologically oriented helping measures can be integrated with social/emotional helping approaches, with humanistic payoffs for both the patient and the helper.*

To accomplish an in-depth understanding of the need for and value of such a model, we have developed this text around a five-stage learning process:

UNIT 1: Contributions of behavioral science to health care
UNIT 2: Defining humanistic health care
UNIT 3: Conceptualizing a framework for analysis
UNIT 4: Applying the advocacy model to health care
UNIT 5: Humanistic advocacy as burnout prevention

To bring the written material to life, throughout the text we have relied heavily on real examples. These examples, referred to as *cases in point,* have been encountered by us and others in a variety of health-care experiences and settings, ranging from traditional hospitals, as stereotyped in television, to storefront clinics, mental-health centers, university counseling centers, home visits, or rapping in Joe's Buffet. The *cases in point* have been purposely selected to dramatize the fact that a defined humanistic helping process is essential, irrespective of where help is required or received. They also emphasize that the essential framework of a helping process is demanded of all health-care workers, no matter to which professional discipline they ascribe. Therefore, examples from the experiences of both aspiring and seasoned physicians, nurses, psychologists, physical therapists, and social workers have been included throughout the text.

Following each chapter, we have included a section of notes, references, and suggestions for further experience. The references are ones we have used to shape our thinking and to test our ideas. Many references are not from traditional health-care literature—an extension of our belief that health-care professionals have a tendency to deny the relevancy of the literature of other fields concerned with the human condition. We have also included reference notes to meet our need to digress from the rigors of developing an integrated text. We hope that our commentary provides not only useful guidelines but also a closer experience with our personal frame of reference:

In researching this book, we traveled back to some of the places where we started. The journey caused many moments of reflection on our own professional beginnings and appreciation for how much we had learned through others. Too many persons from a combined clinical experience of 40 years are involved to be mentioned individually. However, in our struggle to become humanistic clinicians who could yet allow for our culture's rich scientific knowledge, several persons have made unique contributions to our development: Ruth Adams, R.N., Albert J. Glass, M.D., William B. Lemmon, Ph.D., and Martha Stockwell, R.N.

We are grateful for the efforts of Emily Bornstein, M.S.W., Psy.D., Sylvia Lewis, R.N., Mary McAleenan, and Sonya Read, Ph.D., in assisting with the preparation of the manuscript. For valuable researching assistance our thanks go to Louise Leathers.

Jane E. Chapman
Harry H. Chapman

The Psychology of Health Care

Chapter 1

The Psychology of Health Care: An Introduction

During the era in which we grew up in the back areas of rural Wisconsin, one did not hear much about the concept of health care. There were frequent admonitions to "watch out" to stay safe, to "eat all your food" to be strong, and to "stay away from crowds" so as to not catch disease. One knew of doctors through occasions of disease or trauma or when a relative might have to go to the hospital because of impending death. Nurses were fantasy figures in white uniforms whom one heard about from grown-ups who visited people in hospitals. Social workers, identified only as being for those in economic crisis, seemed to have no relationship to health or disease. Psychologists were simply unknown.

With the rapid development of new knowledge and advanced technologies in the treatment of illness and the preservation of wellness, a complex system of health care has developed. Looking back some 40 years, one sees that there was initially considerable emphasis within the field on defining differences between the professions and what each uniquely offered. In the 1970s, health-care personnel began to speak to the professional commonalities that had lain unexplored within the system for some time. In the 1980s, one sees a more formal acceptance of interdisciplinary concepts and practice.

During this evolution within the health-care system, consumers of the system have also been changing. Through the advances of media and higher education of the public, consumers of health-care services have also become more knowledgeable. Sometimes there has been public confusion about health care's professional evolutions and occasional revolutions; sometimes one notes the public's relief at a long-awaited clarity about what the health-care field can and cannot offer. Overall, there has developed a vital, energizing interaction between the users of health-care knowledge and activity, whether they be patients, students, or seasoned practitioners. This text is about this human interaction.

In our examination of the interactive forces within the evolving health-care system, we have utilized a psychological approach. While the text may meet the criteria of a study of behaviors in relation to a particular field of knowledge and activity, the material frequently does not meet the criteria expected in an exact science, as contemporary psychology strives to be; for example, an exact science insists on concrete, empirical evidence and relies on direct, systematic observation and measurement of behaviors. Health care, however, is a dynamic human enterprise richly bound in a humanistic philosophy that asserts the worth of human life and the capacity of people for self-realization—factors that lend themselves poorly to psychology's present methods in the formal study of all facets of human experience.

In spite of these limitations, this text addresses: (1) a general view of the activity of health care; (2) a specific view of the helping process that is transacted within the helper/patient relationship; and (3) a framework for humanistic understanding and functioning within a yet-evolving complex system.

The Helping Process

In keeping with the interdisciplinary health-care-team approach to the helping process, we have developed a multidisciplinary text, using concepts that we believe fit with the similarities of role function repeatedly encountered in health-care settings irrespective of differences between professional disciplines. For example, throughout the book we collectively refer to any preprofessional or seasoned professional as a *helper.* This interdisciplinary term allows students of any profession—whether they be beginning or advanced learners—the means by which to identify and find common ground with their co-workers. We have also used the term *helper* to underscore a central fact of life about which health-care professionals often need reminding—*that the public comes into the health-care system for help.* This text assumes that, regardless of professional discipline, rank, or level of responsibility, those who work in the health-care field *are* helpers, either directly with patients or indirectly in ensuring effective help.

Something about the concept of help, however, baffles everyone concerned with health care. The consumers of health-care services—the patients—seem to believe that after a defined educational process, professionals should know what *helping* means and how it is accomplished. Patients also have expectations about what their experience with helpers should be like. Yet patients are often dissatisfied, as evidenced by their increasing use of advocates outside the health-care system to ensure safe, appropriate help within the system. For example, lawyers are increasingly sought to facilitate malpractice suits, and "Nader's Raiders" have become highly publicized as advocates for the consumer in health and welfare matters. With the spiraling economic inflation of the 1980s, we have also noted that patients are more articulate about wanting more for their money, thereby adding yet another pressure on helpers in under-funded systems.

Health-care professionals and students are often baffled about what the process of effective help involves. Surrounded by some of the most highly sophisticated technology that our world provides, some health-care workers have difficulty appreciating that the receiver of these products still wants something more. Others are keenly aware that something else is necessary to helping beyond buildings, beds, pills, or machines—but they do not know how to isolate that something or to provide it within the system. Some health-care workers attempt to identify their particular brand of help as specific techniques applied only to certain parts of the body; yet they too are increasingly faced with the recognition that some kind of process that involves the total ·person must simultaneously occur.

Patient advocacy   From what consumers and health-care workers are saying, obviously a middle ground of understanding is needed concerning the process of help as it applies to all disciplines and all patients, regardless of their presenting problems. Obviously some form of helping model is required that allows and encourages health-care workers within the delivery system to advocate actively for patients. The question is: What group within the system is willing and able to do something about this need? From our formal and informal observations,[1] we believe that budding advocates for an effective helping process within the health-care system may be found among the multi-disciplinary group of beginning health-care workers. Although we acknowledge the needed efforts of many fine seasoned professionals who have spent a lifetime expressing a humanitarian health-care philosophy, the real power to actualize human, advocacy-oriented health care seems to emanate from the emerging values with which the younger generation struggles.

Cultural values   The cultural values with which beginning students grapple are not readily seen since they are often embedded in expressions of frustration and dissatisfaction with aspects of the health-care system, but they are present. For example, our formal studies of multidisciplinary groups of health-care workers from medicine, nursing, physical therapy, and social work indicate that younger professionals and beginning students still seek out their respective occupations because they place high value on the helping of others. Over 99% of beginning students feel this way and have held this value strongly since early childhood. Yet their experience with actual patients in the clinical setting causes frustration as they attempt to find out how to help in ways that are personally satisfying. Their frustration results in criticism of instructors who are perceived to be "ungiving" and patients who are perceived to be "uncooperative."

The newer values that evolved from the "counterculture" campus movement of the 1960s[2] were and still are brought with the beginning clinical student into the health-care system. For example, those values that emphasize mutual interdependence and a sense of community in contrast to competition and individual achievement, are often reflected in student frustrations concerning overlapping roles, rigid hierarchies, or needing to play the "system game." Likewise, the increasing value placed by youth on direct experience, in contrast to detachment and objectivity, is often reflected in student dissatisfaction with the preclinical delay between theoretical, textbook know-how and the "real thing." This value also may be expressed in students' frustration in wanting to get more involved with patients, teachers, and peers in discussing the helping process, but feeling little system support to do so.

In the following chapters, we have attempted to present material related to experiential values that can be identified, evaluated, strengthened, and actualized within the health-care system. We hope to provide the student with:

1. Acknowledgement of and support for the long-held value of helping
2. An understanding of the difficulties of helping others in ways that provide mutual satisfaction
3. A way of evaluating the health-care system, patients, and oneself in determining the kind of helping process that any given situation requires
4. A way of building patient advocacy and a partnership with patients into the helping process.

Human behavior   At times it seems easier to look on a system as a "thing" and disavow human responsibility for its existence. However, any system is a vital composite of interrelating people whose attitudes, values, goals, and actions to accomplish those goals determine the character of that system. Because this book is about a system, it must be a book about human behavior. Unlike authors of a beginning psychology text, we do not assume that health-care students know nothing about behavior. We have attempted to build on the understanding of the world of behavior—both theoretical and personally experienced—that helpers as motivated, growing representatives of the human race bring with them into the system. We do believe, however, that beginning helpers need supportive reminders that they know more than they think they do and that they can put this valuable experience together with deeper meanings that they need to appreciate.

Our attempts to integrate what people already know with what they should appreciate more broadly may seem like we are talking out of both sides of our mouths from time to time. Particularly if one needs ultimate truths as neat solutions to complex situations, some portions of this book may be frustrating. However, human behavior, in spite of vast scientific and technological advances, remains a mysterious and elusive subject to discuss without reservations. In one situation, behavior seems to lend itself to study, control, generalization, and simplification, only to be resistive to the same generalizations in a similar but slightly different situation. Because of this characteristic of human behavior, a simplistic recipe book that implies generalization across all interpersonal situations would be immensely difficult—if not frankly dangerous—to write. At the same time, we challenge the notion that behavior must be relegated to the world of the occult and become an unknown variable in the helping process. Somewhere between further confusion, flying by the seat of the pants, and neat solutions, we believe that understanding of behavior can be clarified and applied in improving health care.

Overview

The book begins with a broad review of the present state of behavioral science and some relevant universal issues in the history of human behavior. Gradually the reader is carried into situations specific to the health-care field, in which more refined evaluations of behavior are required in understanding the helping process. Unit I, "Contributions of Behavioral Science to Health Care," reviews the several different ways that behavior has come to be categorized by the academic world but also embodies the way of viewing behavior that has worked best for us and our students. We are *integrationists* in that we believe that behavior is determined by many things, that it is a complexly organized product of emotional, social, and physiological processes occurring simultaneously within and without the human being. We also believe that emphasizing any one of these process variables indiscriminately in any given helping situation may be as detrimental as ignoring them completely. We are also *humanistic developmentalists* in our approach. We believe this categorical position is a broad, yet precise posture from which to evaluate, explain, and integrate the complex processes of internal behavioral experience. Such a posture also demands that one attend to the strengths and talents of people, as well as to their liabilities. It is a position that recognizes that people grow, that behavior can and does change over time, and that one can consciously modify one's direction in life—necessary conditions if a helping process is to have any meaning at all.

Unit I also presents considerable philosophical material concerning humankind in general. This content is included in such a preliminary position as a reminder that all of us are historically and universally a greater part of humanity than our narrow perception of ourselves and our life's work might fool us into believing. This material should sensitize those in the health-care field to the fact of their being in an existential area of endeavor, whether or not they wish to recognize it. People do care how they live or die; those committed to health-care occupations must appreciate that those who seek help are trying to work out greater issues having to do with the quality of life.

The ability to evaluate is given considerable emphasis in Unit I. We hold that realistic evaluation of oneself and one's situation is a critical ability that both helpers and patients must employ as they solve problems and develop creative solutions to stressful life situations. Overall this unit is a reminder that helpers of the many disciplines must be concerned with interrelated global issues of philosophy, sociology, and psychology as well as physiology if they seriously intend to understand people.

Unit II, "Defining Humanistic Health Care," has a more specific sensitizing message. It concerns how we, among others, view the present state of the health-care field and some characteristics that contribute to stereotypes, misunderstandings, frustrations, and dehumanization. In Chapter 4, "Humanism and Health-Care Delivery," we take the position that failure of health-care clinicians and researchers to attend rationally to the general process of helping has led to dehumanizing practices that affect patients and caregivers. At the risk of inducing guilt in those already established in the professions, this material speaks to our belief that newcomers into the system— whether consumers or students—often bear the brunt of confused goal directions and inconsistent role behaviors of the "old hands" that they encounter. Tragically, such circumstances contribute to overlooking or devaluing patients and students as a rich source of data about their priorities and capacities to change "the system."

However, this unit does not just snap at the heels of the health-care system and run. It also proposes that something can be done about mobilizing the rich resources within the field, defining humanistic goals, and evolving a structure for a helping process relevant in all heath-care situations. A defined *interpersonal* humanistic helping model is introduced, together with an examination of the critical factors—the setting, the patient, and the helper—that influence the potential for its development and implementation. In examining the impact of this triad of interrelating factors, we focus on the nature of helpers as much as on that of the patients. Highlighted are those aspects of the person of the health-care worker that seem to have the most impact on the capacity to initiate and maintain a helpful relationship.

Because a shotgun approach is all too easy to take in trying to arrive at a better understanding of oneself and others, we thought it important to provide the reader with some kind of structure within which we organize our beliefs and suggestions about humanistic helping. Therefore, in Unit III, "Conceptualizing a Framework for Analysis," we introduce such a structure. In discriminating professional from intuitive helping, the *framework for analysis* can assist helpers to determine what is relevant in any given situation. For those who have found the term *helper* too diffuse, within this unit we sharpen terminology. We propose that utilization of the *advocacy* concept in analyzing the helping process gives health care workers a newfound ability to specify their functions in words and actions that make sense to themselves and to their patients. We detail how, as a health-care *advocate*, a professional helper (1) relies heavily on evaluative functions to determine humanistic goals with patients and co-workers, (2) more succinctly determines what kind of behavioral science input is necessary in any given health-care situation, (3) orders helping actions that are tied to mutual goals, and (4) determines whether the helping process was effective.

Also in Unit III, we introduce one aspect of the framework for analysis that becomes a major emphasis for the remainder of the text: a new set of dimensions by which health-care advocates can evaluate and relabel the primary themes of the setting within which they work and various situations occurring within these settings. These dimensions are (1) *the life-saving dimension,* (2) *the life-sustaining dimension,* and (3) *the life-enhancing dimension.* The final pages of this unit review the characteristics of these dimensions so that the reader can readily appraise the degree of technological expertise and social/emotional behavioral science input that any specific helping situation may require.

Unit IV, "Applying the Advocacy Model to Health Care," discusses the framework-for-analysis material introduced in Unit III. The life-saving, life-sustaining, and life-enhancing dimensions are examined in depth within the context of how they might be utilized in real situations. Because of the many fine texts already available concerning reactions to stress and clinically observed disease syndromes, we by no means attempt to cover these areas comprehensively. What seemed most critical were the situations most commonly encountered, the behavioral approaches most applicable to these situations, and guidelines as to when and how in-depth knowledge might be obtained.

Unit V, "Humanistic Advocacy as Burnout Prevention," is concerned with the phenomenon of burnout. We acknowledge that the concept has become a generalized one in American culture, implying a multitude of negative responses to all work situations. However, among the professionals who have attended workshops on stress, health-care workers seem to know exactly what burnout is in the helping professions. What to do about the syndrome is less precisely understood.

Within this unit, we treat the burnout phenomenon as a stress reaction. We help the reader to be somewhat more discriminating about the concept by presenting two ways of evaluating it: (1) existential burnout as a social/cultural phenomenon and (2) professional burnout as a job-related stress reaction. For beginning and seasoned helpers, burnout is experienced as a compounded stress reaction, a conglomerate of three interrelating factors: (1) stressors that the patient's needs and responses contribute, (2) stressors within the procedural and administrative system of any given health-care setting, and (3) stressors that helpers carry within them from their personal lives.

Throughout the text, much emphasis will be given to patient variables and setting variables. Within Unit V, the major thrust concerns those variables most reflective of the humanness of the helper. We propose that, if the individual helpers, administrators, and educators do not attend to the burnout phenomena prevalent among themselves, co-workers, and employees, humanistic advocacy will break down or become impossible to accomplish. Helpers need to know how to help themselves before they can help others or model adaptive behaviors.

Because we helpers are human beings with much in common with other people, we fall victim like anyone else to boredom stressors, frustration stressors, threat stressors, performance stressors, and so on. Within each of these categories of stressors, we have shared some specific techniques and approaches that are helpful in reducing the negative, deleterious effects of stress and in adapting more optimally. Our workshop experiences have taught us that helpers who attend to their own stress reactions and become skilled in using techniques to manage their own lives effectively are more aware of stress overload in others and are quicker to share stress-reducing approaches with co-workers and patients.

Chapter 11, "Professional Burnout," is a specific challenge to students and educators in the various health-care disciplines. It has seemed to us that the seeds of professional burnout are activated in the early years of clinical education—particularly when educational settings fail to be simultaneously concerned with students' needs to sustain and potentiate personal growth as full human beings. To put our premise into perspective, we have looked at the growth of the professional from preclinical days through the period of becoming a reflective, seasoned helper. Thus we have presented our analysis of surveys and interviews with helpers of all ages as they are personally affected by (1) the culture at large, (2) their educational experience, and (3) the health-care culture, as they attempt to grow and develop within its boundaries over the years. Using a developmental approach to this analysis, we have emphasized that the several "critical periods" of high stress are (1) the period when those who seek to be professional transcend undifferentiated studenthood and must integrate "who they think they are" with what their professional mentors or patients "think they should be," (2) the period when the helper discards student, intern, or resident status and enters a more autonomous occupational world, and (3) the period in the middle years when, on the surface, life seems worked out but uncertainty of goal and function reappears.

We initially focus our attention in Chapter 12 on the beginning student who is just starting clinical practice. It is difficult enough to define oneself as both adult and student and live comfortably in our contemporary culture. It is not easy simultaneously to become a professional in a field that carries heavy responsibility for how others qualitatively experience life or death. We hope that we have not been too harsh on health-care educators in our emphasis on the expressions and analysis of the dilemmas of the preclinical student or beginning professional; but we believe that beginning helpers are truly the hope of the future, and our experience strongly suggests that failure to be responsive to the growth struggles of beginners can only perpetuate burnout stressors and dehumanizing attitudes in health-care practice.

In putting forth our formulations about students' frustrations with their educational experience, we rely heavily on our belief that effective learning occurs in large measure within an interpersonal process. We therefore analyze student/educator dilemmas as they are affected by relations with each other and note how these relationships—or their lack—affect the learning of a desired interpersonal helping process.

In our analysis of student/educator relationships, we trust that educators will perceive the empathy that we have tried to convey as they experience generation gaps between themselves and beginners. A significant shift in values has occurred between the generations over the past ten years and there often can be high stress in the communication gap that this shift creates. Also there appear to be some changes in people's "natural abilities." For example, the older generation seems to have some internalized skills available to them that are lacking in beginners of today. Our experiential and survey data strongly suggest that well-functioning older professionals have more evaluative, critical judgment ability available to them than does the younger generation of students. In contrast, we view "now" students as being least practiced in natural evaluative abilities when they enter the field. We share a concern that, in addition, the concept of evaluation is negatively viewed by them.

We do not believe that the internalized evaluative abilities of the older helper came from professional education or professional experience alone. Rather, we suggest that the era in which older helpers experienced their preclinical growth and development stimulated and required them to use these natural abilities in great measure in daily life. Evaluative abilities were more necessary and more valued in a less technological world. We propose that, in understanding and meeting the needs of the present-day student, educators and students alike must recognize that, in the recent past, the young have experienced their critical development during an era when the need to rely on human evaluative abilities has increasingly diminished.

Summary

Throughout the text, in varying ways, we stress that a well-honed ability to evaluate is one of the most highly valued capacities of helpers in the health-care field; but we emphasize that how evaluation is done and the value context within which it is carried out are the crux of the matter. In the health-care field, our vast technology in the form of sophisticated tests, computerized data, and drug and equipment treatments are fantastic adjuncts to thinking through and solving problems emanating from stress and disease. However, the human imput in the form of determining life goals, integrating outside resources, and evaluating what enhances the humanity of oneself and others is still the real power in the helping process.

We believe that older professionals and the younger generation of health-care students can come together. We believe that technology and traditional abilities and values may be combined with evolving humanistic values in a definable visible helping process that will give patients what they say they want. Helping students integrate technology with psychosocial factors to advocate actively for human rights in any helper-patient situation is what this text is all about.

REFERENCE NOTES

1. One of us (J. C.) began a diary of people experiences as a nursing student at the University of Wisconsin in the 1950s. Both of us have kept anecdotal records of patient, faculty, and student interactions during our graduate work at the University of Washington and the University of Oklahoma. Such diaries are not only helpful in later research work but also are immensely useful in looking back on one's own changes, as well as constancy. In our formal survey work, we are indebted to the participation of multidisciplinary faculty and students from the University of Oklahoma, the University of Missouri (Columbia), the University of Colorado Health Sciences Center, and its affiliated facility the John F. Kennedy Child Development Center. In addition to the formal survey data provided, we are most appreciative and respectful of those students and faculty whom we personally interviewed. They were willing to spend hours "letting down" and trusting us with their hopes, goals, anger, and fears.

2. A suggestion for required reading is Daniel Yankelovich, "Counterculture vs. Conservatism," *The Lamp* 54, No. 4 (1972): 8–11. Yankelovich sees a period of social conflict ahead, even though college campuses are misleadingly quiet and students have turned inward, paying attention to their private lives. He believes that the youth movement has a hidden meaning, a generalization made from his comprehensive survey data. Three themes emerge from these data: (1) students espousing new values emphasize mutual interdependence, pushing competition, individual achievement, and pursuit of personal success into the background; (2) a higher value is placed on sensory experience than on conceptual knowledge, with involvement preferred to detachment and objectivity; and (3) the counterculture of youth stresses the sacred in nature, seeking harmony with it, rather than mastery over it. See also Yankelovich's *The New Morality: A Profile of American Youth in the Seventies* (New York: McGraw-Hill, 1974) and *New Rules in American Life: Searching for Self-fulfillment in A World Turned Upside Down* (New York: Random House, 1981). A superb adaptation of this book can be found in *Psychology Today* 15, no. 4 (April 1981): 35–91.

Contributions of Behavioral Science to Health Care

Chapter 2

Behavior: Knowns and Unknowns

Behavior may be simply defined as "anything that something living does." Yet behavior is a complicated process. It goes on within and around people every second, whether they are aware of it or not. Behavior is orderly and rather predictable as it occurs in plant and animal life. Human behavior, however, is predictable in some forms and extremely unpredictable in others.

Because of the many similarities between humans, no matter how many millions of them are compared, the temptation is to lump them together and make sweeping generalizations. For example, the human fetus behaves in predictable, determined patterns of growth. When something goes amiss in this patterning, the fetus is said to be born with some form of developmental deviation. It is also well documented that consistently expressed, predictable patterns of growth and development continue from infancy through old age. Human beings are also predictable in that internally and externally they all look essentially the same. Their external features and internal organs are expected to be in specified positions and to carry out predetermined functions. Humans also have in common mechanisms by which to communicate vocally and a range of expressive emotions of which all are capable.

Yet just about the time that one becomes comfortable with the fact of commonalities and predictabilities, one must face the fact of vast individual differences. Interestingly, most of these differences can be traced back to another characteristic that all humans have in common: the central and peripheral nervous systems. Of course, all humans have internal and external individual differences, such as size, sex, skin color, or arrangement of facial features; but, in the whole scheme of life, these are subtle compared with the highly significant individual differences that emerge out of the function of the brain, which gives the ability to perceive, to think, to feel, and to express oneself verbally and motorically in unique ways. Predictably, humans group into familiar attachments known as cultures or subcultures, in which certain thoughts, feelings and actions are shared and valued in common.[1] Often these commonalities are referred to as norms, but, even within these groups, the notion of individuality exists. Sometimes the sensation of one's individuality is not felt. The fantastic nervous system, integrated within and in tune with the "out there" world, aids people by carrying out many physiological and social/emotional functions without their awareness; but, simultaneously, this same system allows them to consciously experience themselves both internally and externally so that they feel they are individuals and can make choices about their movement through life.[2]

So, in many respects, human beings are pretty much alike.[3] In other respects, they are individually unique. Basically this paradox can be exemplified in considering the neighbor across the courtyard who is in her third trimester of pregnancy and can be expected to be pregnant just so long. The infant is already one sex or the other. Genetically there are fairly well determined probabilities as to the child's skin color, color of eyes, and eventual stature. When the child is born, it will weigh within a certain range, and the attending physician already has a fairly good estimate of what that will be. The temperament of the child, however, together with the specific emotions that the parents will experience in response to the presence and behavior of a firstborn, are highly unpredictable. The parents may, at this point, verbalize that they want to raise the child in a certain way, but the reality experience of the child will interact uniquely with parental attitudes and beliefs, making what will occur in fact unpredictable at this point. Most certainly, the interaction of the family will be specific to them, even though a first child is not a unique phenomenon throughout the population.

The Dilemma of Behavioral Scientists

Human behavior is also complicated because in its entirety it is difficult to study, to measure, and to report in the succinct ways of technical science. In deciphering and measuring certain aspects of behavior—particularly physiological growth and development—considerable headway has been made through the advances of the chemistries and electronics. From a piecemeal laboratory and case-study approach, much is known about the behavior of muscular and neural tissue at various ages and under varying conditions, as inferred from electrical impulses recorded on a graph. The cellular and biochemical character of the liquid contents of a human being is also known. By putting these bits and pieces of gradually obtained technical measurement together with gross examination of the body internally and externally, the notion of interrelating physiological systems has been arrived at.

Through the development of statistical measurement[4] and analytical techniques, quantitative data that are beyond the scope of individual experience may be better understood. From the orderliness that a statistical approach requires and the rules that govern its use, one can make generalizations with a greater degree of certainty than an educated guess would supply. For example, statistics are highly useful in grasping a clearer picture of the incidence of disease, the utilization of certain health services, or how certain preceding incidents in the lives of persons relate to later occurrence of enhanced growth or defective development. Specific methods of statistical analysis are utilized in ferreting out interacting variables contributing to certain social behaviors or disease processes of groups. For example, the interaction of the variables of age, socioeconomic level, ethnic origins, diet, and stressors can be statistically analyzed in understanding the incidence of coronary disease. Statistical techniques can also be used in delineating which variables seem to hold the most weight in the interaction.

However, for those who rely only on objective technical measurement and statistical analysis as a means of understanding people, an impasse exists: *in science today, methods of measurement that capture all the behaviors of which human beings are capable do not exist.* For example, peoples' subjective internal experience of thought and feeling is also behavior, even though it cannot be objectively measured in the same manner as some physiological functions or disease processes.

Intrapsychic phenomena—one's highly personalized internal behavior, which is consciously or unconsciously experienced—are difficult to quantify. Self-report is a major avenue by which characteristics of this behavior can be obtained; but to put internal experience into straightforward language terms and to translate verbal language about thought and feeling into the symbols required as a part of a statistical analysis are difficult. Self-reports may also be biased by the experimental subjects' giving what they believe to be the desired responses.[5]

A recent article in *American Psychologist* humorously, yet seriously, focuses on the elusive search of science for laws of behavior. Following is a quip from a "conversation" between God and an earthling:

> GOD: You mistake the limitations of your imagination for limitation of the universe.
> EARTHLING: You mean you have not imposed laws on the universe?
> GOD: That is for Me alone to know. For yourself, the existence of natural laws cannot be established empirically owing to (a) the lack of precision in measuring instruments, and (b) your lack of free access to the time dimension. What pass for laws in the sciences are inventions—human artifacts.
> EARTHLING: Anyway, perhaps that is just as well for science—since according to your friend Saint Augustine, the existence of a law implies the existence of a lawmaker. And currently science is disinclined to admit of a lawmaker.[6]

Some researchers of human function resolve the dilemma in attempting to measure and analyze behavior by simply disregarding those behaviors that cannot be observed. Others attempt to study and measure these unseen behaviors by imitating the scientific tradition, which broke through the biological mysteries to provide general principles. For example, objective techniques to study and infer *intelligence, learning, emotions, personality, self-concept,* and *cognitive styles* have been developed. Through the objective approach, much has been learned about these concepts in general ways, but tests to measure these behaviors often hold up poorly in capturing the meaning and variability of human thought and feeling; that is, they must be used with caution in evaluating an individual in one set of circumstances and applying the results to another instance. As yet, no one is entirely certain what some of these concepts mean literally or how to represent them in symbolic statistical terms.

One also must acknowledge that simply measuring physiological function on one side of the behavioral ledger and social/emotional function on the other and adding them together inadequately captures the nature of human behavior. The most complicated behavior emerges from a complex of conscious and unconscious interactions of mind and body that are experienced by the person as a unity. A great deal is learned about human function by studying parts, but one understands people by attempting to grasp their total function. Methodology does not yet come close to measuring and understanding the complexity of the interrelated automatic and voluntary functions involving physiological, social, and psychological systems.

Thus arises the dilemma of the behavioral scientists, who want human beings to stand still long enough to capture the nature of human behavior. Within the field of behavioral science, arguments are prevalent about predictability versus unpredictability, the uniqueness of a person versus commonalities, parts of behavior versus interrelating systems, and objective, technical methods of learning about individuals versus subjective, intrapersonal methods.

Formal Positions of Behavioral Scientists

Those who formally study behavior tend to take one of several views about their subject and the research approaches to be taken.[7] No two behavioral scientists may believe or function exactly alike, even though they may share a smiliar orientation about human behavior and the research approaches to be taken. However, the formal positions assumed by those in the general field of human behavior have certain identifiable features.

One group is referred to as *behaviorists.* Their position tends to the belief that the human being is ultimately predictable. They champion the view that objective, value-free methods of science applied to observable (measurable) behavior come closer to truth in general laws governing human behavior than do subjective, personalized experiences. Skinner, a well-known proponent of the behavioristic position, commented 20 years ago, "The intuitive wisdom of the old-style diagnostician has largely been replaced by the analytical procedures of the clinic, just as scientific analysis of behavior will eventually replace the personal interpretation of unique instances."[8] *Behaviorists* tend to study behavior in a reductionistic, piecemeal fashion similar to that used by early biological scientists; that is, selected aspects of human behavior are studied in absolute terms. The human experience of awareness or of varying states of consciousness tends to be disregarded in formal study. Because of the behaviorists' highly objective approach to the study of behavior, the information gained about behavior is generally presented in quantitative terms.

On the other hand, the behavioral scientists referred to as *phenomenologists* tend to view behavior in a holistic fashion, seeing the human as an integrated being whose behavior is understandable only in relation to other variables. In other words, internal events as well as external sociocultural factors are acknowledged to influence human behavior. Those who hold to the phenomenological view of behavior give value to the subjective expression of experience and to human beings' enduring concern with existence. Because of this highly experiential approach to behavior, the information gained about behavior is presented in more subjective terms. This group believes that human beings are predictable in certain ways, but that human internal capacities and subjective experiences may preclude knowing human beings as total entities. Fromm, a representative of this position who believed that the human aspects of individuals are an unfathomable secret to them and to others wrote, "The further we reach into the depth of our being, or someone else's being, the more the goal of knowledge eludes us. Yet we cannot help desiring to penetrate into the secret of man's soul, into the innermost nucleus which is 'he.' "[9]

Emerging from these controversies is the concept of *humanistic psychology*.[10] Primarily influenced by the phenomenologists, humanistic psychology developed in America under the influence of William James. Within this tradition are found many persons who are concerned with behavior as experienced in real life. For example, the humanistic position is particularly appealing to practicing clinicians. Those who work daily with the dilemmas of a variety of people find that an extreme theoretical view of behavior does not hold up well and that human experience falls somewhere between the behavioral and phenomenological views of human behavior.

The practicing clinician is pressed to use every means available to further problem solving and understanding, regardless of the specific philosophy held by those from whom answers come. Humanistic psychology is empathetic to helpers in real life and acknowledges both the usefulness and the limitations of our presently known objective scientific methods in the study of humanity. For example, humanistic psychology is concerned with what is missed in human understanding and with the dehumanizing attitudes developed when people are studied in a piecemeal fashion and subjective feelings are discarded. Essentially, humanistic psychology views people as persons rather than as animals or machines. Child explains the views of humanistic psychology as follows:

> Man is a conscious agent; that is the starting point. He experiences, he decides, he acts. If there are conditions under which man can be usefully looked at entirely from the outside, as responding to external stimulation with the regular predictability of a machine, a mechanical model may be useful for those conditions. But humanistic psychology

starts with the presumption that such conditions are special cases, that to build the whole of psychology on them would mean an impoverishment of psychology, a restriction that would prevent its general application to the understanding of man.[11]

As with the phenomenologists, holistic *gestalt principles* are also accepted by humanistic psychologists. The gestalt view is that the whole is different from the mere sum of its parts and that the whole can never be understood from a study of its parts. In human behavioral terms, this view would maintain that human nature is (1) organized into patterns or wholes, (2) experienced by the person in these terms, and (3) able to be understood only as a function of the patterns or wholes of which it is made. This implies that behavior is an *interrelated* process system—a process unable to be understood by looking at its "pieces." It is similar to trying to understand why a professional football team loses a game by talking to one player.

The Task Confronting Health-Care Workers

Throughout this text, the basic views of humanistic psychology are integrated. Our emphasis is on health-care workers and patients as persons and their interrelationship in the settings in which they work together. Our concern about individuals is not simply with their externally observed behavior in bits and pieces. Humanistic understanding of behavior involves the human as an integrated being, having the capacity to think, feel, evaluate, solve problems, and assume responsibility for the self and others. It also involves human efforts to stay alive, to discover self-meaning, and to actualize yet-undiscovered abilities.

A humanistic approach seems to have the most meaning to health-care workers in our experience. It offers a view of human behavior and recognition of the everyday circumstances of living that is more akin to what one experiences in health-care settings. For example, the everyday life in health-care settings is different from that in the behavioral scientist's laboratory. Helpers are aware of the differences. Perhaps this awareness is why psychology and sociology texts as well as introductory courses based entirely on experimental laboratory results often have so little meaning to health-care students. As we shall discuss in depth, health-care workers early hold a desire to help, but, as the reality of clinical experience dawns, they quickly appreciate that they have little choice as to who comes through the front door for help or as to whom they may be assigned to care for. "Experimental subjects" cannot be selected, and helpers do not perceive themselves as highly disciplined researchers.

Health-care workers also know that people seek them out because of some kind of problem or because they are motivated to prevent a problem from occurring. A researcher does not need to be concerned about the "human condition" to understand an isolated bit of behavior; but, presumably, health-care workers are concerned about the quality of human existence, that is, the status of a person's health and well-being as these relate to physical and social/emotional factors. Unlike the behavioral-science or physiological researcher concerned with understanding behavior per se, the health-care worker has a more complex task. *The task of the helper is to attempt to understand persons as whole individuals and to do this humanistically within the context of the environment in which help is sought.*

In undertaking this task, health-care workers are required to become highly discriminating; that is, they must acknowledge and welcome the contributions of scientists, but they also must use new knowledge wisely—particularly in appreciating the value and limits of statistical group data about persons or events. Two of the common misuses of group data are (1) stereotyping a person and (2) overlooking how individuals uniquely differ from the group of which they are presumed to be a part. The following interview material from a helper dramatizes a heath-care team's misuse of group data concerning Native American culture.

CASE IN POINT

Maria was brought to the medical center because she seemed to "not be learning right." As a result of an evaluation elsewhere, with which Maria's parents were not happy, they became aware of her epilepsy and learned that her neurological difficulty was caused by a disease that would inevitably be fatal in several years, no matter what was done. The staff at our center immediately developed high sensitivity to this family's being "special," since they were urban Navajo and had a child soon to die. The staff did not know much about the Navajo people and assumed that perhaps the other evaluation center had not fully appreciated that particular culture.

The staff became enthusiastic about formal review of the literature on the Navajo culture[12] and a large workshop conference was held on religious medicine of Native American culture in general and the practices of the Navajos in particular. Native American participants conferred with us, as did several staff members who had worked on an Arizona Navajo reservation. The in-service experience was excellent, and we factually learned much about the Navajo people.

It was a doubled-edged experience, however. Many assumptions we had made about this family went by the wayside, since we now "knew" about Navajos; yet it became clear as we talked enthusiastically about applying our newfound knowledge that we were making new assumptions that tended to perceive the family as a group like "all Navajos." We knew that we had not fallen into the trap of consigning them into Anglo culture. Neither did we feel that we were failing to be "culture conscious." But something was wrong.

Only after we had reflected on why this family had come to us and had begun to struggle with what kinds of helping action they wanted did we realize that we did not have much detail about these particular parents' notion of help, regardless of culture. We retracked with them. Our first surprise was that, although they originally came "from the reservation," they knew less about Navajo culture factually than we did. They both had been separated from their parents at 5 years of age and had spent most of their lives in government schools. They related in an embarrassed fashion that they believed that they knew little of either the Anglo or Navajo cultures. They were lost between two cultures.

They realized that Maria was not going to live a long time. Their anxiety was deep, and they had to cope with her impending death in their own way, but right now they could not live with her happily. She was an overactive, resistive, hard-to-manage child and would allow them to go nowhere without her. She was described as "ruling the roost." Yes, they wanted her to live and learn; but, in the immediate situation, they felt helpless and at a loss as to "how to raise her" or any other child whom they might have.

Another surprise was that they trusted us more than we had assumed. We knew that they periodically used their medicine man when they went back home. We had assumed that they trusted him more and perhaps would not hear us. However, when asked, they stated that they would not have come to us if they did not think we could help, that they could have gone back to the reservation for help anytime but chose not to with their immediate concerns.

In looking back on this experience, I sometimes wonder if we would not have saved a lot of time and have been more effective if right at the beginning we had simply said to them: "We don't know anything about you; we are different; let us spend some time in finding out about each other."

The foregoing example clearly demonstrates that, for a *general appreciation* and as a sensitization experience, data about groups of human beings can have usefulness. In the one-to-one situation requiring *understanding* of oneself and the other person, no greater accuracy is possible than that which can be attained by asking directly, listening, and checking each other out.[13] Assumptions based on literature—scientific or romantic—can lead to blind alleys in face-to-face relationships if they are not put into the proper perspective.

Summary

Health-care students need to appreciate the major arguments within the field of behavioral science. The positions held by clinical instructors and academic teachers will affect how they view human beings and how they elect to treat them in clinical practice. The polarized thinking and opposing theories with which behavioral scientists struggle include phenomenology versus behaviorism and behavioristic versus existential psychology.

The phenomenological model of the human being is on the existential side, more accepting of the notions of free will and the belief that the individual is more than one can ever know. The behavioristic model encompasses the more deterministic posture, seeing humans as predictable and knowable in scientific terms, and is more mechanistic in its approach. Medical science is of the more behavioristic mode, deriving most of its explanations from a scientific disease model. In this model, diseases are "real" and offer the astute observer a predictable course of events. However, if one observes what happens when disease participates with, rather than happens to, a person, a different set of circumstances may ensue. Not the least of the differences may be the different effect that the disease process takes by virtue of someone collaborating with the total person, in contrast to standing back and watching the person trying to confront disease alone.

The pages to follow will clearly show that understanding people, in contrast to understanding discrete aspects of behavior, is no easy task. This is a particularly difficult task for health-care workers because of certain attitudes prevalent within their work settings. In addition, preliminary to the understanding of any one patient is an appreciation of interrelating factors that may be operating within any given helping encounter: (1) the influence of traditional, science-based ways of doing things in the health-care disciplines, (2) the influence of the traditional way patients view health-care problems; (3) the influence of stress at the time that help is sought from health-care settings; and (4) the influence of a disease process on behavior.

All factors that influence the understanding of patients are important. Throughout the text, however, we emphasize the influence of the traditional way of doing things in health-care practice. In part, this emphasis is because, of all the interrelated factors that influence patients' behavior, the way health care is presented is one aspect that health-care workers can modify to reduce confusion. Helpers may not be able to do anything about the attitudes or the physical condition that patients intially present, but they can do something about the setting that patients enter and the responses to which they are subjected.

Because the health-care field has been drastically affected by technology, we challenge the side effects of contemporary science on human behavior. Yet, we emphasize that methods of objective science are highly useful in daily work. A reasonable humanistic position does not demand that scientific methods and generalizations about human functioning be discarded in the process of understanding the unique aspects of people, but a critical factor is missed in exclusively emphasizing so-called value-free scientific methods in diagnosing and treating individual patients. That critical element is the influence of *personal meaning* on behavior. As the seasoned, effective health-care worker comes to appreciate, *whatever people's behavior, it is always a function of highly personalized perceptions and deep meaning that exist for them within the context of what is happening inside and outside of themselves at the moment.* As Combs explains, "behavior, in and of itself, is nothing. It has significance only in terms of its meaning to the behaver and to the receiver."[14]

One who takes a humanistic position in understanding people therefore expects that the available scientific methods and general knowledge of human function will be used in such ways that the totality of a person's experience is taken into account in the process of evaluating and determining what is best for the other and oneself. This approach requires that health-care workers who are steeped in the influence of traditional science broaden their sights. It becomes important that they focus not just on traditional signs and symptoms that converge into a scientific disease-model diagnostic process. It means that additional behavioral concepts, such as attitudes, values, beliefs, potential, and self-concept, be given equal footing in any evaluative and helping interchange. It means that health-care workers must be willing to acknowledge their own human qualities and how these influence the behavior of others.

As will be presented in the following chapters, comprehensive humanistic understanding and responding to people involves multiple approaches. Many approaches to understanding will be highly subjective in nature and unique to any given situation, depending on the persons involved and the situation in which they encounter one another. In many situations, the personality style of the helper is both the primary evaluative and the primary therapeutic tool. In all situations, patients or their representatives or both are rich sources of information, subjective though it may be. After all, human beings were able to communicate meaningfully long before the onset of tests and mechanical evaluative measurement.

REFERENCE NOTES

1. Ethnic subgroupings are not discussed specifically or in depth within this text—but not to negate appreciation for cultural differences. Rather, our view is that cultural uniqueness is best appreciated by understanding that all humans have attitudes, beliefs, and values central to how they perceive the world. Making sweeping generalizations about Blacks, Chicanos, Native Americans, and other groups is not humanistically fair; neither is isolating subgroups because they are so different. Group identification can be so overemphasized that people are set apart from the human race. For a most comprehensive annotated bibliography regarding ethnicity, see Richard Kolm, ed., *Bibliography of Ethnicity and Ethnic Groups.* DHEW Publication no. HSM 73-9009 (Rockville, Md.: National Institute of Mental Health, Center for Studies of Metropolitan Problems, 1973).
2. Gustav Eckstein's *The Body Has a Head* (New York: Harper & Row, 1970) is a must for all beginning students. For those struggling with hard-core anatomy and physiology and how it interrelates with the mind, this book will give an exceedingly fine humanistic understanding. Dr. Eckstein, a teacher in medical schools for more than a generation, states, "The intent of this book is to make the human body more familiar to anyone who owns one" (p. xvii).
3. Bakan talks about one way of understanding people: "After all, we are all pretty much alike. And insofar as we are alike, we might be able to 'understand' one another by referring each other's expressions to our own experiences . . . ." See David Bakan, *On Method* (San Francisco, Jossey-Bass, 1968), p. 84.
4. The basic notions underlying the use of statistics have not changed much over the years. Choose a simplified edition for basic understanding—for example, Robert R. Pagano, *Understanding Statistics in the Behavioral Sciences* (St. Paul, Minn.: West, 1981).
5. Human experimental subjects do not deliberately lie. They may simply want to look good or be socially acceptable. Sometimes people will not reveal their real feelings because they are wary of the consequences of their revelations.
6. John Paull, "Laws of Behavior: Fact or Artifact?" *American Psychologist* 35 (1980): 1083.
7. An excellent book concerning the different views in behavioral science is Irvin L. Child's *Humanistic Psychology and the Research Tradition: Their Several Virtues* (New York: Wiley, 1973). See also William D. Hitt, "Two Models of Man," *American Psychologist* 24 (1969): 651–58. This article is an outstanding piece—concise and easily read. You are also strongly encouraged to read Frank Goble's *The Third Force* (New York: Pocket Books, 1971). This is the story of Abraham Maslow and his ability to walk between the arguments of the scientists and evolve an optimistic humanistic psychology that encompasses the best of both polarized positions.
8. B. F. Skinner, *Science and Human Behavior* (New York: Macmillan, 1960), p. 19.
9. Eric Fromm, *The Art of Loving* (New York: Harper & Bros., 1956), pp. 24–25.
10. A suggested required reading with this text is James F. T. Bugenthal, ed., *Challenges of Humanistic Psychology* (New York: McGraw-Hill, 1967). For beginning readings, see particularly Bugenthal's "The Challenge That Is Man," p. 5, and Charlotte Buhler, "Human Life as a Whole as a Central Subject of Humanistic Psychology," p. 83. See also Buhler's "Basic Theoretical Concepts of Humanistic Psychology," *American Psychologist* 26 (1971): 378–86. The bibliography at the end of the article is one of the finest.
11. Child, *Humanistic Psychology*, p. 15.
12. "Medicine" as integrated into religious, existential experience is unique in Native American culture, as well as within several fundamentalist religions that practice faith healing. Review of this

literature can sensitize one to what one does not know, thereby strengthening the need to share "not knowing" with those from other cultures who seek help. See Robert L. Bergman, "Navajo Medicine and Psychoanalysis," *Human Behavior*, July 1972, pp. 8-15, and "A School for Medicine Men," *American Journal of Psychiatry* 130 (1973): 663-66. Also see Virgil J. Vogel, *American Indian Medicine* (New York: Ballantine, 1973).

13. Scott Morris quotes Gordon Allport as having said, "If you want to know something about a person, why not first ask him?" *Psychology Today* 15, no. 7 (April 1971): 58. See also Gordon Allport, *The Use of Personal Documents in Psychological Science*. Bulletin no. 49 (New York: Social Sciences Research Council, 1942) and Richard I. Evans, *Gordon Allport: The Man and His Ideas* (New York: Dutton, 1971).

14. Arthur W. Combs, "Educational Accountability from a Humanistic Perspective," *Educational Researcher*, September 1973, p. 19.

Chapter 3

Some Universal Issues

In this chapter, we shall briefly explore three interrelated universal issues: *stress, existential anxiety,* and *evaluation.* We refer to these issues as "universal" since, to a major degree, all humans must deal with these issues if they are to maintain their mental and physical health. For example, people need to learn from early on how to recognize and deal effectively with stress in their daily lives. They need to be able to assess their living situations and to learn to value the evaluative processes that are uniquely theirs.[1] When evaluative skills do not produce ready answers to difficult life dilemmas, existential anxiety inevitably results. When existential anxiety occurs, people must learn to avoid the temptation of disregarding their evaluative abilities on the one hand and the temptation of seeking easy external solutions on the other.

All three universal issues are a part of the matrix of the life story that each patient seeking help brings to the professional. The helper's job is to recognize these issues as critical aspects of the biopsychosocial context that influences all illness, since any disorder can be viewed as negatively influencing the "mind/body" system.[2]

Throughout the text is integrated our profound belief in the patient as an essential element in the healing process. All three universal issues require consideration if the patient is to grasp the important role of self in the healing process and thereby gain a greater sense of mastery in coping with life conditions.

Stress

Stress may be defined as anything that requires the body to *change* or *adapt*. Although the term *stress* is frequently used to describe only toxic or negative states of pressure, tension, or frustration, a distinction must be made between normal stress and injurious stress. Since stress is any change to which the body must adapt, stress would include such a simple but necessary act as getting up each morning. Once this task is accomplished, the body adjusts, and the stress involved is rarely injurious to physical or emotional health. Thus it is said that some degree of stress is absolutely necessary for normal functioning and that each individual has optimal stress levels.

Life seems to have become more stressful over the generations. For example, in the anatomical/physiological sense, man stopped evolving 25,000 years ago.[3] People then were adapted to an environment that was largely plains and forests. They usually lived in small groups or bands with cooperative rather than aggressive or competitive interactional modes. There probably were no tribal leaders but rather a loosely knit cooperative unit in which food and tasks were shared. At the time, groups of these scattered bands existed in the Middle East, Africa, Europe, and Asia; perhaps only 2 million people existed on the entire earth, a number comparable to the population of metropolitan Denver.

If one keeps in mind that humans have not evolved further physiologically from the people adapted to the environment described above and then imagines them in the context of the modern world, one begins to realize how stressful contemporary culture is. The evolutionary process that has taken place in the last 25,000 years has been psychological and cultural rather than physical. We have the same inborn mechanisms for adaptation to stress as our ancestors, but these mechanisms are now called on much more frequently, used for longer periods of time, and applied to the solution of more complex problems than were faced by our ancient forebears.

Objective factors in stress   Although there is a general stress level to which all individuals can adapt, there are a number of objective circumstances in which stress becomes specifically detrimental to health. Coleman refers to the following stress factors as objective, since they "are relatively independent of the individual involved or the situational context in which the demand occurs."[4]

1. *Importance of the demand.* Death of a loved one, separation and divorce, and serious personal illness have ranked high on stress-rating scales since Holmes and Rahe's work in the sixties.[5]
2. *Duration of the demand.* Prolonged stress that is unresolved tends to affect people more negatively than temporary stress for which an end is in sight. Lazarus's research suggests that the major problems of life are deleterious to one's health only to the extent that they have enduring effects on day-to-day functioning.[6] For example, Lazarus points out that the death of a brother in a distant city would undoubtedly cause the usual grief reaction, but that the death of a business partner may have a more deleterious, enduring, here-and-now effect than the death of the brother. This

example also illustrates how duration of a demand significantly interacts with its importance.

3. *Multiplicity of demands.* Several major stressors occurring simultaneously, especially if they are of a compelling nature, are even more devastating than if they occurred singly. Even a number of minor stressors occurring simultaneously can have a powerful effect.

4. *Chronic ambiguity of demands.* Uncertainty or lack of definition of the adaptive demand negatively stresses most people since it is a basic need to have order, certainty, and coherence in one's life. Sometimes people have the mechanisms available to clarify stressful ambiguity, but any situation that defies understanding and precludes escape, particularly over long duration, will have deleterious effects.

5. *Strength of conflicting motives.* Decisions are relatively easy to make when one has little invested in the outcome. Situations in which any alternative in the decision process would lead to serious loss are perhaps the most stressful for people. Coleman discusses situations in which one alternative (such as marriage) seems highly positive, yet the ratio of losses and gains (as in a single versus a marital state) may pose high stress in the decision process.

6. *Imminence of expected demands.* Anxiety tends to become intense for people as they more closely approach their goals, particularly in those circumstances in which they must perform tasks that they dread.

7. *Unexpectedness of demands.* Severe stress occurs when an unanticipated event of major proportion occurs and the individual feels inadequate and unable to cope with the situation. Here it is the unexpectedness combined with the feeling of lack of preparation that affects people most severely.

Source of stress   To fully understand the concept of stress, we must be aware that there are three primary sources of stress, which are often interactive: our external environment; our body, or physiological makeup; and our thoughts, or psychological makeup. For example, as I write, my room is comfortably organized, but my environment otherwise is abominable. My neighbor is using a lawn edger, and the noise is extremely distracting and annoying. Since I cannot conveniently escape, my body and mind must adapt so I can write with appropriate focus. Over time, and particularly if the planes begin to come in low on their approach to the airport today, my adaptive mechanisms may fail in shutting out noise stressors from my conciousness. This failure may lead to intense frustration, which might linger as an irritant long past the termination of the noise. My task would then be disrupted not just by the external noises, but also by the subsequent internal feeling state set in motion by the initial stimuli.

Another example of environmental stress is that which comes from externally imposed performance expectations in our work, at school, or in our social roles. At optimal stress levels, performance demands contribute to positive motivational energy. When external performance standards become unrealistic, imposed demands become detrimental stressors.

Physiological stressors can have negative effects whenever we overtax our bodies through physical exercise, overeating, poor nutrition, or illness. Adolescence, when rapid growth spurts are common, is a time when many youngsters are highly stressed. Sleep disturbances, whether in terms of deficits or excesses, are other common negative stressors, particularly when these disorders become chronic.

The third source of major stressors is the way we perceive and think about ourselves and our world. The fact that this source of stress is almost always an intimate factor in any situation is what makes the definition of stress for another so subject to error or misinterpretation. It is because our personal assessment of our ability to cope with an event tends either to relax or negatively stress us that we hear the common phrase "What's one man's meat is another man's poison."

At the interpersonal level, one's unique meaning and sensitivity to others also greatly influence our perception of stress in any given situation. For example, if we see a spouse or loved one frowning, our reaction will be very different if we interpret that frown to mean we have done something personally "wrong" than if we interpret it to mean some other event has occurred to distress the person.

Generally, information and previous experience are profound stress reducers. It is the lack of information and unclear or nonspecific expectations that tend to be stress inducers.[7] For example, health care providers are likely to be stressed to some degree by each new patient, and, indeed, most patients are highly stressed when they seek help from an unfamiliar health-care worker. On the other hand, if we feel adequately prepared and confident from our training or past experience, the negative effects of the stress of such new encounters will be much less.

One group that utilizes this understanding of the subjective nature of stress is the Outward Bound program. Through stressful outdoor experiences, this program gives people confidence that they will be able to handle many emergencies and life crises more effectively in the future. The experience thus contributes to a new perceptual frame of reference concerning one's ability to cope.

Although there are objective characteristics of adaptive demands that are fairly good indicators of events that are stressful for all persons, it is the individual's coping style and interpretation of events that are the most reliable predictors of the deleterious potential of stress.

The stress response: flight or fight   Regardless of the specificity of negative stressors and a person's personality, the body's reaction to many stressors prevalent in our daily lives is fairly consistent. The general stress reaction is perhaps best conceived as a "flight-or-fight" response. Because of our genetic endowment, the human body is equipped in such a way that an automatic set of biochemical responses occurs, similar to those that would occur if one had to confront a dangerous animal. Thus, any time one is confronted with a perceived threat or sudden requirement to adapt, the body is called on to adjust to a change that occurs internally or externally. The following set of biochemical reactions occurs as an individual prepares to confront, escape, or adapt to a threat or change: the pupils dilate to improve vision, and blood is shunted from the extremities to the major muscles of the trunk, legs, and arms so that the hands and feet may feel cold and sweaty. Blood flow is increased to the brain, digestion (peristalsis) is slowed or stopped, and the blood in the digestive system is diverted to the major muscles. Heart and respiratory rates increase. More blood sugar is supplied to the circulatory system through the action of the liver, and the blood flow through the kidneys is decreased. Muscles tend to tense in preparation for dealing with whatever threat or change is demanded.

Certainly one would assume that biochemical changes of such a magnitude would be immediately apparent to the person. Yet, that is not the way we experience the normal stress of getting up in the morning because, for most daily activities and changes, the internal adaptive responses in the healthy person occur only to a moderate degree. When those tasks and activities are accomplished, the body returns, biochemically, to a normal state, and one remains unaware that anything out of the ordinary has occurred.

However, let us assume that, after arising and making the usual preparations for work, you get into your car, turn the ignition key, and hear a dull "clunk" from under the hood. The flight-or-fight biochemical cycle starts anew but with more intensity. There is, in this situation, the perceived threat of being late for work, being without transportation, and other imagined negative consequences. You try the ignition again and nothing happens; anger and frustration in response to feeling unable to cope effectively with the situation are fed back through a complex feedback loop to the brain and endocrine system, which tend to amplify the threat both in psychological awareness as well as in physiological response.[8] When this set of events occurs, if we are not distracted, we do become aware of such symptoms as shallow, rapid breathing, increased heart rate, and so on.

Let us further assume that, at this point, you leave your auto and finally catch a bus to work. In part, you have not completed the task for which your body was biochemically prepared. You have left the basic problem unsolved to move on to waiting work. But your body remains in a state of hyperpreparation because of the amplification of the flight-or-fight response. At the job you are therefore irritable and tense. You may find this behavior and feeling state not only physiologically uncomfortable but perhaps unacceptable to your self-concept and therefore a threat to your self-esteem. These internal psychological responses add to your stress; other systems are brought into play, and biochemical changes occur in the brain that may induce mild depression. Depression, in turn, compounds the stress cycle as, in the depressed state, your efficiency may indeed become impaired.

A classic example of this process was recently reported in newspapers and magazines across the country. It was noted that "air-traffic controllers left their jobs in part, they said, because the daily tension tended to scorch their circuits (the primitive 'flee-or-fight' reaction to danger squirted charges of adrenaline into bodies that had to remain relatively immobile, tethered by duty to scope and computer)."[9]

Since, in the examples given above, there is no dangerous animal to be confronted and nothing that one can flee or fight, the body does not return readily to a normal biochemical state. The insidious and potentially harmful fact about stress is that the effects of biochemically induced changes noted are additive over time. That is, if the body is not permitted to return to its normal state, subsequent stresses, no matter how minor, are added to an already overstressed system, and this accumulation can go on day after day, month after month, year after year.[10] Under these conditions, regulatory centers of the brain, through the mechanism of the feedback loop and amplification, overreact. This overreaction is what eventuates in severe wear and tear on the body, physiological breakdown, and even death. Severe psychological damage in the form of depression, extreme anxiety, and general feelings of misery and despair are also common sequelae.

Unfortunately, most humans are unaware of the source or the presence of chronic stress reactions. Many do not recognize the source of their discomfort until symptoms result in physical and/or emotional illness. Too often, the tendency is for people to dismiss lightly their beginning warning signs as "being uptight," "burned out," "needing a vacation," or simply "having a bad day." Even when physiological breakdown in some form occurs, people may be uninformed as to their unique stress reaction, even if told by a physician that they have to "slow down."

Many physical maladies are known to be related to stress: colitis, chronic hypertension, arthritis, peptic ulcer, certain diarrhea, asthma, sexual dysfunction, muscle tension, heart disease, and cancer. With regard to cancer, it is believed that the mechanism involved in chronic stress interferes with the body's immune system.[11] Not only does stress interfere with the body's ability to destroy abnormal cancerous cells, but also with its ability to check the development of bacteria and other microorganisms responsible for various infectious diseases to which humans are susceptible.

Control of stress   So what can humans do to control stress levels? Most Western peoples do not realize the need to reduce the stresses in their lives, nor are they aware that they do not have to be at the mercy of flight-or-fight reactions. Nowhere is the need to enlist the internal resources of the patient more clearly demonstrated. Education leading to changes in awareness, attitude, perception, and coping styles is becoming increasingly critical. Patients and the people working with them need to learn that the same brain centers that speed up and amplify biochemical processes under stress can be utilized to slow these processes and return the body more nearly to normal levels of reactivity. For example, meditative relaxation, however it is achieved, can normalize physical, cognitive, and emotional processes.

The relaxation response also can be achieved by disciplined vigorous physical exercise, hypnosis or autohypnosis, progressive relaxation, biofeedback, yoga, and so on. The function of these methods is to put the control of the sympathetic and parasympathetic nervous systems and their feedback mechanisms in the hands of the stressed individual. It was once thought that these systems were beyond voluntary control, but, due to recent advances in mind/brain research, we now know that they can be controlled. It is essential that appropriate methods be initiated and used daily if stress management is to be achieved. It is particularly essential for persons in high-stress occupations, whose experience will be discussed in Chapter 11, "Professional Burnout."

Existential Anxiety

The majority of people who seek health services are anxious and stressed. They are seeking answers that will reduce their sense of discomfort. They usually try to derive explicit meaning from both the internal sensations and the external experiences that motivated them to seek help. Some of the stress reactions expressed by patients represent conditions health-care workers can alleviate. Some anxiety, however, must be recognized as an integral part of life itself—a response to the dilemma of being human in a world that has never been completely understood. Such existential anxiety is normal, historically inescapable, and part of the fabric of life stressors to which everyone must adapt.[12]

At any point in time, including the present, humankind has struggled with understanding the meaning of life and with the inability to control the world. Not comprehending or being able to control the central mystery of human experience results in generalized uncertainty. The anxiety of uncertainty is humanity's enduring discomfort, but, paradoxically, it is also the motivating force for exploring new dimensions of experience. For some, existential uncertainty leads to maladaptive resolutions, such as neurotic anxiety,[13] avoidance through drugs, or self-induced death. For some, generalized uncertainty leads to overreliance on others in the form of attachment to soothing, but dictatorial, leadership.[14] For still others, existential anxiety leads to creative responses to uncertainty, such as the development of tools that increase understanding of the unknown. As Hoffer wrote:

> Nature attains perfection, but man never does. There is a perfect ant, a perfect bee, but man is perpetually unfinished. He is both an unfinished animal and an unfinished man. It is this incurable unfinishedness which sets man apart from other living things. For, in the attempt to finish himself, man becomes a creator. Moreover, the incurable unfinishedness keeps man perpetually immature, perpetually capable of learning and growing.[15]

Overall, in the search for relief from existential anxiety, humankind has developed belief and value systems to anchor meaning.[16] Beliefs and values may be considered the cultural structure within which humanity has been able to evaluate its maladaptive, adaptive, and creative responses to life at hand and to cope with its fears of the future. Many beliefs literally guarantee higher degrees and rates of survival since they are related to what today are called "health practices."

Beginning helpers as well as seasoned professionals, like their patients, are not immune to existential anxiety. Enticing as it may be to identify with a professional discipline and to use it to seek answers to the enigma of life, individuals will not necessarily be reassured merely by stepping from the culture at large into a subsystem of that culture, particularly the subsystem of health care. Health care is a value-laden business, within which the historical, immediate, and future struggles of humankind converge and demand answers. Nor do beginning health-care workers leave behind their unique reflections of the general culture as they move into a profession.[17] Just as fingerprints are common to humanity but also unique to individuals, all persons coming into the health-care field bring their own complex integration of the common culture within which patients, peers, and teachers are embedded.

Individualistic as we may be or strive to be, we are all bound together in coping with the world, which today offers little of the peace and constancy that humanity has always been presumed to desire. Persons at all levels, particularly the young, experience existential anxiety along with heightened consciousness. One nursing student, keenly sensitive to the shifting and often uncertain values of the nursing school, individual instructors, medical students, physicians, social peers, patients, and other elements of the health-care world, clearly put it on the line: "In view of everything changing and the turmoil I see, where am I to find myself? How much simpler if someone would just say 'This is where you start, this is it, and this is what will be when you are finished.' " How close to the sum essence of the whole history of humankind is woven into the student's existential question and plea for a panacea to make the pain of uncertainty disappear. How easy it is to consider the student's question as one of many similar expressions heard over the years and give pat answers. How easy it also is to reassure patients by offering stock solutions. Unfortunately, glib reassurances do not work so well with people anymore—if they ever really did.

The nature of contemporary existential anxiety   Existential, or diffuse, anxiety in response to the "human dilemma" has always been present. Tracing its historical footprints can give insights into what is happening today; but, as with any behavioral phenomenon, existential anxiety must be evaluated within the context in which it occurs. Essentially, contemporary Western peoples are experiencing an extraordinary dilemma. They are in the middle of a collision between their traditional values and beliefs and the influence of their technological products.[18] There is a circular Sisyphus aspect to the existential conflict presently experienced.[19] It is confounding to acknowledge that the very technological solutions devised in response to the basic existential dilemma have created even more problems. While contributing to the comfort of modern life, the automatic washer and the automobile present problems of pollution from phosphates and carbon monoxide. An energy crisis exists at the same time that much energy is contained in destructive nuclear weapons. Some medications once touted as miracle cures are later found to have negative side effects that cause alarming concern. Frustration rises with the awareness that technologies have often failed to solve those problems for which they were intended. Teaching machines, hoped by many to solve learning problems, have not exactly fulfilled their promise. With all the automated help in accomplishing household chores, women still feel that something is missing from their lives. As many health-care workers can appreciate, all the benefits of automated services within hospitals to "free them for other things" often leave old problems unsolved or introduce new problems.

In the midst of this circular dilemma, contemporary people often think that there is little help available that feels supportive and enduring. Rapid transitions facilitated by sophisticated communication systems have altered the pace of social evolution and the quality of interpersonal relatedness. Anxiety in response to the threat of loss of personal identity is heightened by uncooperative herd living in the population crush and multiple places called home.[20] Traditional values have been disrupted, dispensed with, or thrown into flux. New knowledge about old phenomena has shattered many beliefs that once seemed to explain life "perfectly." Today, little of the childlike faith that tomorrow will automatically bring a brighter day remains. Within a few short years, recognition has come that, in the here and now, human beings are in the middle of profound alterations in their concepts of (1) survival, (2) their relative place in the universe, and (3) time.

Long preoccupied with harnessing natural forces to strengthen the slender thread of human survival, people have begun to realize that, within recent generations, they have created forces from their own knowledge with a higher probability of destroying them than is found in a natural event. Accustomed to historical beliefs that the end of the world might come about by the hand of God, humankind is taking an anxious peek at the possibility that the end just might occur as a result of their own misguided willfulness. Lack of reliance on an outside God to be the "bad guy" who may destroy them is difficult for many persons: it makes humans so much more accountable and places responsibility closer to home. When this insight is coupled with increasing lack of reliance on an outside God who will save them from the consequences of their acts, further generalized anxiety is created.

Whether one personally has had to cope with the disruption of the concept of God, it seems useful to reflect on humankind's early development and to appreciate that people have always had their gods. Belief in gods was critical and integrated within belief systems to explain events of the past, present, and future. Always the gods were related to forces of nature and to critical survival issues. Gods were experienced as elements beyond oneself, but present and close by.[21] God in nature and in the heavens was an affordable explanatory concept when people believed their small life space to be the center of the universe. As the twinkling star became a planet, then was conceptualized as being larger than the planet earth, perhaps replete with life, and as the heavens were explored by human beings, God was pushed further out into infinity. The notion that knowledge per se has replaced the concept of God is not fully adequate. Increasing knowledge and the technologies that depersonalized the heavens also ravaged psychological interpretation of an "out there" as humans conceived it to be and thereby altered the manner in which God and humanity had related for centuries.

It is important for health-care workers to remain sensitive to the impact of a disrupted concept of God. Many persons in physical and social/emotional crises meaningfully call on their God, *as they have come to perceive the concept.* The public arguments about the existence of God in the face of scientific explanations have, for some, threatened their faith in a greater power to carry them through bad times. Some patients wonder if it is appropriate to talk with the professional about "those things" and suffer silently with the stress of their uncertainty.

What most separates contemporary human beings from the experience of their forebears is their relation to time. As progress in scientific technology has taken a quantum leap forward in the past century, the rate and direction of change have had to be accommodated with a rapidity and urgency never before witnessed by humankind.

No longer does humanity have the luxury of reflecting leisurely on what has happened. Instant feedback forces on us the knowledge of what is occurring everywhere almost at the moment that it is happening. At a time when a calm, thoughtful appraisal of what to do about precarious personal and world survival issues of the future is crucially needed, most human energies go into trying to understand the present. How ironical it is that, at a time when human knowledge has contributed to physical longevity, the meaning and enjoyment of extended life are blurred either by our not wanting to think about the future or not having time to do so.

Some individuals look to the past for solace and solutions, but many people are not convinced that "the good old days" were much better. Technological media that bombard people with communication about "right now" also gives people a comprehensive view of history, reflecting more accurately the trends of the past, in contrast to romanticized, biased myths. Although this more realistic view is advantageous, people continue to wonder whether history, in spite of so-called advances, is not merely repeating itself.

Ironically, even though there are significant changes in social/cultural contexts, contemporary people resemble their counterparts of millennia ago: we sense that we are up against something big, and we do not exactly know what we are going to do about it. Unlike our historical counterparts, however, we have few traditional beliefs that reliably dispel anxiety. We must face survival issues realizing that we have failed to prevent death while at the same time knowing we have perfected tools to prevent life. As humankind has assumed many functions that formerly were ascribed to God, we remain disturbed by resolutions that God is dead or that God may have to be reconceptualized to include humanity in greater proportion than ever before. Increasingly seen in health-care settings are persons who feel alienated from the group while struggling to develop a selfhood with which they can feel comfortable.[22] Not only is there a search for new values that are meaningful, but people increasingly seek help in maintaining the values that they presently hold.

Human problem-solving capacities   Any student of the humanities or the behavioral sciences knows that humankind has a number of enduring attributes of long historical standing. Some of these attributes lead to salvation, some to self-destruction. These attributes are important for health-care workers to understand if they are interested in helping people achieve behavioral change.

A basic characteristic of Western culture is that people have generally looked outside themselves for answers and sources of strength rather than to the unexplored depths of their internal experience. Regardless of the fact that all human accomplishments have emerged from the brilliance of the human mind, a stubborn denial of this fact remains. It has not been easy for humankind to view human qualities as the hope of the future, never having trusted them much. Perceiving themselves frail, has not humankind spent centuries dealing with natural forces, knowing simultaneously that they will die regardless of anything that they do? Neither have human beings automatically trusted the internal workings of others.

Early humans understandably attributed most of the power over life, death, and safety to an external-god system. Later, as new knowledge and technology developed, the tendency was to deify, or make such happenings "godlike." As an elitist group of knowledgeable humans developed, common people came to rely on their benefits. To the extent that knowledge and skill were attributed to human beings per se, those who held these abilities stood side by side with the gods. This phenomenon strengthened people's perception that good things came "from the outside." To the extent that the power conferred by knowledge and skills was not openly shared or that common persons needed to make knowledgeable individuals godlike, the masses continued to see themselves as powerless by contrast.

As discussed earlier, human beings commonly experience a state of generalized anxiety that causes us to ask the same existential questions: "Who am I? Where am I going? What will it be like when I grow up? What is after death? How are we to survive forces that seem beyond our control?" If anything, in the contemporary super-dilemma, the pangs of uncertainty are more keenly felt. How tenaciously humanity has developed science and technology to counteract perceived frailties; how ironic to find that, in the attempt to stay away from inner experience, one comes closer to the self, about which so little is known that does not frighten. Although perhaps for different reasons, human beings are still highly vulnerable to the controlling effects of exploitative, manipulative, and competitive power [23] in seeking answers and relief from anxiety. Even today, this persistent susceptibility can limit the human capacity to achieve solutions that are humanizing—self-satisfying *and* growth enhancing.

Humankind, however, has also always had the attribute of awareness. Forced on us though it may be, more of that ability is being used by people today as a first step forward out of the existential mire. Awareness can reduce people's need to deify others and accept unquestioningly the knowledge that lies beyond their present comprehension. People can learn to trust their own intellect, their judgment, and their opinions. Those in positions of "knowledge power"[24] can reevaluate their status in relation to others, thereby becoming more aware of tendencies to be caught in power plays used either to keep away one's own anxiety or that of others. This awareness must become part of professional helpers' concern for how knowledge and its technological products are used in combating the existential anxiety expressed in the halls of helping. Professionals must also keep aware of the specific effects of new knowledge on their own rapidly shifting values and those of their patients. They cannot evade the development of new values. Those who function in a field that deals with the issues of living and dying have a responsible contribution to make, and they must be highly aware of the effects of those values that they come to espouse or impose on others. Professionals must be highly cognizant of what the people of flourishing past civilizations discovered, to the detriment of humanity: *to the degree that technological knowledge becomes a source of power greater than that of the prevailing beliefs of the common people, it is seductive for humans to be viewed as mechanistic objects to be controlled.*

In learning, as well as in the application of helping skills, it must be kept in mind that, as knowledge comes to be viewed as a blindly accepted "god," it is all too easy to control or be controlled without thought. It is not only the common people who are inclined to pay homage to knowledge beyond their understanding. Even high-powered scientists are vulnerable to making the present status of their knowledge a "god-out-there" that cannot be challenged. How easy for patient, beginning helper, or seasoned professional to fall victim to the notion that anything that does not fit "science" is not to be trusted as useful knowledge.

Human beings have several other enduring attributes that they are capable of bringing to bear on existential crises. Historical development of civilization demonstrates that, vulnerable as humankind may be to avoidance of dilemma through devices ranging from opiates to rigid dogma, they have done things other than run. The individual has, in spite of all foibles, been an "active guardian of his existence."[25] For example, humans have demonstrated repeatedly that they do not like being "boxed in" for long. Deprived of adequate food and shelter or the stimulation of novelty and creative expression, they can emotionally, if not physically, succumb. Most human beings before reaching such a point are motivated to do something about their predicament. Although the spirit can indeed be killed, a human being has a potential for reacting against forces that foster subjugation and overreliance on outside control.

Although capable of destructive power, the internal human capacities also permit the use of nutrient and integrative power, [26] such as the ability to be assertive for and with others. This attribute of humans allows us to join together, to form partnerships, and to approach crises with a sense of cooperation, thus constructing an enduring defense against an existential dilemma that is greater than any one person.

Overall, the motivations that long ago gave birth to creative ways of keeping the tiger from the door remain attributes of humankind. Our ever-present human evaluative capacities can help us reexamine values and the purpose of life. We can change the direction of certain of our follies by using the capacity of humanity for reason and judgment. Technologies already developed can be controlled and disallowed for destruction. Stockpiled technologies unused for humanitarian purposes can be equitably freed. Above all, humankind is capable of even greater technological breakthroughs, having hardly begun using technology to enter the arena in which we believe that future discovery will occur—namely, the uncharted universe of internal human experience.

Human Evaluative Capacities

One of the underlying themes throughout the text will be an emphasis on people's ability to evaluate their own circumstances and to trust that their subjective feelings, thoughts, and perceptions can be as valid as those coming from the outside. Certainly, for a humanistic helping process, the attitudes that the health-care worker and the patient hold about each other's capacity to evaluate are highly significant. As previously discussed, this is an era of high reliance on mechanistic evaluative procedures to provide answers, and the health-care field uses such procedures in great measure. These procedures are of high value in assisting people to solve problems, but overreliance on them can have negative effects. It becomes easy to disrespect what humans can still do in analyzing, integrating, and coming up with subjective data that are not only relevant, but sometimes more accurate in given situations.

Because of our commitment to a humanistic helping process, we highly value people's evaluative abilities; but our concern grows that, as a culturally valued human capacity, these abilities may be going out of style. The decline of evaluative abilities has been most apparent as we have observed the last several generations of students struggle with the mind-versus-machine dilemma. Particularly characteristic of this struggle has been their expressions of doubt that they have anything subjectively worthwhile to offer a technologically oriented society. Along with these questions about personal worth, it is significant that the younger generation of health-care workers seems to be (1) not as aware or respectful of their own critical thinking or evaluative abilities and (2) often frankly hostile to the concept of evaluation as it might apply to an appraisal of themselves made by others.

We propose that the blind spot concerning critical thinking and evaluative abilities is in large part a result of subtle, but powerful, cultural changes. In a realistic sense, contemporary human beings do not have to "use their heads" as much in many problem-solving situations. Educational settings at all levels reflect the emphasis of our culture at large on technological progress and the manipulation of its products, but life situations continue to exist in which all one has to rely upon is one's own or another's innate human capacities. In our opinion, educational settings for youth have not kept abreast of the need to provide environments that simultaneously help students to value and use the vast resources of the human mind as well as those of the machine. As with any human function, understimulation and underutilization of the mind deny its usefulness and wither its growth potential.

At the same time that contemporary life contributes to a devaluation of the human evaluative capacities, the approaches and tools utilized in appraising other human beings have become increasingly mechanistic and objective. The youth of today are openly strident about appraisal methods that have been applied to them over the years within the educational system. Grade symbols, percentile ranks, and assorted group categories in which students see themselves placed after a series of objective tests are increasingly resisted. The tests are perceived as inadequate in deriving a meaningful profile of who one is or is struggling to become. Dissatisfied with the usefulness of mechanized outside evaluation as applied to themselves, many students have become wary of taking on evaluative roles with respect to others.

A third cultural characteristic also reduces the appreciation of one's own evaluative abilities—the rapid shifts in values about almost everything. It is tempting to assume a posture that says "What is there to think through about anything? It all changes so fast anyhow."

The interactive effect of the rapid shifts in general values, the diminuation of one's critical thinking abilities, and the avoidance of an evaluative stand about oneself and others can lead to several behavioral phenomena. For example, people often respond to this existential dilemma with a chaotic feeling of having a structureless, valueless existence or with an unthinking passive conformity to any prevailing outside influence. In both situations, one becomes increasingly insensitive to one's ability to influence one's own destiny in any way. A feeling of helplessness ensues that belies the person's potential, and one's self-concept suffers in the most dehumanizing way. Not only might one respond with lowered self-confidence in one's ability to direct one's own life, but one might also feel no confidence in others or in being able to lend assistance to another person.

What we have just described happens to thousands of people, many of whom become patients. Therefore, part of understanding patients as persons must be accomplished within the context of the learned helplessness derived from sociocultural forces. Many of the persons thus inhibited in their growth and development also become health-care students. To understand helpers as persons, one must attend to how they, too, are responding to the culture at large.

Within the student group, in contrast to the general public, people are observed to be more restless and vocal about these sociocultural influences. Even though at times they question their own judgment and become less vocal, these youth are communicating something vital. They seem to be saying "We want the best of technology but much more. We also want to be human and need help to do that right now." Health-care students, in particular, additionally want to help others humanistically and require assistance from their health-care culture in order to to that.

This book's final chapter presents our view of what health-care students are saying and not saying about what they see as their goals and what they want to happen in accomplishing them. Although beginners tend to shy away from the concept of evaluation, we find them to be more sensitive critical evaluators than they perceive themselves to be. We have contrasted their views with the commentary of older professional helpers. We have chosen this method of presentation so that (1) similarities between them might be understood as enduring adult developmental tasks in any generation and (2) differences between them might be understood as having essential implications for new directions in the educational process.

For both beginning helpers and older professionals, essential similarities are most apparent in the fact that all are human beings. All have had their developmental roots involved in coping with and working through similar growth tasks. One significant developmental task that all of them have in common, even before coming together in the health-care culture, is that of learning to evaluate significant others and themselves. Let us briefly review the developmental roots of an evaluative process that all have had to learn in order to cope and achieve individual resolutions. Throughout this review, it should be kept in mind that one's ability to evaluate is the critical skill underlying the eventual ability to make accurate definitions of patient problems, develop appropriate treatment plans, and be reasonably accurate with respect to prognostication and follow-up.

Roots of the evaluative process   From our earliest postnatal beginnings, evaluation is a process that one must learn in order to put reality into meaningful perspective. Evaluation starts completely outside oneself in the form of feedback from parents and other caretakers. Parents must analyze, order, and evaluate the total life space for their infants, making choices relating to security, comfort, safety, and stimulation. Children increasingly operate motorically on their world but lack the necessary judgment to avoid certain dangers. As a result, adults continue to analyze the life space of children and evaluate it as to whether it is safe to explore or experience. Through the outside evaluative input of parents and significant others, children gradually learn the parameters of the universe with respect to physical survival, as well as the social conventions prevalent within their environment. They also learn that there is a world of fantasy and dreams with no fences.[27]

Through internalizing aspects of the appraisals of others, which seem to integrate with an apparent innate willfulness, an analytic, evaluative thought process begins to develop within the child. This cognitive thinking process provides an important intermediary step between an impulse and acting indiscriminately on the impulse to plunge ahead.[28] Aided by the development of symbolic language, the child further acquires a rudimentary basis for ordering, classifying, and valuing new phenomena as they are encountered, including the emerging feeling of "self." Very early, therefore, the child develops a beginning base for anticipatory planning and hindsight appraisal in terms of what worked or did not work. Such an internal evaluation process provides the growing and developing child with a set of meaningful judgmental operations that allows both child and parents a feeling of who the child is and promotes increasing trust that the child can survive greater distances from the input of the family and the supervision of adults.

It is these very reflective evaluative capacities that separate human beings from other forms of life that are dominated primarily by reflexes and instincts. These capacities allow human beings creative thoughts, fantasy, and the ability to set personal/social goals for future action. They allow one to develop values, to attach symbolic meaning to feelings, and to choose between courses of action, and they provide built-in deterrents to one's being treated like an object or a machine. These reflective, evaluative capacities eventually allow humans to solve problems of high degrees of complexity and to develop autonomous functioning without total dependency on the group. These capacities make possible a frame of reference within which internal and external events are uniquely organized. Evaluative abilities allow one to mediate between one's own highly personalized needs and feelings and those of others.

Just as human beings seem to have patterns of physical growth and development that approximate points of chronological age, so is it with the development of these analytical, evaluative thought processes. They begin early and, with a certain degree of predictability, can be observed to develop complexly and integratively over time.[29-31] The general capacity exists in all persons, barring serious cerebral deficit or impairment. Each individual develops a stylistic way of utilizing those capacities that emerges out of a host of critical interacting factors, including basic genetic endowment.[32] Equally important are the environmental factors of how parents and significant others respond to the child's independent evaluative judgments and how overpowering or responsive the outside world seems during those critical periods when one needs to rely on others, as opposed to relying totally on oneself.

CASE IN POINT

Theresa, age 8, was observed by her mother to be playing in the backyard with two neighborhood boys who were in the delight of discovering how an old motor might work. When they were frustrated in understanding how they could get the fan to rotate, Theresa ran into the house to ask her mother whether the old fruit jar opener in the kitchen drawer would help them to move the resistant part. Her mother responded with an unsupportive admonition: "Theresa, that's a crazy idea! Besides, you shouldn't be playing with that kind of thing. You don't understand a motor; that's boys' stuff." Theresa returned to her friends and said, "Mom said I couldn't use that jar opener. Let's not play motor anymore." Her mother's disapproval transformed an enjoyable experience into a joyless one as Theresa accepted her mother's value judgment.

As any series of similar observations will reveal, a "cognitive style" tends to cohere quite early.[33] One observes that early on, some children seem overall more inner-directed, or self-reliant, whereas others seem more outer-directed, or conforming and dependent on external guideposts. Another way of talking about this phenomenon is to speak of someone's appearing to be more field-independent or more field-dependent.[34] Coopersmith discussed style of relating within the broad concept of self-esteem. His work showed that persons with high self-esteem have been reared in an atmosphere of acceptance, clear limit definition, respect, and parental self-esteem, in contrast to one of rejection, ambiguity, and disrespect. He found that individuals with high self-esteem who are reared under strongly structured conditions tend to be more, rather than less, independent and creative in contrast to persons reared under more open and permissive conditions. Apparently, in environments that are more clearly defined as to limits, standards, information, and cues, children experience cognitive clarity that early enables them to evaluate for themselves whether they have achieved a goal, are making progress, or have deviated. Coopersmith explained:

> A psychological world that provides sparse, ambiguous, or inconsistent information makes it difficult for the child to make rational decisions—that is, decisions with predictable outcomes—and increases the likelihood that he will either continually seek aid in interpreting his environment or will gradually withdraw from it; in neither case will he come to believe that he can, by himself, interpret his environment and guide himself through the thickets of ambiguities.[35]

All human beings, regardless of individual tendency to one style of functioning or the other, will from time to time be more inner-directed or more creatively "their own," given certain circumstances. Conversely, at other times, one's own discriminative sense may consciously or unconsciously suggest more reliance on the judgment of others as temporarily one functions in a more outer-directed, or field-dependent, mode. Particularly in stressful situations of high environmental ambiguity or in the face of feeling that one has few internal "structures" (e.g., beliefs, values, and guidelines for action) on which to rely, one may develop a more outer-directed collection of behaviors. It is as if humans intuitively know that some kind of structure and organization brought to a new, frightening, or complex experience will relieve it of its mystery and render it more understandable. For example, as will be seen in our overview of the helper as human being, there are critical periods in personal/professional growth when the desire (almost demand) is expressed for structure in the form of feedback from others about how one is doing. Yet, as will be seen in other chapters, those persons who are unable to be verbally insistent on structure from others, often show coping behaviors that are passive, conforming, and helpless appearing.

As the preceding view of evaluation suggests, it is a process that is essential to survival. All have a profound investment in their own ability and in the ability of others to evaluate in a way that provides growth-enhancing structure. At the same time, evaluation holds an interesting paradoxical meaning for human beings. It opens doors to new discovery and creative ideas, yet it is often feared, as if some dark mystery or undesired piece of reality will be revealed. Whenever it is directed toward oneself, evaluation retains a measure of discomfort, both when it is asked of others or when it takes the form of introspection into one's own feelings and behavior. From childhood through adulthood, individuals are responsive to what others may feel or know about them that may deny or facilitate their acceptance into significant relationships or allow them to maintain relationships they already have. Periodic uneasiness about one's own beliefs, feelings, or knowledge, as contrasted with those of others, continues as an ebb and flow in life.

The paradoxes within the evaluation process operate between people in the health-care culture in abundance, even though the paradoxes may not be recognized as such. In listening to health-care students and practitioners, one is particularly impressed that they do not want to let go of this evaluative ability. They say that they very much want outside evaluation structure, expressing an understandable desire in a highly ambiguous field at the same time that, like any other human beings, they are ambivalent, sensitive, and even defensive about the evaluation methods utilized, who employs them, and what the outcome will mean.

Summary

The foregoing material we consider highly relevant to all health-care workers. These universal issues are important to all of us in some measure for they affect how life is perceived and the personal meanings that are derived from those perceptions. Health-care workers need to appreciate that they are a part of a greater humanity and not just members of the particular discipline with which they identify. Our discomforting observation is that the professional disciplines that provide the vital tools of health care have tended to ignore this greater context during the current era of science and specialization.

The health-care field is comprised of human beings and therefore is vulnerable to all the foibles of humankind. Collectively, the health-care field is particularly vulnerable to setting itself apart with its own traditions, knowledge, and gadgetry. Often loath to share its rich knowledge or admit its lack of knowledge to those asking for help or those wishing to learn to help, professionals in the field are highly susceptible to controlling others.

Many, including ourselves, believe that the field requires a broad reevaluation, with changes in its emphasis and actions in carrying out its purpose. We believe that the health-care professions need to develop interdisciplinary sensitivity to and responsibility for the power that they hold in influencing people's lives. Whether one speaks of patients or health-care students, the professions do hold power over how persons learn to live and what they come to believe about their potential to become effective, healthy human beings. This power of the health professions can be used in negative ways, but many natural resources can be found within the health-care field, along with room for this power to be used in growth-enhancing ways.

Essentially, the field of health care exists for only one reason—to help people live longer and better. This reason often becomes unclear to health-care workers, or they behave in ways suggesting that they alone know what "longer" or "better" means for others. Ideally, evaluation and determination of the central values of the health-care field are jointly decided by givers and consumers of the services, but mutual goal setting is not always easy. Since people in need tend to abdicate responsibility and let someone else be their god, consumers sometimes simply let others do it. In the face of this tendency, professionals often find expediency in taking over because they believe they "know better." In many aspects of the helping process, professionals do not actually know what is better for the other person. In some matters, no ultimate truths, magic cures, or fast answers exist. The time has come for health professionals to confide that fact to those seeking help and to begin to share the responsibility for answers with them. Growth enhancement begins by letting other persons know that they are capable of assisting in the solution of their own dilemmas.

Basically, health care is a very human enterprise. Made up of persons from all walks of life, the health professions nonetheless share common aspects of humanity. Health care is a field within which human interdependence must be recognized in the struggle to survive and find personal meaning. Whether in the world at large or within health-care settings, mutual resourcefulness is needed. By helping each other to accept ultimate mortality as a natural process and to acknowledge human capacity to enhance—not merely destroy or control—significant humanistic values can be revitalized. Perhaps, when life can be seen more clearly as a mutual challenge and aging as a privilege, death can be afforded natural dignity and new respect can be offered for the circumstances in which death occurs.[36]

REFERENCE NOTES

1. David W. Ewing, "Discovering Your Problem-Solving Style," *Psychology Today* 11, no. 7 (December 1977): 69–73, 138. Ewing discusses the Harvard research of McKenney and Keen concerning four cognitive styles in problem solving: systematic-perceptive, systematic-receptive, intuitive-perceptive, and intuitive-receptive.
2. Kenneth R. Pelletier, *Mind as Healer, Mind as Slayer* (New York: Dell, 1977). For any serious student in the health-care field, this is a "must read" book. Pelletier, who espouses a holistic humanistic philosophy, elucidates the intricate relationship between the individual and his psychoso-

cial environment. Probably one of the best sources for the understanding of stress, its consequences, and its treatment.

3. Richard Leakey and Roger Lewin, *Origins* (New York: Dutton, 1977). Leakey uses hard scientific data and theory to present a fascinating story of the genesis of modern man. One of his notable commentaries concerns the evolution from purely anatomical change to psychosocial and behavioral changes in the development of *Homo sapiens*.

4. James C. Coleman, *Abnormal Psychology and Modern Life*, 5th ed. (Glenview, Ill.: Scott, Foresman, 1976), p. 112. Chapter 4, "Personality and Adjustment: An Overview," is a must for the understanding of stress as it is related to personality development. It is easily read and well researched.

5. Thomas H. Holmes and Richard H. Rahe, "The Social Readjustment Rating Scale," *Journal of Psychosomatic Research* 11 (1967): 213–18. See also Thomas H. Holmes and Ninoru Masuda, "Life Change and Illness Susceptibility," in *Separation and Depression* (American Association for the Advancement of Science, 1973), pp. 161–86. This is a comprehensive report on Holmes's Social Readjustment Rating Scale and its use in predicting the time and nature of disease onset following a clustering of life changes or crises.

6. Richard S. Lazarus, "Little Hassles Can Be Hazardous to Your Health," *Psychology Today* 5, no. 4 (July 1981): 58–62.

7. Lazarus takes issue with the helping professions regarding *indiscriminately* encouraging patients to "face facts" in certain situations (for example, serious illness and surgery). He discusses that, in some cases, the maintenance of illusion and denial allow hope and contribute to a person's psychological economy in stressful situations, even as he recognizes instances in which denial can be dangerous. With regard to what to tell patients, he states, "Most of the time you want to present the facts as they are, but in ambiguous enough terms to allow for the preservation of some hope. And that's sticky." Richard S. Lazarus interviewed by Daniel Goleman, "Positive Denial: The Case for Not Facing Reality," *Psychology Today* 13, no. 6 (November 1979): 48. See also Ethel Roskies and Richard S. Lazarus, "Coping Theory and Teaching of Coping Skills," in *Behavioral Medicine: Changing Health Life Styles*, ed. Parke Davidson (New York: Brunner/Mazel, 1979).

8. See Pelletier, *Mind as Healer*, pp. 46–48, for an excellent description of the neurophysiology of stress.

9. Lance Morrow, "The Burnout of Almost Everyone," *Time*, 21 September 1981, p. 84.

10. Meyer Friedman and Ray H. Rosenman, *Type A Behavior and Your Heart* (New York: Fawcett Crest Books, 1974). Friedman and Rosenman present their research on personality types and behavior, and explain how these psychosocial variables have long-term deleterious effects on health.

11. O. Carl Simonton, Stephanie Matthews-Simonton, and J. L. Creighton, *Getting Well Again* (New York: Bantam Books, 1978). An excellent presentation of the holistic approach to the treatment of cancer, with particular emphasis on the patient's role in the treatment of disease. See pp. 34–38 for discussion of the impact of stress on the immune system. Also see Maggie Scarf's "Images That Heal," *Psychology Today* 14, no. 4 (September 1980): 32–46. Scarf reviews not only the work of Simonton, but also that of Cousins, LeShan, and Pelletier.

12. See Rollo May, *Psychology and the Human Dilemma* (New York: Van Nostrand, 1967). For those just beginning to explore the concept of existentialism, this book is a good place to start. Classic authors who explore the subject in depth are Buber, Heidegger, Kierkegaard, Sartre, and Tillich. An excellent review of existentialists and their influence on the practice of behavior change can be found in the last two chapters of Edith Weigert's *The Courage to Love* (New Haven: Yale University Press, 1970).

13. May, *Psychology and The Human Dilemma*, p. 41. In evaluating anxiety, as one will often have to do in health-care settings, it is important to be able to differentiate between existential anxiety and neurotic anxiety. Existential anxiety all persons experience; some experiencing this anxiety together with highly specific social/emotional or physiological crises, or both, develop neurotic anxiety. May describes neurotic anxiety as destructive, "the shrinking of consciousness, the blocking off of awareness; and when it is prolonged it leads to a feeling of depersonalization and apathy."

Other characteristics of neurotic anxiety are immobilization in both thought and action and inability to take risks in altering one's self-concept or relationship with the objective world. Existential anxiety one has to learn to live with; neurotic anxiety one has to learn to live without.

14. The syndrome of attachment to dictatorial leadership has been written about extensively, particularly since World War II and the terrifying example of Hitler's rise to power. For further reading try Eric Fromm's *Escape from Freedom* (New York: Holt, Rinehart & Winston, 1941) and *Man for Himself* (New York: Holt, Rinehart & Winston, 1947). Silvano Areti's *The Will to Be Human* (New York: Quadrangle/New York Times, 1972) is excellent.

15. Eric Hoffer, *Reflections on the Human Condition* (New York: Harper & Row, 1973), p. 3.

16. Milton Rokeach, *The Nature of Human Values* (New York: Free Press, 1973), pp. 3–25.

17. Survey work to support this commonsense truism can be found in Earl Babbie's *Science and Morality in Medicine: A Survey of Medical Educators* (Berkeley: University of California Press, 1970). This text is one of the finest that we have encountered; it is provocative and humanistic. We suggest it as required reading for instructors as well as students of all health-care disciplines.

18. Alvin Toffler, *Future Shock* (New York: Random House, 1970). Toffler just about said it all with respect to Western society in the "here and now." Also see Warren Bennis, "A Funny Thing Happened on the Way to the Future," *American Psychologist* 25 (1970): 595–608.

19. For displeasing Zeus, Sisyphus was required by the Greek gods to spend eternity rolling a stone up a large hill only to have it skip back down every time that it just about reached the summit.

20. See Vance Packard, *Nation of Strangers* (New York: Pocket Books, 1974).

21. Loren Eiseley discusses this concept eloquently in "Cosmic Orphan," *Saturday Review*, 23 February 1974, pp. 16–19. Eiseley was a prominent anthropologist with a humanistic orientation. Poetic literary skill is characteristic of all his writings. We also suggest his personal expressions in *Night Country* (New York: Scribner's, 1971).

22. See Chapter 10 for a discussion of existential burnout.

23. Rollo May, *Power and Innocence* (New York: Norton, 1972), pp. 105–9.

24. Willis Harman, "The Coming Transformation in Our View of Knowledge," *The Futurist* 8 (June 1974): 126–28. Harman presents a hopeful perspective on the ability of persons to use knowledge morally, inclusively with everyone, eclectically, and hospitably to all forms of human experience—not just those that are observable and measurable.

25. Heidegger sees humankind not as victims of biological forces over evolutionary time but as active guardians of their existence. There is a subtle point here relevant to the influence of how one views a problem or what one feels able to do about it. Although oversimplified, the following examples illustrate the point: the passive-victim posture leads to a form of sour, paranoid pessimism; an assertive willingness to preserve what is precious leads to a more hopeful idealistic optimism. In grade school, it was always more fun to join the team that thought that they could win against all odds, rather than those who believed that the jig was up before they started. We suspect that people really don't want to think that the jig is up and tire of being told that it is. For more about Heidegger, see Martin Heidegger, *Being and Time*, trans. John Macquarrie and Edward Robinson (New York: Harper & Row, 1962).

26. May, *Power and Innocence*, pp. 105–9.

27. Parents are powerful in setting the tone for the development of evaluative abilities of the growing child. For the best compilation of research on "parent power" and its relationship to the development of self-esteem, see Stanley Coopersmith, *The Antecedents of Self-Esteem* (San Francisco: W. H. Freeman, 1967).

28. An excellent discussion of this point can be found in Arieti's "From Spontaneous Movement to Responsible Action," in *The Will to Be Human*, chap. 2.

29. Between 18 months and 2 years of age, children develop symbolic functions that allow them to do other than explore and manipulate motorically. Children develop language, mental imagery, and imitative abilities. Observation of these behaviors suggests that symbolic functions allow representation of events that went on before. They allow the internalization of actions into thought. Piaget describes this state as that of "preoperational thought," a stage that children experience until ap-

proximately 7 years of age and in which they are still struggling with accurately understanding relational concepts, such as dark*er*, bigg*er*, and *better* than. Intuitive, highly personalized explanations of world phenomena are characteristic of this stage. For an overview of Piaget, see Hans Furth, *Piaget and Knowledge* (Englewood Cliffs, N.J.: Prentice-Hall, 1964).

30. More logical thought processes, such as thinking of things and persons in terms of classes and relationship to one another, and the ability to integrate these operations into dealing with numerical concepts, develop increasingly between the ages of 7 and 11 years. Piaget refers to this stage as that of "concrete thought." Children experiencing this phase of development have some tools of reason and objectivity that they did not have before. They can reason out part/whole relationships. They can better order their world, particularly around things that can be quantified.

31. From the age of 12 years onward, the Piaget model speaks of the stage of formal operations. This is a delightful age for children; they begin to develop hypotheses and test them against previous experience and gathered facts. They can deduce and infer. Their explanations of phenomena are not just intuitive anymore. Children at this point have internalized evaluative abilities that allow them to use both their subjectivity and objectivity. The self alone no longer needs to be the central reference point. As Piaget suggests, it is well to appreciate in working with children that not until approximately 12 years of age are they capable of understanding or using this "adult logic."

32. For an overall grasp of the early development of "style" see Sybil Escalona, *Roots of Individuality* (Chicago: Aldine, 1968). Research support is increasingly for the notion that from birth a child has a distinctive style—a unique activity level. This early discernible style is powerful in effecting how adults respond to the child.

33. Cognitive style was defined by Klein in 1951 as the way that someone could be observed to deal with reality. See George S. Klein, "The Personal World Through Perception," in *Perception: An Approach to Personality*, ed. R. R. Brake and G. V. Ramsey (New York: Ronald Press, 1951).

34. See Herman A. Witkin, *Personality Through Perception: An Experimental and Clinical Study* (Westport, Conn.: Greenwood Press, 1972). The tempo of cognitive style also deserves attention. Kagan speaks of a reflective/impulsive dimension in how children approach tasks. See Jerome B. Kagan, et al. "Information Processing in the Child: Significance of Analytic and Reflective Attitudes," *Psychological Monographs: General and Applied* 78 (1964): 1–37.

35. Stanley Coopersmith, *The Antecedents of Self-Esteem* (San Francisco: W. H. Freeman, 1967), pp. 238–39.

36. A most poignant essay on aging is found in Eve Merriam's "Conversation Against Death," *Ms.*, September 1972, pp. 80–83.

OTHER SUGGESTED REFERENCES

In developing expertise in evaluating and understanding oneself and others, it is almost imperative to contrast one's knowledge of healthy human development with that available in the literature. Following are two excellent handbooks:

Paul H. Mussen, John J. Conger, and Jerome B. Kagan, *Child Development and Personality*, 3d ed. (New York: Harper & Row, 1969).

John Nash, *Developmental Psychology: A Psychobiological Approach* (Englewood Cliffs, N.J.: Prentice-Hall, 1970).

SUGGESTIONS FOR FURTHER EXPERIENCE

Persons of all ages openly or subtly express their existential views, their definitions of stress, and their unique style of adaptation and coping. In sensitizing yourself to commonalities and uniqueness, consider the following experiences:

1. Ask your parents what their greatest personal urgency in life was when they were your age. By contrast, explore with them what they perceived the large-scale world scene to be like at that time. Talk with them about what they did to cope with their anxieties about the world future and their personal goals.

2. Arrange to talk an hour a week with a lonely aged person in a nursing home. Converse about "how it was back then." Explore together those things that had deep personal meaning in life then and those that do now. Ask what it is like to become older.

3. Interview a number of 7-year-old children of both sexes. Ask them what they want to be when they grow up and why; what they think the world will be like when they get big; what they think is their biggest problem in life. Ask them what they think the biggest problem in the whole world is right now.

4. In interviewing your next new patient, ask what things in life in general are the most stressful. Ask how the patient goes about solving a problem situation. Compare the data obtained from the patient with the material suggested in reference note 2.

5. Try to live through the character of Dr. Bernard Rieux as he experiences existential crisis in Albert Camus's *The Plague*, trans. Stuart Gilbert (New York: Random House, 1948). Compare Rieux's mode of adaptation to the epidemic with those of other characters. Also compare Camus's treatment of existential crises with that of Hermann Hesse in *Narcissus and Goldmund*, trans. Ursule Molinary (New York: Farrar, Straus & Giroux, 1969).

Defining Humanistic Health Care

Chapter 4

Humanism and Health-Care Delivery

Many have been pleading the cause of distributed justice to ensure that health-care services that are available to a few in one part of the country be available throughout the nation.[1] Encouraging as the signs of serious planning and legislation might be on the surface, we are concerned about how well any broadly conceived system will provide the kind of care that people say they want.

We are concerned that several notions, critical to understanding what it means to care for people, be included in the development of a delivery system: (1) recognition that delivery of health-care services is not necessarily the same as the delivery of health care; (2) recognition that, although, historically, "helping" is the presumed outcome of efforts in the health-care field, actually little is known about helping; and (3) recognition that a set of humanistic values effectively applied to the human interactions that occur within any health-care system has been desperately needed.

Helping[2] is a practice that may or may not take place within a system. Helping per se will not occur simply because the number of personnel, clinics, and technological products increase or are coordinately available to all citizens. These are content aspects, or tools of the trade, that can be critical to a helping situation but cannot be relied on exclusively. Although these tools are impressive to the public and highly sought, ultimately the interpersonal actions and reactions that occur during their utilization determine if helping has occurred.

As you will see, *effective helping is ultimately defined by the patients.* Whether they have been helped is decided perceptually—by how they perceive themselves "to be" after the interventions sought from another. The helper's personal nature, through which knowledge and technological products are made available to the persons seeking help, is a part of patients' perceptions of whether they have been helped. Apparently, therefore, actually helping patients is intimately tied to value assumptions that are held by both health-care workers and those to whom services are provided.

Health-care delivery is a human enterprise. To be a successful helping operation, it is important that any model of health-care delivery allow a high degree of integration of humanistic assumptions that apply to both helpers and patients. Assumptions vital to a humanistic orientation are: (1) that all human beings have a right to dignity; (2) that to respect this dignity is to view persons as they normally see themselves—as whole, consciousness-experiencing persons, neither animals nor machines; and (3) that humankind has as a life goal a satisfying, self-actualizing, and committed existence.

To many, these assumptions seem obvious statements, as everyday evidences of humanism are apparent in those who seem to be intuitively so inclined. For example, those who extend themselves with respect and courtesy for the stranger who inquires directions show humanism, as do those who offer childen appropriate choices, rather than telling them what the degree of their appetite or the nature of their preference should be. For instance, one of our students thought that defining humanism was not a big deal: "You just believe in humanism, and then certain things come automatically. You just believe that both you and the other guy have brains in your heads and feelings about everything." However, because these basic assumptions so often go without saying and without being acted on, there is a high risk of overlooking how devastatingly human beings often respond to each other. Thus, rather shaky assumptions are made that everybody knows how to be humane. History is punctuated with destructive actions carried out for people under the guise of being the "humane thing to do."

Unfortunately, within health-care institutions, complete humanistic disregard is often observed to affect both patients and staff. Patients are often induced to cooperate through staff threats and intimidation. Environmental factors contributing to depression, as well as overuse of drugs to ensure patient placidity, are circumstances well known to health-care workers. Dehumanizing warehouses of the aging population abound, while business operators amass profits. Personnel in these circumstances often "just get used to it" or, if they become vocal about their observations, are told to stay in their place or lose their job.

Increasing numbers of these examples are finding their way into the public media.[3] Even without these strong reminders about what goes on in hallowed halls, it is certain that new buildings, equipment, supplies, and increased numbers of health-care personnel will not seriously influence how persons appreciate and treat one another. Following is an excerpt from a recent magazine article widely circulated to the general public.

CASE IN POINT

Cook, in expressing his concern for humane medical practice, states: "What's more, I can testify that physicians' personalities can be quite different from those presented on TV. Temper tantrums in the operating room, fierce in-fighting within the hospital, and inappropriate arrogance are all too common. More than once I have seen physicians become so enraged because a patient refused to submit to a particular operation—and incidents in which the physician blew up because the patient refused to get well on the treatment he prescribed. But the public still prefers to watch Marcus Welby, M.D.—and dream."[4]

Stevens, writing to enlighten humanistically both the professional and the public, speaks to distinctly contrasting experiences in being physically ill. Following are excerpts from her reflections on how being a patient has influenced her both negatively and positively.

CASE IN POINT

When a medical treatment is harmful to me, I can know this before it can be apparent to others, but I am required to go on with it, and am 'troublesome' and 'unreasonable' if I refuse. I am subtly or unsubtly punished for my disobedience. I am placed in a position of having to fight when what my body needs, to put itself in order, is to be at rest.[5]

On the other hand, Stevens can speak of growth-enhancing experiences with helpers:

This doctor and I went through some very troubling times together. At one time in the hospital, I wanted to give up. It seemed so much easier to die. He didn't let me. At another time, he lacked confidence in himself and offered to turn me over to any other doctor whom I chose. I didn't let him. Between us there was *agape*—and mutual understanding.[6]

As Stevens's various accounts exemplify, every highly dehumanizing incident can be countered with helping examples that have deeply positive meaning; but the question of why highly negative dehumanizing experiences happen remains.

The deterrents to helpers' being able to implement humanistic goals and feel satisfaction often directly relate to chaotic conditions within health-care settings or to complex social conditions experiencd by the population that a setting serves. It is difficult to feel appropriate concern about whether another is helped when one is working daily in an environment that is physically abominable and short of staff.

CASE IN POINT

The downtown mental-health center was located two flights up and then down a long hallway maze. The crowded waiting room reminded me of the sitting rooms in the large mental hospitals that I had worked with so long ago to "humanize." The patients seemed more depressed and hassled than I remembered them looking in the institutions that I had thought were abominable. One fellow about 50 was singing "My Country 'Tis of Thee" too loudly, but nobody seemed to care; a young man about 20 insistently asked the secretary how he could get to Texas. I sat next to an old woman who was wearing only galoshes and a heavy coat and was picking invisible lint off herself. Periodically she increased her distance from me, and she bolted away when I moved my arm too fast in getting something out of my purse.

One by one, different staff members emerged and called people to come in for medication checks. They stayed only moments, it seemed, and left. The whole place smelled like sour old clothes and unbathed skin. It was soon to be my turn, I hoped. I had so little time to do my interviewing with staff in between my own patients. The director came out and talked briefly with the secretary, only to be interrupted by the young man who wanted to go to Texas. The director yelled at him to shut up and sit down, telling him this wasn't a travel bureau and, in any case, he'd have to wait his turn.

In talking to the director behind the safety of his closed office door, I found an extremely sensitive, conscientious man who was tormented at the impossibility of using his knowledge and carrying out his ideals. The city was soon to close the center, and these patients would then be roaming the alleys and streets. The football stadium and its improvements now seemed to have the city's top financial priority. The state legislature was nonreactive. The staff was discouraged and threatened by the prospect of having no place to work.

I live ten blocks from where this center used to be. It pains me and sometimes frightens me as the alley behind my home becomes filled with ex-patients making their daily inspection of our garbage cans. The other day, an older chap encountered me in front of my garage and was furious because he heard me talking about him (he thought). He warned that he was going to call the FBI about me and proceeded to open a shoe box he was carrying and pull out an old phone on which to call. I've worked with people like this in a helping way for years, but, in my alley, I could do nothing. There was not even an available place to call to get help for him.

Increased personnel and technical equipment help in certain areas, of course, but these external solutions can be an avoidance of the real issues. Throughout our many consulting experiences, we have encountered the phrase "If we just had the money or the power to change things, all this would be different." However in many of these situations, our unfortunate appraisal has been that money and power would help not one bit. More often than not, increased staff funnels ineffectively into tasks to keep the bureacratic aspects of the system going—never reaching patient involvement.[7] Sometimes concern is not even felt or articulated about what goes on under one's nose. So many functions in health-care settings now are splintered into pieces for "increased efficiency." It is easy not to feel responsible for what goes on beyond a delimited area of function.

Our observation has been that our culture in general and our health-care culture specifically have become increasingly prone to conceptualizing an impersonal super-system to hold responsible, for example, the American Medical Association, the hospital administrators, or the "feds." Blaming "the system" has become a national pastime; yet, simultaneously, that very system is looked to for on-high direction in matters that an impersonal system can never help. Persistence in this approach is not only ineffective but also shrivels human potential. It leads to the misperception that a system is constructed of something other than live humanity, of which one is a part and for which one is responsible. It leads to a feeling of helplessness or blaming "the other." Displacement of blame onto the system also extinguishes both the sense of personal risk taking and the healthy struggle to define what is really valued.

Of course, there is a group of people in any organization that holds more power than others. Certainly this is so in any health-care system; but what are "they" being held responsible for by we who are also a part of that system? We believe that our health-care culture requires strong commitment to humanistic values. It is these values and the means to carry them out that health-care workers and consumers should be demanding. We would like to see legislative proposals carefully and emphatically artic-ulate humanistic goals for any evolving health-care delivery system; but, at the same time, we would also like to see the powers-that-be, patients, and helpers within any health-care system openly acknowledge that such goals are not going to be met simply by saying so. We believe that, ultimately, the essence of humanism is experienced between people in a dynamic interpersonal process and that it cannot be politically and financially mandated. To be humanistic is more than talk. It is to hold both an attitude and a set of behaviors that allow one to express visibly the dignity that one perceives in oneself and others.

Humanism as Defined Action

Some people behave in humanistically inclined ways in their everyday lives regardless of occupation. Others can be observed to commit themselves consciously to carrying out humanistic goals through such means as volunteer work, the Peace Corps, and civil rights projects. The well-meant intentions of these people are admirable. We breathe a sigh of hopefulness that there are those who maintain such values in an era when respecting the dignity of the other is sometimes difficult.

However, health-care workers must be more than well meaning. They are in a serious business, requiring roads that are paved with more than good intentions. When humanism is professed in a publicly recognized social role that gives one the privilege of lending formal assistance to another by being a helper, considerable responsibility ensues as to (1) what one's beliefs are about one's fellow human beings, (2) how one acts on those beliefs within a helping process, and (3) what the outcome of those beliefs might be for the other person. One cannot simply abide by embedded routines and policies and not know why. As pointed out previously, becoming insensitive to the commitment to being humane can be subtle. Following is an excerpt from an interview with a public-health nursing instructor at a large university medical center.

CASE IN POINT

It was back in the early 1960s—I guess when everybody was feeling like crusading for something. . . . One of the Kennedy sisters had been through the ob/gyn service as a part of a nationwide tour concerned with pregnant women. Word got back through the rumor mill that one of the back-East papers said that we were one of the places treating women "like cattle." Everybody was pretty defensive. I decided to put on my street clothes and go over and sit in the outpatient clinic all day. At 8:30 A.M., a woman who had been on the bus from downstate all night walked in; she said she had had six pregnancies and was here to see the specialist. She looked 50, and she was only 28 years old. I think she had three kids at home, which was a small ranch she and her husband were working. Every month she came up to the clinic because she had "sugar in her blood," as she said.

Five hours later, she was still waiting for her turn; she said she was afraid to get a sandwich or go to the bathroom lest she lose her turn in line. I went into the exam room with her when her name was called. She had yet another rotating doctor she hadn't met before. She had a pelvic, some blood drawn, a pat on the shoulder, and a friendly quip that she was doing "just fine." A nurse bruskly told her that she would be notified if there was "anything in her blood" and that she should try to keep her weight down. Ten minutes later she was on her way to the bus depot.

I talked to the staff afterward. No one remembered her from before, and no one knew how she got started coming. Everybody thought it was just sheer dumbness for a high-risk mother to come all that way, but nobody felt the responsibility to do anything about that. For sure, nobody felt they could do anything about the waiting-room situation. The whole episode was crazy; then it hit me that there was something about me, too; I got so caught up in trying to pick up what was wrong with everybody else in that system that I didn't even think to offer to go get that woman a sandwich.

In this situation, the public-health nursing instructor thought that her hands were tied in acting on her observations and personal insights. She explained that her efforts to raise concern about the quality of care were seen as threatening to the administration of the obstetrical service. She believed that she was "put off" as intruding in areas in which she did not have direct responsibility or authority. The best that she thought she could do in the face of a value clash was to utilize the experience in sensitizing her students in her own area of teaching responsibility.

In contrast, consider the example of Charlie, in regard for whom a hospital unit staff developed a willingness to explore its values and to define what help might be indicated in his particular case.

CASE IN POINT

Charlie was brought in from down in the Larimer Street area—a section of the city that had been his narrow life space for the many years that he had been a "street alcoholic." He had recently been "on the outs" with his buddies, and they could not care less about his not having the booze he wanted (and needed) to stave off the dt's. Charlie was having a hard time since he never had been one to share and the chickens were coming home to roost. He was also having a hard time talking clearly; he had a "thick" throat that did not go away. He would not go near the Wazee neighborhood center any more, since his old gang would only "come down on him." The police found him in the gutter one night with the dt's and brought him into the hospital.

It was a struggle to keep him alive, much less deal with his irrational behavior. As he became physically more intact, his hallucinations seemed to become worse. He was not pleasant. Just about the time that he was ready for discharge, he was discovered to have laryngeal carcinoma. Surgery was scheduled for the following week after what was to be a complete appraisal of his physical ability to survive a major procedure. He would stay on his present unit until after surgery.

After weeks of Charlie's having been a difficult patient to care for, I was asked to consult about this "obnoxious, cantankerous man who wouldn't cooperate with anything." Hardly a professional referral statement, but telling, in that apparently the staff wished him to be pleasant and cooperative.

Interviewing Charlie was a hard task; he *was* obnoxious and cantankerous, and his first utterance was to demand that I leave the room. I said that I would but asked when it was more convenient to come back. He said that he did not know what the hell I was bothering for anyhow. I explained that it was because he was blowing up everything here and I was supposed to straighten out the mess. He was aghast that "an old lush like me could stir up any such thing." I explained that he had more power than he thought, to which he immediately retorted, "If that is so, then why is it I can't have my cigarettes anymore?" We had got down to brass tacks. Charlie indeed did not know why he could not have his cigarettes, but neither did the staff "really" know when we conferred later.

At one level, everyone agreed that, if Charlie smoked, it would not help his throat, but this reasoning was countered with "Well, he's got cancer anyhow; so what does it matter?" But did Charlie know that he had cancer? No, he did not. Did they think that Charlie's dignity should be acknowledged by extending this information to him? Some thought that telling him would not change Charlie's attitude about smoking, since he "never seemed to care what happened to his life anyhow." On and on we went, indirectly working on the task of whether Charlie should be allowed to smoke. Beneath it all we were exploring how staff values were challenged by the nature of Charlie's life up to then and what Charlie's behavior meant in view of the hard work that had been put into saving his life.

To make a long story short, the staff was able to look a few facts straight in the eye. At the outset, they realized that they had chosen to struggle with what *they* wanted for Charlie. Only secondarily did they "listen" to what Charlie was saying: (1) Charlie placed high value on running his own life the way he saw fit and was more cooperative when people played it straight with him and when he believed that he had the power to make choices; 2) Charlie did not want to make all the decisions, since he had proved to be amenable to the proposal of surgery; and (3) Charlie had some different notions about how he wanted to live than the staff would have liked him to have. However, Charlie did want to live.

The problem came down to approaching Charlie about what *he* wanted to do about smoking in view of the fact that he had cancer of the throat. Charlie thought that he might as well keep smoking, since he did not have a great many satisfactions in life. He complained, "I can't even have a few good stiff belts." It was also explained to Charlie that a general anesthetic was less stressful to the lungs if heavy smokers quit for awhile before surgery. Because of his need to survive, Charlie agreed that two days before surgery he would quit smoking. Some of the staff were able to reflect with Charlie about how much they had wanted him to live when he had the dt's: "Guess we got sort of uptight when it looked like all our hard effort might go down the drain." One staff member apologized to Charlie for being an old bitch about his smoking. She later reported that he had said, "That's okay, honey; I used to have a wife like that a long time ago. She never used to ask either, and I showed her. You just ask— even an old drunk like me—and we'll get on just fine."

Charlie's example shows that to become an advocate[8] for humanistic values requires sensitization to some personal issues about oneself. Second, it requires openly defining some ethical issues about extending help, the answers to which require the making of value judgments. Answers to three critical questions are essential to defining the posture from which to operate in the helping process.

1. *What are the desired outcomes of any particular helping process?* For example, will the result of this help be just the maintenance of life, or is the patient's right or desire also respected? Will this help be focused on one aspect of the person's life, or will the helper attempt to appreciate the totality of the patient's present life space?
2. *What are the actions necessary in accomplishng the desired outcome of help?* For example, if certain treatment services are known to be available somewhere but not in the present circumstances, what does one do to make them available? What actions will be taken that are specifically related to help as defined by the situation and the patient's goals, in contrast to "scientific curiosity" or "routines?"
3. *Who assumes the responsibility for making the judgment as to the goals of help and the actions to be taken?* For example, when a person seeks help in a conscious, rational manner, who in the helper/patient dyad has the power in saying what will be the goals of the help? When persons are not capable of participating in what will happen to them, who becomes the advocate of the patient's rights?

Values Affecting Humanistic Helping

In response to the previous questions, a number of our students and colleagues have issued challenges about a health-care worker's right to get into the value-judgment business at all. Such challenges suggest that a helper is perceived as a robot. It is as if the overused professional motto "Be wary of imposing your values on others" has come to be interpreted as "Do not make any value judgments at all." The fact remains that everyone does make value judgments. What is important is to recognize (1) what one's values are, (2) how they are utilized in carrying out a practice believed to be helpful, and (3) how sensitive one is to their impact on others.[9]

We agree with Menninger,[10] who pointed out clearly that, in the formal study of values in the research sense, one must avoid posing as an expert on ethics. However, he recognized that those who help foster change in individuals from sickness to health cannot avoid making at least tacit value assumptions. Consider those values of which Menninger speaks and evaluate the potential impact that they might have on helping outcomes and the actions that a health-care worker might take: that health is better than illness; that pain hurts and its relief is good; that reality adaptation is better than retreat into a world of fantasy; that productivity and creativity are better than laziness; that love is better than hate; that constructiveness is to be preferred to destructiveness.

Few persons in Western culture would disagree with the value statements put forth by Menninger. They are articulated often in a variety of health-care settings and are responsible for many positive aspects of health care, but other values that often undermine humanistic value statements lurk in these settings under the guise of traditional ways of doing things. For example, countering a patient's complaints about treatment with the response that the professional knows best; insistence that it is safer, more efficient, and ultimately less trouble for the patient not to be allowed personal belongings; or discounting students' viable input about a patient because they have not yet had "enough experience."

Unfortunately, the subtle devaluations of human potential and right of choice in one's own destiny, as reflected in the foregoing examples, are likely to become an institutionalized set of beliefs held in common by all. How easy it is for exploitative, competitive, and manipulative power[11] to reign under the cloak of helping and learning. How difficult for such attitudes to be altered when the values become embedded within a subculture in which the receivers of help are incapable of doing much about such attitudes. People, when they become patients, cannot collectively revolt in the face of values that do not reflect their best interests. When seeking help and experiencing stress, patients are highly individualistic in their view of their life space. Often they become extremely dependent in their struggle against real or feared threats to their survival. For such patients to rally together and become a force powerful enough to counteract the collective power held by the helpers is nigh to impossible.

The values of helpers expressed through the power that they hold are critical if humanism is to exist in health-care settings. Values are important at more than one level of professional development: (1) seasoned professionals who, in failing to evaluate themselves with respect to their own values, can subtly contribute to a set of global standards that disallows a wide repertoire of behaviors of patients, students, and multidisciplinary peers and (2) students and beginning health-care workers who, in failing to evaluate and appropriately challenge, easily come to embrace prevailing systematized beliefs that perpetuate dehumanizing practices. At any level, if helpers choose not to go along with the values of the system but also fail to struggle consciously with their own values, they encourage passive rebellion to a point of "letting everybody do their own thing." Thus, they fail to recognize that no value structure at all may be as devastating as that which is discarded.

Particularly relevant to a humanistic helping process is the issue of deeply embedded policies about who makes decisions with or for the persons who come for health-care services. For example, increasing emphasis is being placed on participatory decision making in defining the goals of health as these involve patient and helper. Informed-consent procedures and patient bill-of-rights movements are in vogue at this time, but beneath the concern about patients' having an increased voice in goal setting and determining the helping actions to be taken, it is still argued that it is the medical profession's sole right to make judgments about helping processes engaged in by any discipline.[12] Although the physician holds considerable power over persons who seek help, helping as ultimately perceived by the patients comes in many modes and through a variety of personages. Once health-care workers of any discipline have become committed to the notion of the patient's having an equal share of responsibility in goal setting, value clarification as to what is better for whom comes rapidly to the fore.

Summary

In any formalized helping process, value judgments are unconsciously and consciously made. Sometimes these judgments are made with no concern for their power in affecting the attitudes and perceptions of patients and health-care colleagues. In the health-care field, so responsible for life-and-death results, we believe that value judgments must be openly acknowledged and defined. Forethought must be given to their effect on groups and individual patients. Not to do so is frankly unethical. At minimum, ignoring the impact of values present in the helping process leads to wasted effort on the part of health-care workers who are vaguely trying to help.

We also believe that, in the helping process, no one person is god, including the patient. Making critical value judgments regarding goals in this process is a jointly held responsibility between the helper and the patient or the patient's representative. When the patient requires the services of many people and a team effort, responsibility is always a multidisciplinary issue, in contrast to a unidisciplinary one.

Our concern is great that both the consumer and health-care workers continue publicly to express their discontent with subtle and gross inhumane practices and conditions within which human beings are being cared for and work. We are just as strongly concerned that, although the majority of health-care workers across the disciplines sincerely want to help others, they really do not know much about how to do so effectively. Follow-up studies increasingly show that, even with technological knowledge and under the best of physical conditions, health-care workers may not really be helping those who come for their services. A repeated theme haunts those who ask the empirical question "What is it to help?" Apparently not only is the essense of humanism expressed in a dynamic interpersonal process, but the essence of any kind of help in the health-care field must be experienced in a value-laden interpersonal process if help is to occur at all.

REFERENCE NOTES

1. For a service-oriented review of the American health-care system, read Stephan P. Strickland, *U.S. Health Care: What's Wrong and What's Right* (New York: Universe Books, 1972) and Lawrence Corey, S. Saltman, and M. Epstein, *Medicine in a Changing Society*, 2nd ed (St. Louis: C. V. Mosby, 1972). In *Life and Death and Medicine* (a *Scientific American* book) (San Francisco: W. H. Freeman, 1973), see the following: Martin S. Feldstein, "The Medical Economy," p. 112; James L. Goddard, "The Medical Business," p. 120, and Ernest W. Saward, "The Organization of Medical Care," p. 129.

2. *Helping* has many meanings, depending on the context in which it is used. Part of the purpose of this book is to evolve a more useful working definition of *helping*. For initial purposes, the structural definition by Maier may be useful: "A series of socially engineered interventive activities in which the practitioner deliberately introduces into the experience of an individual specifically structured means of preventing or treating deviant development." See Henry W. Maier, *Three Theories of Child Development* (New York: Harper & Row, 1969), p. 229.

3. Roger Rapoport, "It's Enough To Make You Sick," *Playboy Magazine* 20 (September 1973): 120ff.

4. Robin Cook, "My Turn: The New Doctor's Dilemma," *Newsweek*, 14 May 1973. Also see Cook's *The Year of the Intern* (New York: Harcourt Brace Jovanovich, 1972).

5. Carl Rogers et al., *Person to Person: The Problem of Being Human* (Lafayette, Calif.: Real People Press, 1967), p. 255.

   Ibid., p. 134.

7. For a discussion of professional/bureaucratic role-conflict theory, see Marlene Kramer, *Reality Shock: Why Nurses Leave Nursing* (St. Louis: C. V. Mosby, 1974), pp. 27–66.

8. To be an advocate usually means more than quietly holding to a value; it requires an active, visible position. One can advocate for an idea or for other persons through acting in their behalf. Chapter 6 discusses helpers as advocates in more detail.

9. For a pungent reminder of value-shirking behaviors of health-care workers during the Nazi regime, see Leon Uris's novel, *QB VII* (New York: Doubleday, 1970).

10. Karl A. Menninger, with Paul W. Pruyser, "Morals, Values, and Mental Health," in *The Encyclopedia of Mental Health*, eds. Albert Deutsch and Helen Fishman (New York: Watts, 1963), vol. 4, pp. 1244–45.

11. Rollo May, *Power and Innocence* (New York: Norton, 1972), pp. 105–8.

12. The right of the medical profession to make judgments about helping processes engaged in by any discipline is a controversial and touchy, but nonetheless real, issue. Many professions other than the medical make judgments about the helping process in various health-care settings. The issue is who makes ultimate decisions or can work without the supervision of a physician? Nurses, in their struggle for autonomy as a profession, encounter such controversies both legally and in everyday work with medical peers. A particularly hot debate in this regard has occurred in congressional committees between the American Medical Association and the American Psychological Association with respect to the National Health Insurance regulations. See Russell J. Bent, "A Professional Issue: The Psychologist Supervised by Medical Doctors," *Professional Psychology* 3 (1972): 351–56. In the 1980s, the debate continues.

SUGGESTIONS FOR FURTHER EXPERIENCE

1. Contact the administrative offices of the hospital or clinic in which you work and request from them all the written material available concerning the following:

   a. Policies regarding standards for patient care.

   b. Formal statements concerning a "patient bill of rights."

   c. Informed-consent contracts for patients, as well as release-of-information forms.

   d. Personnel policies as they apply to all levels of staff.

   These materials, when collectively reviewed, ideally should reflect the belief-system basis from which the health-care agency operates. Within a group seminar, evaluate these materials from the following standpoints:

   a. *Adequacy of materials available.* Such materials generally must be available to accrediting agencies. However, how immediately available these are to consumers and front-line staff is a first test of whether the administrators of a system mean what they say in writing.

   b. *Weight of concern.* Many policies and standards in health-care systems were created more to "protect" the staff than to respect the rights of patients. Evaluate carefully whether, collectively, all the materials present a balanced concern.

   c. *Avenues by which to express oneself formally.* An open system that is committed to the rights of others provides visible mechanisms by which humanistic concerns can be raised. Evaluate whether such mechanisms exist for patients and all levels of staff.

   d. *Values that the materials suggest.* Embedded within policy and procedure statements are the values to which a system holds. Attempt to ferret out a series of value statements that you believe the written materials to reflect.

2. Review pages 246–48 of Marilyn Ferguson's *The Aquarian Conspiracy: Personal and Social Transformation in the 1980s* (Los Angeles: Tarcher, 1980). Study her simplified comparison of the prevailing paradigms concerning health and medicine. Discuss which of the paradigms seem to be reflected in the health-care setting in which you are presently working and learning.

Chapter 5

Humanistic Helping and the Interpersonal Process

We have proposed that the humanistic intentions of health-care workers are actualized in interpersonal behavior. We have also proposed that, no matter what is known about highly scientific technology, effective *helping* will not occur unless the importance of interpersonal happenings between helper and patient is acknowledged. The elusive, quicksilver nature of the interpersonal process is the major difficulty in putting humanistic helping into action.

Shlien states, "What's to say? I have the feeling that everybody knows everything as far as human interaction goes."[1] Yet, people feel like novices when they try to formalize enduring human-to-human phenomena that transcend "book learning." For students and practicing professionals alike who are trying to apply what has been formally taught, this attempt is highly frustrating. When one is energetic in discovering what helping is all about or actively engaging in problem solving, it is discouraging to be told that health care's Gordian knot cannot be cut with bold, hard scientific knowledge. How frustrating to appreciate that one must unravel the interpersonal process slowly and examine the "something" that affects learning, helping, coping, resisting, conforming, searching, and even dying. How ironic to be told that one can look *outwardly* only so far in modeling the behaviors of other professionals, since much of helping requires an *inward* look and acceptance of one's identity before one can begin to appreciate the views of others.

Frustration with not being able to pin down and predict the exact nature of the interpersonal process is often expressed by students in bursts of diffuse anger. This frustration is exemplified by a Phi Beta Kappa social-work student who, before going into her first "professional" interview, exclaimed, "Five years of college and straight A's; I feel like I'm going on my first blind date!" We assured her that going into the situation as if it were a blind date would undoubtedly hold her and the patient in good stead. Obviously we were confronting her with what she already knew well before college: that she was entering into a process within which she and another person, as two "unknowns," would try to learn something about, and hopefully like, each other. Having been through innumerable new encounters in her social development, she needed reminding that she had indeed survived that process; but, at the same time, we were confronting her with a situation of potentially high anxiety—that the experience of her expensive preclinical education suddenly felt useless in providing the structured technical direction that she thought was needed.

For students in fields requiring a hard core of technical skills in addition to interpersonal prowess—nursing and medicine—the demand to be a safe, effective helper is even greater. Pressured to apply techniques accurately and master equipment at the same time that patients are met face to face, beginning students not surprisingly become vulnerable to reliance on stereotypical procedures to carry them through the elusive interpersonal process. How much easier it becomes to view patients as "cases" who have to respond to a helper's imposed structure with enforced dependency.[2]

The Elusive Nature of Helping

Because helping is largely an interpersonal process, the concept of helping is not an easy one to grasp immediately. Look further, then, at the concept of helping as it is set forth in the health-care field.

At the informal level of trying to determine how the health field defines helping, one is confronted with hints suggested by slogans and professional jargon. For example, on the walls of one collegiate school of nursing appeared attractive posters acclaiming "Helping is to care"; yet, interviews with the students to whom the posters appealed revealed that they were not at all certain as to how to carry out that message in a meaningful way. Similar statements, such as "Meet total patient needs," also suggest that this mandate has something to do with "really" helping. Clearly, meeting the patient's total needs is difficult to do, and some patients do not want that much involvement. On the other hand, the equally admonishing motto of helping, "Don't get involved with your patients," is easy to follow, although many patients do want involvement. Although such slogans suggest that an ultimate truth exists somewhere within the health-care culture, the derived messages are conflicting and provide diffuse guidelines.

Little written material has been available to health-care workers until recently on the specific subject of *helping*. This lack was exemplified in our travels when we found that the libraries of two prestigious medical centers did not even have the subject heading in the card index. On the other hand, the subject heading *therapeutic* often contains myriads of references, primarily those reflecting drugs and various forms of mechanistic procedures. Not only is the broad literature short on the subject of helping, it is also overwhelmingly one-sided in its descriptions of patients, in contrast to those of helpers. There is a sparse number of case histories of helpers, depicting those who were successful and those who were not, against which others might evaluate themselves.

The lack of firm knowledge about the process of help or the nature of the helper, as contrasted with the emphasis on technological products, in large measure reflects the value placed on exacting procedures and on "things." It also reflects the lack of a research orientation within service settings as to what "treatment" includes in addition to the results of laboratories or research wards—both of which are often distant from where realistic helping action occurs.

The dearth of people/action research concerning helping is understandable. Service-providing personnel are generally not educated in research techniques, and, in the need to provide services to large numbers, accountability as to outcomes of their efforts has been difficult to obtain. When researchers do appear on the scene, those on the "front lines" often believe that researchers know little about the human interactional problems that are experienced day after day. Many times the researcher is not concerned with the same issues that plague health-care workers. Often those within the eye of the hurricane are frankly hostile to persons "from the outside" who attempt to carry out formal studies about helping.

CASE IN POINT

Talking to the clinic staff after the Research and Evaluation Team left was an angry team leader: "I've got enough to do right here without talking with some smart aleck, wet behind the ears, who wants to find out if we're worth it. So what if they find out we didn't do any good— there's more coming in the front door, baby. I'm paid to do the best I can do inside—right here."

Researchers who are able and willing to tackle human-interaction problems are not in abundance within the broad health-care field. This also is an understandable situation. Study of any form of interpersonal process entails tedious research. The subject·matter is not easily encapsulated. Present scientific models of research are designed primarily to explore quantifiable entities that are easily transposed into symbols that computers can analyze. Helping, presumably an interpersonal process, is seemingly as resistant to our present methods of research design as is the concept of love— one that many argue might best be left to the poets. Also, in an era in which "hard" science research is in vogue and in which one ascends the status ladder by doing the kind of thing that is "in," material that does not meet these qualifications tends to be unexplored and disregarded. For better or worse, the reality is that material presently available in understanding the helping process is still highly subjective. Perhaps it always will be. Maybe the task of the future is to explore everyday complexities not by forcing them into existing research models, but rather by devising more creative research models that not only capture, but also preserve, the forces that operate between persons.[3]

Helping is an elusive concept, even for researchers of social behavior and human development. For example, the understanding of helping at even the most primitive level involves consideration not only of why someone becomes a helper but also of how motive interacts with what a helping person considers to be a necessary payoff for actions.[4] More complicated is understanding why, in certain circumstances, helping does not occur, even when the need for "help" seems obvious, and individuals are seen to retreat to the point of view of another's "right to be left alone" or the principle of "why me?" For example, for individual neighbors to withdraw from aiding a street victim who is undergoing a gang attack is one matter; for these same neighbors to refrain from calling the police is another matter.[5] More difficult to unravel is the dilemma of Vietnam veterans who found themselves initially motivated to help the fringe victims of the war, as did the GIs in World War II, but instead involved themselves in the ruthless killing of women and children, behaving as if they had no conscious control.[6]

How someone develops into a helping person is not yet clear.[7] B. F. Skinner, writing about the ethics of helping people, stated that we presumably help others, in part, out of concern for survival of the species, stemming from a genetic endowment or behavioral disposition that is culturally reinforced. He pointed out, however, that our capacity to learn is the critical factor:

> It is more obvious that we *learn* to help or do good and that we learn because of the consequences that follow. We may find the helplessness of others aversive and help them to reduce our own discomfort. We help those who help us in return, and we stop doing so when they stop—when, as we say, they are ungrateful. The importance of reciprocal action is clear from the fact that we often fail to help those who are too weak to reciprocate or to protest effectively when we fail to help. The very young, the aged, the infirm, the retarded, and the psychotic are classic examples of people who have often been not only not helped but mistreated.[8]

Our survey of multidisciplinary groups of health-care workers shows that, somewhere in childhood, the notion of wanting to be a sharing, helping kind of person had its origin. Dare one go so far as to believe that humans are born that way? We often think not when we consider the behaviors within the egocentric, narcissistic developmental levels of early childhood, which make parents question whether their offspring will ever learn to share or to be empathetic. On the other hand, our society has not given high priority to teaching or maintaining children's concern for the welfare of others.[9] One wonders if some form of innate altruism eventually becomes lost within the violent visual and auditory stimuli to which youngsters are increasingly exposed. It is encouraging to note that research is emerging to study how one learns to be concerned for others.[10]

What help means to one's patients is also slippery to grasp at times. In situations in which patients' conditions allow them little choice in what is going to be done to them, what was done in a technical sense to prevent death or to bring patients to a state of orientation may be easy to define. However, what one did in helping a patient who seeks care consciously and voluntarily is more difficult to explain. One may receive feedback from such patients that they were helped a great deal during their crisis. Often the furthering of understanding stops at that point. Positive platitudes and thanks are the desired messages, and so, content with that music to the ears, one often fails to ferret out those specific activities that the patient thought to be helpful.

At other times, after receiving one's best-defined efforts and skills, patients believe that they were not helped at all and proceed to seek another professional or to find "help" from proponents of nonsensical gadgetry.

CASES IN POINT

Alva and Mary had been to two major medical centers for the evaluation of their 6-year-old son. The staff at the Developmental Center was committed to full exploration of parent goals before beginning a third appraisal. The center team spent a number of hours talking with the parents about their previous experiences, how they wished to be responded to, and major concerns that they wished addressed. All through the course of the sessions, Alva and Mary were asked if the team was proceeding as they had anticipated. At the completion of a comprehensive evaluation, six hours of parent feedback sessions were held.

Three months after the final parent conference, Alva and Mary were asked to fill out a follow-up form that would assist the Developmental Center to learn whether help had been successful. Their response was that everyone had been warm and responsive to what they wanted. However, they felt that all they had learned was that their child was "atypical," and they said that they had known that before they came.

Lori and her husband had both been heavy heroin users and became members of a couples' rehabilitation group at the Methadone Clinic. Part of the program was to assist clients to begin utilizing broad community resources instead of relying entirely on the drug program. Lori was having a number of gynecological complaints. She was encouraged to seek out a private specialist, whom she could now afford. After the initial visit, she returned to the group and furiously explained, "That dumb so-and-so. All he did was get a history, examine me, and tell me I needed a D and C. All I wanted was something for pain, and I couldn't even con him for a lousy codeine. I used to cop those birds for stuff at least twice a week, and I get ahold of a guy that's straight."

As the following cases show, sometimes both the patient and the helper initially believe that help has indeed been experienced, only to find later that something was occurring that had unique meaning to the patient but was not shared openly with the helper.

CASES IN POINT

Betty and her husband had worked hard with the therapist in learning to live effectively with their mentally retarded and often emotionally distressed son. Periodically, when the helping process was reviewed with them, both parents expressed their satisfaction with the results. Help was always defined in terms of the progress of their son and a less chaotic home situation. After formal termination of the helping process at the clinic, Betty was interviewed as to what had helped her most. She explained, "No one told me what I really wanted to hear. Who wants to hear that their child has damage in the brain? Sure I was upset, but you let me be upset without jumping in and putting me on tranquilizers. That was the first thing they wanted to do at that other place. They knocked me out. How can you manage two kids and a husband if you are a zombie? But more important, when they immediately suggested drugs, it made me feel like an idiot. It helped so much when you people didn't do that to me. It helped me feel like I really was a strong person and like I had a right to be upset. I couldn't say that to you at the time. . . ."

From a nursing diary is recorded a painful experience of a helper's feeling "left out." Sylvia had been discharged from the hospital two weeks previously, after a long stay. She had been in a horrifying car wreck. . . . She had been driving, and her sister and two little nieces had been killed. Tonight I was called down to the emergency room, and there was Sylvia in terminal condition from a suicide attempt. She was still able to talk and I just had to ask her how this could have happened. When I had seen her last, she had praised the staff for 'all we had done.' Tonight she said we had all helped her a lot, but we had been 'too good' to her. She felt she didn't deserve to live."

A 55-year-old widow was interviewed after surgery for a complete hysterectomy. She was asked about the most important aspects of the helping process as experienced with her physician. She responded by relating her thoughts and feelings prior to seeking help. She explained that, at the onset of heavy vaginal bleeding, she instantly thought that she had cancer. She became preoccupied with the word to the extent that, if she even thought of it, she experienced an attack of anxiety (i.e., increased heart rate and breathlessness). She also could not tolerate having anyone else say the word out loud. When she sought out her physician, she told him that she wanted to know what she had—the full truth—but did not want him to use "that word" in telling her if she had "it." After surgery, the first thing that her physician told her was "You don't have 'it.' " She summarized what she perceived as help by explaining, "He did a skillful task with that surgery, I'm sure, and I'm grateful for his skill. I told him that, but what helped me the most—which he probably doesn't appreciate—is that he automatically respected my wish for the word *cancer* not to be used. I was raised to value dignity. I was so fortunate to find someone at this time who also respected that. I suppose I should tell him about that, too."

A further difficulty in understanding the helping process is that multiple confounding factors often do not grant the helper a clear-cut place to begin. When some patients come for help, their stress level prevents them from being specific about what is happening to them or about the kind of help they want. Often, what patients say they want does not seem to fit with the helper's intuitive sense about what is happening. Following is the beginning episode in what came to be a long course of a family helping process.

CASE IN POINT

Jerry, a 15-year-old high school dropout, was brought to the mental-health center by his mother. Obese, disheveled, and markedly uncomfortable in response to being in tow by his mother, Jerry initially spoke little. His mother thoroughly dominated the initial interview. She was a worn-out-looking woman, exasperated with everyone and mistrustful of anyone who tried to help her. "The school is picking on Jerry; they always have." "He's such a good boy, but he's lazy and won't listen to me anymore." "I want someone to make the school let him back right now." The mother's agenda was clear: she wanted someone to defend her perceptions of her son against those persons whom she saw as misunderstanding him.

Jerry's view was not at all comparable to that of his mother. He did not want to be in school. He thought that it was a drag and wanted to go to work. He did not think that he was lazy. He thought that he was "sick" but would not elaborate. He expressed verbal aggression openly against his mother and wanted to talk with someone alone. His mother initially refused, making vague references to something "crazy" he would talk about "that was nobody's business."

Where to go from this point of strong impasse was difficult to know. Who needed the advocate in a situation involving a minor child? Jerry's mother clearly had the power. The decision was made to share the conflict openly with Jerry and his mother. The following question had to be resolved *with* them: where does one begin if two people have different ideas of what they want to happen and one is in control of the other? Fortunately, the mother did allow Jerry to be seen for one interview by himself, but she agreed to it only if he would allow her the same privilege. Jerry complied.

He rambled during his interview. Periodically he would express vehement anger at what he perceived to be a "busybody" mother and an "alcoholic slob of an old man." He wanted them to leave him alone. The only thing he wanted from the center was a blood test for syphilis because he thought that "something is crawling around in my brain." He mumbled from time to time, particularly as he ruminated about the blood test. When he spoke of it, he interspersed comments that his mother "really thinks I'm crazy." Several times he related being crazy to what obviously had been a terrifying homosexual experience that had occurred when he was 8 years old.

It was impossible to sort out anything that he wanted from the center other than the blood test, and about this he said, "Yes, *I* want it," but "No, my mother won't allow it to happen." It seemed best to start with exactly what Jerry wanted, but within a broader context of what his mother might accept. Jerry agreed to be cooperative with a full physical examination and not to do battle with his mother if she agreed to the suggestion.

To Jerry's surprise, his mother agreed to a complete physical examination as a place to begin. She was able to accept the idea partly out of relief at not being rejected. As she said, "I thought you people would put me off right away like all the rest." In addition, she thought that starting there made sense, since "he hasn't had a physical since he was a kid" and "maybe it's a good idea to make sure there's nothing else besides being just lazy."

The physical examination revealed no syphilis. Jerry's fear had been stimulated by his learning about venereal disease in school and had been misapplied to the memories of his homosexual attack and had become a way to explain his felt neurological symptoms. The neurological examination revealed a slowly growing brain tumor that no one had expected to find.

As the above cases emphasize, to understand a helping process fully, one should be highly sensitive to the fact that any particular patient/helper dyad is highly susceptible to each other's values and personal perceptions. How true is the old saying "One man's meat is another man's poison," or the more modern phrase "Different strokes for different folks." How difficult it is to accept the truism that, if patients say that they have not been helped, they have not.

Critical Ingredients of Helping

Much research has been done on the effectiveness of certain drugs on a disease process. That certain drugs work with most patients but have idiosyncratic effects with other patients has been documented for centuries. Most of these cases involve highly sensitive physiological differences within individuals that contribute to special isolated reactions. Recently, it has also been found that certain therapeutic procedures do not have the desired effect—not because of physiological idiosyncracy—but because of social/emotional variables interacting with disease processes or one's feeling of well-being. These variables can range from the patient's simply not taking the prescribed medication because Aunt Martha had something that felt better and worked faster, to the patient's attitude about living or dying.[11-15] Out of such insights, it becomes clear that (1) helping cannot be confused with the treatment of disease; (2) helping will not occur simply because the physician says that it will; and (3) helping is a process supplementary to what patients already have going for them—emotionally, socially, and physically.

In isolating the critical ingredients of a helping process, we will explore what is generally obvious to some already working in the field. In the annals of research on the effective outcomes of professional helping, within the health-care disciplines that practice psychotherapy, much work has been done.[16] As to psychotherapy (a helping process that relies almost entirely on the quality of interpersonal relationship), it has long been demonstrated that the personal nature of the therapist is a critical variable. The therapist's beliefs, values, and philosophy about human beings influence the particular behavioral approaches that will be taken in problem solving with the patient.[17] These personal characteristics, integrated with the clinical knowledge that the helper has learned, influence effective helping according to whether these "fit" with the person of the client. This fact seems to hold true in less formalized "psychotherapy" settings as well. For a number of years, through studies in the institutional care of the "mentally ill," attitudes of mental-health workers who are less authoritarian, restrictive, and custodial have been known to be perceived as more helpful.[18]

Although not as systematically researched as to helping outcome, studies done in other health-care fields reflect the historical insights that medicine and nursing have always intuitively "known": something in the doctor/patient or nurse/patient relationship effects a "healing" process. Innumerable studies have been carried out on attitudes of the nursing or medical student-practitioner in response to certain kinds of patients.[19] Most of these studies imply that characteristics selected for study include certain attitudes and behaviors that are more critical to helping than others—for example, sensitivity versus insensitivity; honesty versus avoidance; warmth and acceptance versus hostility and aloofness; involvement with patients versus isolation of them; and belief in a patient's ability to change versus belief in inability or resistance to change.

In comparing the better-researched outcome studies found in psychotherapeutic literature with attitudinal studies carried out in other health-care situations, the critical ingredients as defined by Rogers[20] seem to have the highest utility in application across all health-care settings. Rogers has long held that, unless a high degree of positive regard, congruence, and empathetic understanding exists between the helper and the patient, effective helping will not occur. These ingredients will be explored in depth, since they seem analogous to what many health-care experts say "should" be occurring, what students say that they want to learn to do, and what patients say that they want in all health-care encounters with professionals.

Positive regard   From divergent viewpoints in the health-care field, the ability to express positive regard for the patient is stressed. Through this ability comes the effort to provide a nonthreatening, safe, trusting, or secure atmosphere for the patient.[21] At its most simplistic level of definition, it concerns an underlying respect for another, regardless of the behavior at hand. Rogers describes positive regard as caring "for his client, in a nonpossessive way, as a person with potentialities. It involves a willingness for the client to be true to whatever feelings are real in him at the moment—hostility or tenderness, rebellion or submissiveness, assurance or self-depreciation."[22] To this description, we would add respect for what patients say they want for themselves, regardless of whether it seems to fit at the time with the helper's notions of what the patient should want.

Admittedly, positive regard is a difficult attitude to maintain with all patients. In our everyday life, prior to becoming formalized helpers, we were aware that some people we "simply don't like"; some we are afraid to "get close to"; and, with others, we find that we have to "work at it." In informal social relations, it is easier to disregard persons that we do not like and go about the business of building involvements with those that we do. Some people initially reject for themselves what we see their potential to be. It is hard to accept the feelings of persons who insist that they want to die in the face of a social/emotional crisis or a physiological disease for which we feel another "treatment" might help; but, regardless of what people say, their feelings must be respected as real and meaningful to them. In health-care settings within which we have little choice as to who enters our life space for help, the challenge of developing humane, positive regard is not easy; yet it is critical that all patients find someone who can feel that way about them.

As a review of the attitudinal literature about health-care workers reveals, there is much need for attitude change in the direction of acceptance and willingness to become involved with patients experiencing certain behaviors or disease conditions. For example, those who do not seem to be "ill," those with widely deviant behavioral patterns, those with chronic physically disabling conditions, and the dying may require change in the helper's attitude toward involvement. Devaluing these patients by staying away from them or responding to them as "cases" because of dislike, low satisfaction, and fear denies these patients a *helping* experience, even though a realistic helping model cannot demand that everybody like everyone. Through conditions of congruence and empathetic understanding, helpers can develop ways of overcoming both their initial reactions and those of the patient.

Congruence   Rogers[23] explained that helpers are more congruent when they are what they are—genuine and without a front or facade. This is in contrast to helpers who seem to be playing a role or to be operating behind a front. Sometimes we refer to these people as "fakey," "stuffy," "too cool to approach," or "phony." Such persons are described as exhibiting incongruence; they are not in touch with themselves in a way that convinces others in their life space that they are genuine in their interactions. No one is totally congruent at all times, but there appears to be a critical element of realness about oneself that is revealed to others before helping is perceived by them to be effective. Jourard clarified congruence as he responded to students who knew that they faced situations in which they must be both "professional" and "real." "It is a difference between *taking* a role and *playing* a role. To take a role is a commitment to a task; to play a role is a charade."[24] Coles, reflecting on his beginnings in trying to "get with" people, described what being more congruent is like:

> I wasn't good at it at all at first. . . . I was stiff and nervous and very much being the important doctor. . . . We'd get home, Jane and I, after a day of that sort of interviewing, and I'd realize that people of the family really liked Jane and were chatting like an old friend. But they were stiff and formal with me. And one day Jane said, "For heaven's sake, Bob, stop doing that. Stop being so stuffy." And gradually I got better at getting acquainted with people.[25]

Congruence is not just a helpful attribute in relating to patients. It also can assist health-care workers in honestly acknowledging some aspects of themselves—for example, openly facing whom they believe that they can or want to work with.

CASE IN POINT

Missy is a nurse practitioner in a private, holistic family-health clinic. She was asked if there were some people who used the clinic to whom she simply could not relate comfortably. She promptly said yes. She explained: "When I was a student and until the past year, I totally recoiled inside whenever I was confronted with a middle-aged woman who had chronic head-aches. I would perceive her complaints as 'whiney.' I felt only aversion—no empathy at all. . . . Visions of my mother lying on the couch for hours with a wet rag on her head. I sought counseling about it briefly so I could understand my feelings better—at least to keep my inter-nal state somewhat more under control. I had so much leftover little-kid rage at Mom for not 'being there' for me when I felt I needed her." When Missy was asked if she could now relate helpfully to such a person, she replied, "No, I still could not be a primary helper. We here at the clinic understand we all have some form of hang-up like that. We don't press guilt buttons. We don't walk on water, you know. . . . We grow into facing such things in our own time, whenever that is. We help each other. That is comforting to me."

It is better for health-care workers to determine early at what point they have difficulty in relating to others, choosing either to grow in relating to a broad variety of people or to dispense with the goal of working in a people-oriented profession. Every-one has the qualifications to be a patient at one time or another. Not everyone has the personal qualifications to be a helper. It is not a sin to acknowledge that one's abilities may not fit an occupation requiring a high degree of close involvement with other persons.

For those who choose to stay in the helping professions and work through an interpersonal process, the quality of congruence will be struggled with again and again. How real is "real"? How many of one's honest feelings can be revealed? As will be shown, deciding how real one can be or should be depends a great deal on the pressures of the work setting and one's respect for and knowledge of the patient.

Empathetic understanding   Within the helping process, one's ability to be con-gruent is intimately related to the ability to develop empathetic understanding. Empa-thy is a concept that has been treated in a vague way that often misses the point. It is more complex than "walking in another's moccasins." Helpers who are not very open to their own values and attitudes or who share little of these with others tend to view the other person's world primarily in terms of the helper's, not the patient's, experi-ence. Empathy is more objective than just pretending to be other persons and imagin-ing what their lives would be like. It is a combination of listening for another's particular feelings and sharing the humane concern that one would want one's own feelings—whatever they might be—respected if one were in a similar situation.

The critical outcome of empatheic understanding is to be as accurate as possible in understanding the subjective moment-to-moment perception of the patient without get-ting in the way.[26] Literally, it means attempting to infer as clearly as possible the other person's private world and to understand those personal meanings without losing ei-ther one's separateness or the capacity to imagine how it would be for oneself to be "the other guy." To learn maximally about how patients perceive their schema of life and thereby be constructively empathetic, helpers must be maximally congruent. To the degree that they can be real, helpers will generally find patients developing in-creasing trust and thereby disclosing more about themselves.[27,28]

If one is real and empathetic and if patients trust and disclose more about themselves, then what? Carkhuff[29] explains that then one can get at patients' *frame of reference* and thereby their goals. This understanding, however, can retard the helping process if it is used to make categorical generalizations.

Frame of reference is a concept that has been around a long time in the field of psychology—especially social psychology. In modern terms, it is similar to what is meant by "getting on the same wavelength" or "knowing where someone is at." The term cannot be used to explain behavior simplistically, as by saying "Oh, he just has a hippie frame of reference." It is a useful concept that can helpfully analyze specific influences operating both within and outside a person at any given time.

Sherif and Sherif[30] refer to the totality of external and internal factors operating in an interdependent way in a person's life space at any given time as a frame of reference of the experience and behavior of the person or group in question. The external factors are those stimulating situations outside the individual, such as objects, events, other persons, groups, and cultural products. The internal factors are motives, emotions, attitudes, general states of the body, and effects of past experience. Sometimes these internal factors are experienced consciously; sometimes they are not. Both internal and external factors in dynamic interrelationship form a unity of experience and behavior. They influence how the person will structure situations psychologically and subsequently respond.[31]

The fact that both internal and external factors within a person's frame of reference may have different weights or degree of influence at any point in time is what makes the interpersonal process so elusive to grasp at times. That is why it appears so important to evaluate empathetically and congruently in the patient/helper relationship where the other is "at" in the here and now. Certain internal factors (such as beliefs, attitudes, and values) lend constancy or consistency to the way that one tends to view or react to a situation. However, these factors may change over a period of time or be denied temporarily because of interaction with external circumstances or internal physiological events. Human beings are capable of assuming many modes when it is critical to do so, resulting in a person's suddenly not acting as usual. This kind of behavior change is most dramatically observable when people see that their survival is at stake. An example of painful, public, forced denial of privately held values is aptly described by Grier and Cobbs in *Black Rage*:

> A boy lived with his uncle, whom he adored. Their particular pleasure was spending Saturdays in town together. One such afternoon while walking along a street, they met a white man with his son, who was larger than the dark child. Without ado the white man kicked the black child and ordered his son to beat him up. The white boy beat him thoroughly while the uncle stood aside and sadly watched the proceedings.[32]

As in this example, helpers in every health-care setting experience persons who respond contrary to their normal everyday behavior, particularly when the reality of a threat to physical survival from disease or injury rushes into awareness. Sensitivity to alterations in a patient's frame of reference *or* to the struggle to maintain a view regardless of reality can assist helpers in understanding the patient. In the following case, consider the importance of understanding where Arthur "was at" if any helping intervention was to fit effectively with his individual style, which he needed to maintain staunchly.

CASE IN POINT

Arthur had always been a successful hustling businessman. He equated money and status with power in his profession. Both he had achieved. He shared little of himself with his family and employees, except for material goods and insistence on loyalty to the organization. He took much pride in being a self-made man who did it alone.

At the onset of hospitalization for stomach pains, Arthur was alternately jovial and demanding. He thought that he deserved the best, stating "I have the money to afford it, and I expect it." However, stomach pains were found to mean gastric malignancy with metastases to the pancreas, and the course of his progress did not meet with his expectations of easily overcoming the "little intrusion." As time went on, rather than maintaining his buoyant, demanding style, he became increasingly quiet and seclusive.

At the time that Arthur was interviewed, he did not know the actual diagnosis, but he had suspicions. What he did know was that his usual style was ineffective in controlling his progress. He did not view others as failing to come through. He believed that "I should be able to do anything" and could not accept the fact that he could not rise above "whatever this damn thing is" alone.

Summary

Dehumanizing practices exist in the health-care field; however, such practices do not always occur. In attempting to understand this disparity, one is impressed by the fact that it is "something" occurring or failing to occur *between persons* that makes the difference. A further impressive fact is that a particular characteristic of this "something" causes patients to perceive that they have been helped. Review of the kind of interpersonal process that spells help to patients suggests that it is not limited to any particular kind of health-care setting or professional discipline. If this "helping" does occur so widely, where are the guidelines to what this mysterious process is all about? And why have those in the health-care field not already attended to where the answers might lie?

In part, the interpersonal process in helping has taken a backseat in the recent years of enthusiasm for the technological products of science. As an extension of technological progress and the knowledge boom, the era of specialization has in part obliterated the awareness of where some of the knowledge about helping might lie. For example, until recently, the valuable results of research about the effective ingredients of a helping process as learned from psychotherapy have been either ignored or compartmentalized by the general health field. For many years, understanding human behavior and applying interpersonal skills have been given a secondary position as an "art" for health-care workers to acquire mysteriously along the way.[33] If the "art" was defined and specifically taught, it took place during a psychiatric rotation when the student was "older" or "more mature."[34]

However, the picture has been changing. Helpers of all professional disciplines are questioning why certain procedures and techniques do not work; and, much earlier in their professional development, health-care students are asking for input concerning what can be done when patients do not "act like they should." Health-care workers in settings other than those with a primary psychotherapeutic emphasis are listening to patients and reporting that patient dissatisfaction lies within interpersonal patient/ helper communication.[35] It is also beginning to be learned that those students who make more effective helpers—as perceived by patients—can be carefully selected or educated to be effective beyond their intuitive inclinations.[36] Such personal characteristics as the capacity to have positive regard for another human being, to evaluate another empathetically, and to be a congruent, open person are salient in the profile of an effective helper in any setting.

At this juncture in our analysis of helping, several messages seem to emerge: (1) all the hard-earned technological knowledge and mechanistic procedures so essential in providing safe physical care in certain situations may be worthless unless simultaneously people come to grips with the "nature" of each other; (2) coming to grips with each other must occur in an interactional communication process, the critical core of which is each person's frame of reference, reflecting a view of life in general and of each other specifically; and (3) the individual natures of the helpers and their interpersonal abilities are factors of major impact if an effective, humanistic helping process is to occur.

In the previous material, we have emphasized that health-care workers must learn a great deal about the individual nature, or "person," of their patients. They must know their complaints, their goals for help, and the personal meanings that they attach to what is happening to them. Not only does this knowledge ensure safe care, but also, what one chooses to know about another forms the basis of humane care. With as much emphasis, we stress the importance of the person, or nature, of the helper. It is increasingly apparent that, as a person, the helper is a powerful therapeutic "tool." Appreciation of one's power as a helper cannot be gained by standing back from the situation. Helpers must come to feel it is okay to be about the business of "knowing thyself," not just for one's own personal/social growth, but as a professional responsibility.

To continue to ignore the person of the helper would overlook the power of the health-care worker—both as a vital positive resource and as the key to the dehumanizing conditions so often observed in health-care settings. In addition to the internal capacities for positive regard, empathy, and congruence, the values that helpers hold or come to hold through experience with the health-care culture are critical variables in the helping process. For example, we maintain that the belief system of helpers will ultimately allow or disallow patients to be "who they are" or to articulate "who they wish to become." Confronted with thoughts, feelings, or overt behaviors of others that go beyond the values held by helpers, helpers tend to do what is safer for themselves.

In becoming a helper, conscious evaluation of where one stands (i.e., awareness of one's own frame of reference) is a highly important process. This awareness is central to appreciation of what not imposing one's values on others really means. It is not simply withholding one's views about politics from the patient who holds an opposite argument or refraining from challenging a patient's assertion that there are spiders on the wall. It is understanding how one's own and others' behavior contributes to why patients act the way they do. It is appreciating that some of the values that one consciously or unconsciously assumes in becoming a professional may interfere with being effective with a patient.

The more that health-care workers at any level consciously and comfortably understand their own frame of reference, the more definitively they can appreciate to what extent they have become part of "the system." In a general way, this process can assist in defining how unique one is, thereby reducing the requirement to buy a herd philosophy unreservedly before feeling like "somebody." More specifically, helpers can come to appreciate, rather than deny, both the limits and the breadth of their helping ability in certain situations and with certain kinds of patients. This kind of "knowing" prevents much wasted effort, forced energies, and guilt-ridden breast-beating in trying to be all things to all persons. To understand oneself more consciously can also be a valuable guide in defining for oneself when creative assistance is needed from others in expanding one's helping capacity for patients who seem unreachable or intolerable to be near. This consciousness can reduce the need to rely on rigid, institutionalized practices to solve problems.

A further reason for emphasizing the helper portion of the interpersonal helping equation is that a fuller understanding of oneself seems to increase one's ability to appreciate quickly who the patient really is. Our experience is that helpers who have a realistic awareness of where they stand with respect to themselves, their peers, their ideas about life, and their helping practice are ultimately more efficient at reaching the patient in ways that result in help being brought to bear more quickly. For example, on initial entry into a health-care setting, patients may not be able to be congruent or "real." Their distress may be such that empathy with others is impossible. They may not be able to state their goals or aspirations in a way that the helper can immediately understand. The less the helper is caught in a similar quandary, the more quickly a helping process can get under way. All helpers potentially have access to and time available for knowing themselves more fully than any other human encountered in life—including the patient. With the trend of increasingly short-term contacts with patients, it is even more critical that at least one party in the helping dyad "know" who he or she is to the maximal possible degree.

Overall, a major message in placing as much emphasis on the helpers as on the patients is that all of them are people. We believe that helpers also must be viewed humanistically, lest they become mechanistic and perpetuate this attitude. Helpers deserve high value and respect, just as do patients. They must be listened to as individuals and as groups and assisted in every growth-enhancing way to know and actualize themselves more broadly. Only then do we believe that helpers can more comfortably allow and assist their patients to express who they are and what they seek.

Ultimately, we believe that helpers have to appreciate that patients have strengths as well as weaknesses in life's struggle, just as they do themselves. Allowing the strengths of another person to exist or grow is perhaps the ultimate humanistic tribute. To believe in the helping relationship is to trust that the burden of helping does not have to be carried out by the helper alone: the power is shared.

As little as we know about the exact nature of helping, the following definition of humanistic helping is believed to be a valid basis for further exploring the process as it might be actualized across all health settings and as it can apply to all disciplines: *humanistic helping is a variable interpersonal process between helpers and patients, or their representatives that integrates technological knowledge and personal/social experience in an interdependent way so as to provide both parties (1) a satisfying, self-actualizing experience and (2) movement toward those life's goals to which both helpers and patients are committed.*

This definition of helping will be utilized throughout the remainder of the text. In Unit III the definition will become the basis on which is built a formal framework for analysis of the helping process and the various real life situations in which health-care workers find themselves. A vital core of the framework is that of an advocacy model of helping within which both patient and helper can more consciously evaluate their values, primary concerns, and jointly established goals.

REFERENCE NOTES

1. Carl Rogers et al., *Person to Person: The Problem of Being Human* (Lafayette, Calif.: Real People Press, 1967), p. 275.
2. Robert E. Reynolds and Thomas W. Bice, "Attitudes of Medical Interns Towards Patients and Health Professionals," *Journal of Health and Social Behavior* 12 (December 1971): 307–11.
3. See Abraham Maslow, *Motivation and Personality* (New York: Harper & Bros., 1954), p. 353.
4. References cited in notes 4 and 5 can be found collectively summarized in *Mental Health Digest* 5, no. 6 (1973). This issue was devoted in large measure to the topic of helping, coming to be known in the literature as "prosocial behavior." See D. L. Rosenhan, "Learning Theory and Prosocial Behavior," *Journal of Social Issues* 28, no. 3 (1973): 151–63.
5. John Kaplan, "A Legal Look at Prosocial Behavior: What Can Happen for Failing To Help or Trying To Help Someone," *Journal of Social Issues* 28, no. 3 (1972): 219–26.
6. Peter Marin, "Living in Moral Pain," *Psychology Today* 15, no. 11 (November 1981): 68.
7. Robert Hogan, "Moral Conduct and Moral Character: A Psychological Perspective," *Psychological Bulletin* 79, no. 4 (1973): 217–32.
8. B. F. Skinner, "The Ethics of Helping People," *The Humanist* 36, no. 1 (January/February 1976): 7.
9. Otto Kernberg, interviewed by Linda Wolfe, "Why Some People Can't Love," *Psychology Today*, 12, no. 1 (June 1978): 55. This is the most concise, simple-to-read description of the narcissistic personality that you will find. It will help you to understand the impact of developmental roots and their interaction with our contemporary culture. It may also assist in further understanding the nature of certain people who are profoundly difficult to help or who are so difficult to teach to help or love.
10. Marian Radke Yarrow, Phyllis M. Scott, and Carolyn Zahn Waxler, "Learning Concern for Others," *Developmental Psychology* 8, no. 2 (1973): 240–60.
11. R. A. Ramsay, E. D. Wittkower, and H. Warnes, "Treatment of Psychosomatic Disorders," in *The Therapist's Handbook*, ed. Benjamin Wolman (New York: Van Nostrand Reinhold, 1976), pp. 451–519.

12. A. H. Schmale, "Giving Up as a Final Common Pathway to Changes in Health," *Advances in Psychosomatic Medicine* 8 (1972): 20–40. This is one of the single finest articles that can be perused in understanding the psychosocial aspects of disease. The bibliography is extensive (68 references) and comprehensive of the classic, as well as contemporary, literature.

13. Edward A. Suchman, "Social Patterns of Illness and Medical Care," in *Patients, Physicians, and Illness*, ed. Egbert Gartley Jaco (New York: Free Press, 1958), pp. 262–79.

14. Eberhard H. Uhlenhuth and Eugene S. Paykel, "Symptom Intensity and Life Events," *Archives of General Psychiatry* 28 (1973): 473–77.

15. James H. Young, "The Persistence of Medical Quackery in America," *American Scientist* 60 (1972): 318–26. This article is particularly good from the standpoint of understanding the patient's motivation for becoming involved in quackery. It covers the "miss-no-bets" syndrome as well as the "rejection-of-authority" complex.

16. The one single text to seek out for a comprehensive review is Allen E. Bergin and Sol L. Garfield, eds., *Handbook of Psychotherapy and Behavior Change: An Empirical Analysis* (New York: Wiley, 1971). Also see Garfield's "Psychotherapy: A 40-Year Appraisal," *American Psychologist* 36, no. 2 (February 1981): 174–83. The bibliography following this article is excellent.

17. Many references pertain to this statement from the previous text. A short reference that makes the point clearly is Steven L. Weiss, "Differences in Goals, Interests and Personalities Between Students with Analytic and Behavior Therapy Orientations," *Professional Psychology* 4, no. 2 (1973): 145–50.

18. George M. Carstairs et al., "Ideology, Personality, and Role Definition: Studies of Hospital Personnel," in *The Patient and the Mental Hospital*, eds. Milton Greenblatt, Daniel J. Levinson, and Richard H. Williams (New York: Free Press, 1957), pp. 197–230. This text is a classic in its entirety and still highly relevant.

19. In addition to the studies cited in note 16, the following studies are representative: C. M. Crow, R. M. Mowbray, and S. Block, "Attitudes of Medical Students to Mental Illness," *Journal of Medical Education* 45 (1970): 594–99; Russell Eisenman, "Creativity in Student Nurses and Their Attitudes Toward Mental Illness and Physical Disability," *Nursing Research* 20 (1971): 503–8; Amasa B. Ford, Ralph E. Liske, and Robert S. Ort, "Reactions of Physicians and Medical Students to Chronic Illness," *Journal of Chronic Diseases* 15 (1962): 785–94; Jack K. Genskow and Frank D. Maglione, "Familiarity, Dogmatism and Reported Student Attitudes Toward the Disabled," *Journal of Social Psychology* 67 (1965): 329–41; Sharon Golub and Marvin Reznikoff, "Attitudes Toward Death: A Comparison of Nursing Students and Graduate Nurses," *Nursing Research* 20 (1971): 503–8; Malcolm L. Meltzer and Haikaz M. Grigorian, "Effect of Psychiatric Education on Attitudes of Medical Students to Mental Illness," *Psychiatry* 35 (May 1972): 195–204; A. F. Muhlenkamp, "Attitudes of Nursing Students Toward Eight Major Disabilities," *Psychological Reports* 29 (1971): 973–74.

20. Carl Rogers, "The Interpersonal Relationship: The Core of Guidance," in Rogers et al., *Person to Person*, pp. 89–103. Also see Rogers' *On Becoming A Person* (Boston: Houghton Mifflin, 1961). Research investigations concerning the three conditions for effective helping can be found in Bergin and Garfield, *Handbook of Psychotherapy and Behavior Change*.

21. Charles B. Truax and Kevin M. Mitchell, "Research on Certain Therapist Interpersonal Skills in Relation to Process and Outcome," in Bergin and Garfield, *Handbook of Psychotherapy*, p. 302.

22. Rogers, "The Interpersonal Relationship," p. 94.

23. Ibid., p. 90.

24. Sidney J. Jourard, *Disclosing Man to Himself* (New York: Van Nostrand Reinhold, 1968), p. 70. Any serious student of the helping process will find this text a must.

25. Tony Hillerman, "Robert Coles: The People's Voice," *Human Behavior*, December 1973, p. 20. Reprinted by permission of *Human Behavior Magazine*, © December 1973.

26. Rogers, "The Interpersonal Relationship," pp. 92–94.

27. Jourard, *Disclosing Man to Himself*, pp. 18–34.

28. Zick Rubin, "Lovers and Other Strangers: The Development of Intimacy in Encounters and Relationships," *American Scientist* 62 (1974): 182–89. See also Sidney M. Jourard and Peggy E. Jaffe, "Influence of an Interviewer's Disclosure on the Self-Disclosing Behavior of Interviewees," *Journal of Counseling Psychology* 17 (1970): 252–57.

29. Robert R. Carkhuff, *Helping and Human Relations* (New York: Holt, Rinehart & Winston, 1969). See also Carkhuff's "Black and White in Helping," *Professional Psychology* 3, no. 1 (1972): 18–22.

30. Muzafer Sherif and·Carolyn Sherif, *An Outline of Social Psychology* (New York: Harper & Bros., 1956), p. 41.

31. "Some Principles To Be Applied," ibid., pp. 77–116, is particularly helpful in understanding the frame-of-reference concept.

32. William H. Grier and Price M. Cobbs, *Black Rage* (New York: Basic Books, 1968), p. 147.

33. Nursing has moved further than the medical profession in the direction of acknowledging the vital need for integration of the behavioral sciences in their practice. See Hildegard Peplau's text, *Interpersonal Relations in Nursing: A Conceptual Frame of Reference for Psychodynamic Nursing* (New York: Putnam's, 1952). It was a masterpiece then and still is now; it has yet to be discovered or accepted for its relevance in all the disciplines, including some schools of nursing.

34. See Sidney L. Werkman, *The Role of Psychiatry in Medical Education: An Appraisal and a Forecast* (Cambridge: Harvard University Press, 1966).

35. Barbara Korsch and Vida F. Negrete, "Doctor-Patient Communication," *Scientific American* 227 (August 1972): 66–74.

36. Truax and Mitchell, "Research on Therapist Interpersonal Skills," pp. 337–41.

SUGGESTIONS FOR FURTHER EXPERIENCE

Understanding another person's frame of reference does not occur in just one interview. One builds a knowledge about another through multiple inputs and over a series of contacts. In the following experience, several ways of getting at patients' internal perceptions of help are suggested. Contrasting what patients say in various ways with what you thought that they felt can give further appreciation for why one is not always on the same "wavelength" with others.

1. Conduct a simple written poll of the patients who are presently staying on the ward in which you are working or of those who come into your clinic. Ask them to respond to three open-ended questions:

   a. What was the problem for which you wanted help when you first came to the hospital (or clinic)?

   b. What was your most helpful experience the first time that you came to the hospital (or clinic)?

   c. What do you want to happen *now* that would help you more?

When conducting any form of research, one should obtain *informed consent*—that is, let the person know what you are doing, why, and how the results are to be used. The responses that you obtain may not correspond exactly to the patient's feelings. People tend to give socially desirable responses, particularly when they fear that presenting the truth will lower their chances of getting a fair shake. Interviewing a select few of the patients after they turn in their written responses can assist in testing out how "socially desirable" they were attempting to be. Verbal interviewing generally obtains more information about the patient's frame of reference than do written responses.

2. Evaluate the patients' individual responses against your own perceptions of their situation. Following are some questions that you may utilize in self-evaluation:

   a. Do the reasons for seeking help given by the patients coincide with what you thought they were?

   b. Do the patients' perceptions of what has been most helpful fit with your notions about your professional helping responsibilities?

   c. How realistic do you perceive individual patient desires to be for the help that they want now?

   d. If it is not possible to come through with what the patients say they want, what factors seem to be getting in the way?

3. Suggest to your instructor that your group of fellow students hold a formal discussion regarding their early motives and present notions about becoming a helper. Use the following questions as a discussion guide:

   a. At what age did you decide to become a _____ (doctor, nurse, social worker, and so on)?

   b. What else had you considered being when you grew up? Why did you not pursue that career?

   c. When you help someone, in any sphere of life, what seem to be the rewards for you?

   d. What kinds of behaviors in others are "turn-offs" for you when you are trying to help?

   e. Are you presently satisfied that you have chosen the right career for yourself?

   f. How do you see yourself functioning as a helper five years from now?

Conceptualizing a Framework for Analysis

Chapter 6

A Framework for Analysis

Overview

In the previous unit we attempted to sensitize you to a number of facets of the health-care field that are basic to understanding the behavior of patients. Throughout this appraisal, a number of concerns were raised. An overall concern is the need for humanistic values to be more visibly emphasized in the health-care field.

We support the advancement of science in furthering improved ways to detect and respond to human ills; but we believe that all service-providing settings must reexamine their attitudes and practices for the effects of mechanistic, technical scientism and gaps in humanistic goals for people. Simultaneously, the educational arm of the health-care field, which provides service-giving personnel, must evaluate whether it is both emphasizing humanistic values and developing methods by which students can learn to act on them.

For the foregoing to be accomplished will require the responsiveness of the present leaders in the major health-care disciplines, but consumers of the health-care system—patients and students—must also take responsibility in influencing change. Unmet needs in both experiencing and learning a humanistic helping process can be individually and collectively expressed to the administrative powers that be, but this expression is not enough. Without waiting for the "world at the top" suddenly to change, we believe that health-care staff and students can also effect humanistic goals at the grass-roots level.

Health-care workers can begin to reconceptualize their function and behave with patients and each other in many ways that are more humanistic and do not require permission from above. For example, no health-care commandment denies concern about a patient's increasing "bitchiness" during treatment at the same time that one is being technically accurate about the administration of an intravenous solution. If so motivated, one can be observing of other behavior that accompanies technical contacts, and humanistic follow-up can be carried out. As another example, a unit staff or clinic group does not have to wait for administrative mandates to carry out self-appraisal and redefinitions of their functioning. Many administrators would welcome this initiative. Those who bristle at their staffs' appraising themselves might be reminded that a group that can commit itself to evaluative questioning shows signs of being a maturing, humane group. As Hoffer explains, "Humaneness comes of age when man asks the first question. Social stagnation results not from a lack of answers but from the absence of impulse to ask questions."[1]

Questions as to what health-care delivery is about ought to be many as helpers within the system are faced with increasingly complex factors: (1) innumerable requests for help that are confounded with intricate social/emotional variables; (2) diffuse role functions that overlap disciplines; and (3) ethical issues about life, death, rights, and responsibilities. However, lest this complexity cause panic, remember that some health-care situations have been around a long time.[2] Ponder how much a blind spot in taking time to think can subtly influence what helpers fail to do in situations that are not new and require reaffirmation of common sense. In evaluating the following case, consider the various points in the sequence of events at which high degrees of scientific knowledge and administrative permission giving were *not* required to "do right by" the patient.

CASE IN POINT

Judith, age 39, was seriously injured in a car wreck at 7:10 A.M. 5 miles from the hospital to which she was taken. In conscious shock, she was initially more preoccupied with the fact that her wig had slipped off during the accident than with her bodily condition. Nonetheless, she had enough discriminative sense after the police came, to inquire if an ambulance was on its way, since she felt that "something was slipping away inside her."

In the emergency room, she recalled beginning to fear that the staff were not going to be concerned about *her*, since, for two hours, the taking of x-ray films and history and interrogation by the state patrol over who was at fault had superseded any response to her expressions of severe pain. At 11 A.M.., almost four hours after the initial injury, she was admitted to her two-bed ward room. She again mentioned her severe pain and repeated her request for something to be done about it. She had been informed by the emergency room staff that she had—so far as they knew at the time—fractured ribs, a collapsed upper lobe of the left lung, and questionable internal injuries to soft abdominal tissues. She thought that these injuries, together with the severity of her pain, made her request legitimate. The helper who was carrying out the ward admission procedure ignored her question and instead asked for her height and weight. Judith remembers that she thought this response to her question was "so dumb," but, even more, it frightened her that concern for herself was not shared by those who were supposed to help her.

An hour later, she received medication. She related that, during the waiting time, she felt increasing apprehension about getting lost in the rush and the need to steel herself "to stay sharp." She believed that she needed to double-check that what they brought to her was neither morphine nor codeine, to which she was allergic. She remembered telling them those facts in the emergency room but indicated that she lost confidence that the message had been received upstairs or would be attended to if it had.

After two days of encountering a series of ward staff who entered her room presumably to help her, Judith called long distance, saying "Everybody except my private doctor comes in and acts like they just discovered me. They are nice but they ask *me* how I got there and what I'm there for. How can someone come in here and try to help if *they* don't know what's the matter with you?" We suggested that she muster if she could the same critical judgments that she utilized in her daily life as head of an industrial health program, wife, and mother of four vivacious children. We supported her acting obnoxiously if necessary to get the staff to know her and listen. Judith said that she did not know whether she had the energy.

With respect to Judith, it was known to us that she had strengths on which she might rely in coping with her frightening situation and her perception that she had to act almost totally alone in her own behalf. Historically, she had had an assertive, self-reliant style; we remembered that, several years previously, when she sought help for a troubled son, she could confront clinic personnel with her feelings that she was "being treated like a ding-a-ling." In both the past and present situation, it was fortunate for Judith that she had assertive functions available to her. Later, these would be invaluable in her adapting to a long postaccident recovery; but how unthinking of those involved in the initial circumstances to require her to utilize high degrees of energy in keeping "on top of the situation" at a critical time when all energies would have been better utilized by the body in bringing curative processes to bear on the effects of trauma, pain, and shock.

Judith is not a rare type of person, but neither is she representative of all people whom one will meet within the health-care system. Many persons, like health-care workers themselves, are variably affected by sociocultural factors that foster passive, conforming coping styles. Many persons do not have assertive, self-reliant functions readily accessible to them, and they appear to take anything, neither trusting their own perceptions nor believing that speaking up will do any good. In the process of seeking help, situational physical or social/emotional stress or both can even further obliterate a person's natural assertive coping potential.[3] A high degree of sensitivity to what a health care worker evaluates when people initially enter a health-care system is required; patients need to know that the helper is competent to focus on what will spell the difference between life and death and between suffering and its relief. However, *how* one empathically evaluates and responds will determine how much energy the patient has to expend in defending against the insensitivity of the helper versus utilizing that energy to cope with the stress of the initial mind/body insult—real or imagined.

On an ongoing basis, in the evaluation of helping situations, continuing appraisal and shifting priorities must be valued and flexibly applied. Within both new and ongoing encounters between helper and patient must be awareness of the heavy responsibility in "diagnosing" situations *and* the patient's coping abilities: finding a disease is simply not adequate, and one may not even exist to be treated.[4] Unless health-care workers come to (1) value their critical thinking abilities and (2) learn to utilize these discriminatively in the context within which they are working, the helping process too easily becomes the blind leading the blind.

In our attempts to assist health-care workers to enhance their critical thinking abilities concerning health care and the helping process, we have asked ourselves innumerable general questions: What kind of evaluative framework should be used in either individual or group self-appraisal? On what bases can the general health-care field and the process of help be reconceptualized so as to preserve their essential purposes? How can preclinical students and beginning helpers make better choices as to the kind of setting that best fits their need to help and their personal styles? How can patients be assisted to be more discriminating in choosing those who are best suited to help them with their particular problems? How can help be more clearly discussed so that students and patients have a realistic set of expectations about health settings, helpers, and the process of help? How can patients' human rights be preserved when their condition fails to allow them to seek or participate in the help of their choice?

In the following pages, we speak to these issues. The goal is to provide a framework for analysis of the health-care field, the settings in which one works, and the specific helping relationships that one may encounter. Central to the framework is an advocacy model within which we have reconceptualized the helping role of health-care workers. We hope that this advocacy-oriented framework for analysis provides for helpers an internal evaluation model[5]—that is, a way of looking at one's professional life space that becomes integrated with the internal frame of reference and thereby capable of being flexibly applied to various situations.

In the summary of this chapter, we pose a number of evaluative questions that either an individual or a group of health-care workers might utilize.

The Helping Role Reconceptualized

Central to the framework for analysis is an overall goal. A goal is an objective that one works to actualize in reality. It does not necessarily tell how to do something. Rather, a goal is like a destination on a road map: there may be many ways to get there, but it is at that spot that one desires eventually to arrive. Our task in this chapter is (1) to establish a goal concerning help that we believe ought to be central to the health-care field and (2) to make suggestions as to how to get there. The goal that we have selected is identical to a concept introduced in Unit I—the goal of humanistic helping:

Development of an interpersonal process between helpers and patients or their representatives that integrates technological knowledge and personal/social experience in an interdependent way so as to provide both parties with (1) a satisfying, self-actualizing experience and (2) movement toward life goals to which both helpers and patients are committed.

Another characteristic of goals in general is that they reflect values. As can be quickly realized, the preceding goal is loaded with a number of humanistic value statements. For example, the goal of humanistic helping is concerned with what goes on between people and interdependency. This goal implies the value placed on shared function and respect for what both individuals contribute to the process—not on one telling the other what to do. The goal also implies that a positive value is placed on the total realm of experience in the helping process—for example, the personal/social experience of people, as well as the technical aspects of knowledge. It is a goal also concerned with self-actualization and movement toward goals held for existence in general. This concern implies a belief concerning the potential of persons to become more than they are as a result of their experience—not simply being returned to some former state. The goal also implies that helpers as well as patients are valued for their humanistic needs and concerns.

However, humanistic values have a way of appearing, or becoming, diffuse, or they often are carried out in wishy-washy, although well-intentioned, ways. This goal could easily become the victim of such fuzzy thought or action if left at that. This pitfall can be avoided by means of a definitive statement of ways in which this goal may be actualized. We will begin by reexamining the general concept of helping and placing the concept in a new light that can give it more formalized substance and the potential for directing humanistic action.

Helping revisited   As previously reviewed, the concept of helping has been embedded in vagueness. It has characteristically been thought of in terms of doing something for or to someone so that something "good" will happen to that person. Presumably, by doing something helpful to or for someone, the helper will thereby feel more meaningful.

Informally, people experience helping encounters throughout most of their lives. In some situations, what is desired is specifically defined by the other: "Would you help me move this weekend?" "Would you give to this fund to help needy victims?" "I have a problem; can I come over and talk?" Another form of need for everyday helping is sensed intuitively. One may read another's situation in such a way that spontaneous assistance seems to be called for without anyone's making a direct request. For example, the person in front of one slips and falls; a child alone on a street corner cries and wanders as if certainly lost. Parents, combining intuition and child-rearing knowledge, have long been natural helpers in facilitating growth and development through doing-for and doing-to actions, as well as by withholding assistance at critical times.

All these examples of informal helping have their counterparts in situations encountered in health-care settings. As you have seen in previous examples, the intuitive, commonsense abilities gained in everyday life are extremely valuable in formalized helping situations. Through increasing life experiences, one becomes more trustful of one's own thoughts, feelings, and intuitive judgments. At times, within informal helping encounters, they may be all that one has to rely on; but, in formalized helping, common sense and intuition alone cannot suffice. These abilities must be combined with an appreciation for the responsibility that one takes in assuming a publicly acknowledged helping role. Following are some specific dimensions around which formalized helping in a professional role differs from informal, natural helping:

1. In everyday life experiences, one may choose whether to help another when one is asked. In accepting a role as a health-care worker, one's purpose as a helper is preordained. Whether or not one is asked directly or appropriately for help in health-care settings, it is important to recognize that people come to helpers because they want to receive something. It is a formal helping responsibility to stick with it or see that persons find the help that they are seeking with resources more fitted to their expressed needs.

2. Informal helping tends to be based primarily on subjective, commonsense knowledge and a high degree of reliance on what one thinks is best to do at the time. Formalized helping requires helpers to have both common sense *and* specialized helping skills that they discriminatively bring into the situation. For example, "talking it out" is a basic psychological repair mechanism that people use within informal and formal helping situations. It is a process that allows one to put more form to garbled feelings and thoughts that pressure one's internal experience. "Just listening" often assists the help seeker to organize thinking and be relieved of internal stress. However, specialized interviewing skills are necessary for the professional helper not only to "hear the patient out," but to keep the interaction guided so that the critical problem is understood and appropriate therapeutic interventions can begin.

3. The seeker of informal help is not so demanding or expecting of expert knowledge and actions from the helper. In contrast, persons seeking help in health-care settings do expect that those who are publicly acknowledged as helpers will have more formalized helping skills and some expertise in the problem that confronts them.

4. The end result of informal helping is vulnerable to being what the helper wants for the other person. Even the parent who can stand back in appropriate objectivity from 'time to time is tied to highly personalized needs for the child to develop in ways that fit the parent's frame of reference. Formalized helping requires care in respecting and protecting the views of help-seeking persons as they are assisted in coping and in actualizing undiscovered strengths and potentials.

Advocacy: a way to look at formalized helping   A formalized helping model that seems to have the highest potential for actualizing the humanistic goal is that of *advocacy.* As it applies to helping functions, advocacy is an old term that recently has received new recognition. A review of advocacy by Kahn and associates states the following:

> Historically, advocacy has existed as long as there have been powerless groups in need of a champion. The self-advocacy of suffragettes and the class advocacy of social reformers are as integral parts of American history as the more traditional form of legal advocacy. Recently consumer health and family advocacy programs have mushroomed. Among these, child advocacy is perhaps the latest manifestation.[6]

Advocacy is a form of helping, and those who ascribe to its basic meaning refer to themselves as *advocates*. In common with the term *helper,* the concept of advocate can have different meanings, depending on in what branch of helping one functions (e.g., law, education, or health). However, unlike the term *helper,* the word *advocate* has a somewhat clearer meaning across disciplines that propose to help within any given area of concern. For example, advocacy is an activist concept and implies that the helping activity is in behalf of another person.[7] Advocates publicly put themselves forth as helpers of those who cannot, or perceive themselves as unable to, solve their dilemmas on their own.

As reviewed previously, within informal helping situations and, unfortunately, within many formalized health-care situations, helpful processes are often obtained only after someone specifically asks or demands. Also, in these situations, helping may not be tied to a goal that is concerned with the ultimate welfare of the help seeker. However, advocacy requires (1) the statement of a humane goal or cause, (2) assertive action to accomplish the goal, and (3) an attitude of concern that the best be obtained for those for whom one advocates. In its traditional meaning, advocacy involves concern for, and defined actions in behalf of, another at both the individual level and the system's organization level.

Advocacy in Action:
A New Style with Patients

In utilizing an advocacy model of formalized helping, one gives the terms *health-care worker, helper,* or *caregiver* more active meaning by substituting the term *health-care advocate.* This new terminology, together with its specific meaning, provides more succinct guidelines against which representatives of a variety of disciplines can consciously (1) evaluate their attitudes and beliefs about helping, (2) check their role relationships with patients and each other, (3) define what one needs to know about the other to advocate appropriately, and (4) more meaningfully define the order of priorities of their helping actions.

Within an advocacy model of humanistic helping, (1) the goals of the health-care advocate are established *with* consumers of help, and (2) actions are taken in behalf of these consumers when it has been determined that, on their own, the patients (or their familial or legal representatives) cannot bring to bear resources that facilitate healing or problem solving. This formulation demands that the health-care advocate, from the beginning to the end of therapeutic contact with the patient, function *with* patient interest if humanistic help is to occur at all. Consider how clarifying the initial contact between helper and patient might be if the following position of health-care advocacy were conveyed at the outset.

I am a health-care advocate. You and I will determine what things I may do in your behalf. I am prepared to share with you any of my knowledge, skills, and therapeutic administrations that you may require in your present circumstances. Some skills and knowledge I may not hold, and I may not be able to provide all the resources that your specific situation requires; but, for those resources that we cannot muster between us, my responsibility is to put you in contact with those persons or services that you may require.

I am prepared to be an evaluative person and to assist you in defining and interpreting your problem. I am prepared to sensitize you to the aspects of your central concern of which you may not be aware. I am also prepared to sensitize you to your inner strengths, of which you may not be aware, that will allow you to act in your own behalf.

To the extent that I am needed to act in your behalf, I will do so; but I will not go beyond my bounds. In those circumstances in which you have the ability or in which it is your right and responsibility to make humanistic ethical decisions, the consequences of which you and your family will have to live with long after your contact with me is ended, I will clarify your rights and encourage your taking of responsibility.

Overall, if our helping relationship is productive for both of us, you will have a broader view—particularly with respect to the options that you have available to you and your own capacity to cope with your life space.

In an advocacy model of helping, the behaviors of the health-care advocate are primarily dependent on the patient and the situation in which both encounter one another. The actions of patients or what happens to them are not necessarily dependent on the whims or particular bias of the helper. Reinforcement of helpless, voiceless dependency behaviors of patients can be avoided as the assets, or strengths, of patients are acknowledged and utilized in growth-enhancing ways from the outset. An advocacy model also strongly implies action and interaction of *both* parties in goal setting: it calls for defining in what circumstances responsibility realistically can and cannot be taken for another. Open communication with patients or their representatives concerning power and mutual expectations is thereby possible within such a framework. Helping can be formalized around a "contract," and specified transactions can ensue. Helping thereby becomes a partnership.

Informed-consent procedures within an advocacy framework are not simply separate, additive legal procedures transacted in isolation. Informed consent is an ongoing, integrated part of an advocacy helping process. It is carried out in highly individual ways in keeping with the needs and concerns of the patient—not simply in "canned messages" and signatures on a form to protect the agency or its personnel. Following is a description of a patient's experience in consenting to major surgery. The two helping situations as experienced back to back exemplify both the personalized struggle that patients often experience when faced with a health crisis and the effect of explanations not focused on total patient concerns.

CASE IN POINT

Martha, 39 years old, had been experiencing deep lower left quadrant pain for some months. It seemed to vary with her menstrual periods. Repeatedly she checked with her gynecological specialist, but no tangible cause for the pain could be found. After her fall vacation, the pain became intense, and she made another visit to her physician. A large ovarian mass was found, and immediate surgery was recommended. Martha was told the possible consequences: it might be a benign cyst, or it might be a malignancy. She understood that, if the mass were malignant, she would lose not only the ovary involved but also the remainder of her reproductive organs. She recalls being overwhelmed by the thought of a possible malignancy and wanting it taken care of. Verbally she agreed to the surgery.

Two days before surgery, she returned for an outpatient preoperative examination and further information about what to expect. Since her first visit, she had had time to rethink the situation. She now asked what she could expect if the mass were not malignant. She was concerned with keeping as much of her reproductive system as possible. Silently she harbored the question of whether immediate major surgery was the best alternative without a second medical opinion. Openly she admitted to being "scared stiff" of major abdominal surgery in general. She explained to her physician that this seemed particularly realistic in view of a history of chronic respiratory problems in the form of childhood asthma and many adult experiences with pneumonia. She therefore asked if she could possibly have a "spinal" anesthetic instead of having anesthesia induced through her respiratory system.

Martha's perception of how she was responded to was negative. She found her physician glib and not understanding of her true feelings. Initially he responded that she simply had "cold feet" and assured her that this was common with everybody. She believed that he was not listening to her specific concerns and was merely putting her into a general category of "how everyone acted." Specifically she went down her list of questions again. If the mass were benign, could her uterus and right ovary be left intact?

Response: At your age, what do you need them for? Having it all out now will prevent later trouble.

Question: Have you decided on the kind of anesthesia that will be administered? What about the status of the request for a spinal?

Response: The anesthesiologists at the hospital are separate in their function. I can talk with them about it, but it is all up to them.

Martha remembered being angry and scared. She told her physician that she was canceling surgery. She remembers feeling frightened in making that decision so abruptly, since she knew no one to seek out immediately instead. She also wondered about her judgment. However, she thought that she had done the right thing after her physician responded to her cancellation of surgery with anger at "the inconvenience this will put the hospital through." She told him that she was not, at this point, concerned about the hospital's inconvenience. She was concerned about herself and could not understand why he was not.

Shaken and feeling alone, Martha went back to work that afternoon. She asked various persons who was a "good" gynecologist who would be understanding of her concerns. She also wanted someone who could see her right away. She was afraid that, if she were walking around with a malignancy, she might not have done right by herself to walk away from treatment; but she also remained concerned about what would happen to her in the event that the mass was benign. She decided to make an appointment with someone that a medical friend of hers recommended—someone whom his wife had utilized and who sounded like the kind of person that Martha could trust to listen.

Martha called and received an appointment for the next day. She explained her situation with some chagrin. She was not altogether certain that she would not be written off as a "kook" or a "shopper." However, she was reassured from the outset by the physician, who told her, "Don't feel apologetic about seeking another opinion. When I recommend surgery, I expect my patients to obtain one. If they do not wish to, I encourage it nonetheless. I lay out the facts and the choices as I see them. I want my patients to make the best decision for themselves."

Martha was also encouraged because this new physician seemed to her to be empathetic with her desire to avoid surgery if possible but, if not, to respect her desire to keep whatever organs were not afflicted. She also felt reinforced about being a competent person by the physician's sharing with her a diagnostic hunch that she might pursue if she chose. Martha believed that full details had been shared with her as to risks and choices. She decided to go along with the suggested medication. Within five days, the mass was markedly reduced in size, and, within ten days, no trace remained.

In looking back, Martha describes her experience as a "nightmare." She does not focus on who was the better physician in terms of scientific know-how because, as she said, "I never got that far in knowing my first doctor." Rather, she emphasizes how fortunate she believes herself to be to find someone who could put humanistic concern for a patient together with solid scientific knowledge and make her seem to be a full participant. She thinks that, had surgery been once again recommended, she would have been less fearful with this physician, since "I felt the second doctor was on my side. He was working with me *for* me." She also emphasized how much more she had learned about her own body from the second helper. She angrily commented that, with her first experience, she learned more about "the system" than herself.

Signs that at last there is substantial medical-organization concern about situations like the one above were notable at the 1981 62nd annual session of the American College of Physicians. In a seminar on "double diagnosis," codirected by Shochet and Lisansky, it was stressed that there are two levels of inquiry of the patient that enable a comprehensive, exploratory diagnosis:

1. The level of physical symptoms
2. The level that holds the elements within the patient's psychosocial environment that influence or provide a background for the illness—for example, "feelings, moods, opinions, judgments, fears, hopes, attitude toward significant others, attitude toward self, money, and sex"[8]

In implementing the "double diagnosis" interview, Lipansky pointed out four principles:[9]

1. Development of an effective relationship with the patient, keeping it more professional than social

2. Goal-directed planning and management of the interview toward meeting the desired goals
3. Focusing the patient's attention on topics relevant to the goals by selective indication
   of interest
4. Minimal activity on the part of the physician, utilizing maximal initiative of the
   patient

We agree with Lipansky in the attitude that "the patient has come for a specific
purpose and with a specific problem, and we need to keep our sights on why the
patient is here, and by showing the patient that we are sincerely interested in a professional way in their complaint and then as a person we can effectively develop the kind
of relationship we need to carry on this exploratory type of diagnosis."[10] Clues to the
"kind of relationship" as a "person" that is necessary to carry on the helping process
are found in the advocacy model. Within this model is clarified the meaning of the
critical ingredients of a helping process: *positive regard, congruence,* and *empathy.*[11]

In our experience, positive regard is easier for helpers to gain or retain when they
hold an advocacy point of view. As the previous case in point shows, the potential for
patients to hold positive regard for and trust in the helper is also increased. When
mutually discussed and jointly established goals are part of a humanistic helping process, advocates can avoid unconsciously contributing to patient behavior that later
comes to be disliked. For example, advocates who establish treatment goals through a
process of negotiation with the patient will avoid the bind of overdependency, in which
the patient expects the helper to carry the full load. Neither do they get into so many
power plays, against which patients often react in growth-retarding ways.

In the advocacy model, patient resistance to information-sharing or to what indeed
may be appropriate treatment procedures is reduced. To the degree that resistance is
reduced and cooperation with helpers increases, health-care workers feel more satisfaction and therefore more positive attitudes toward the patient. Professional helpers,
through an attitude and style based on advocacy principles, know more about resistance *to what* and cooperation *with what.* If resistive behavior is encountered in the
advocacy helping process, advocates discuss it or renegotiate with the patient directly.

Congruence, or being more real with the other, is built into an advocacy model
from the beginning of contact. Through clarifying what patients can expect from the
beginning, health-care advocates essentially convey to them the following: *This is who
I am. This is what you can expect from me. I will not try to kid you by playing the role
of being more or less than I am as a helping person.*

Clarifying reality for patients is important in terms of ultimate patient satisfaction. As has been seen in innumerable preceding examples, patients enter health-care
settings with highly personalized meanings attached to what is happening to them.
These preconceptions may or may not be accurate. For example, some patients ascribe
an almost magical power to those whom they perceive as controlling factors influencing life and death. On the other side of the coin are also encountered those patients
who may be highly mistrustful of anyone who is helping them. Health-care advocates,
in clarifying what they can and cannot be expected to provide, set the tone for realistic

expectations. Later disappointment and false inferences can be avoided. Within such an atmosphere, help seekers also have more potential for choosing to pursue help with any given health-care worker in any setting.

In other words, health-care advocates allow others to know them. They recognize that their humanism, together with the technical skills that they have learned, is a powerful therapeutic combination. To the degree that this is more openly shared, patients can more easily determine with advocates the limits of dependency and how their own sources of strength can be utilized. The helper does not have to play God or reinforce the patient's need to make the helper God for hope to be maintained and help to be obtained. It is difficult for patients to relate to godlike, all-knowing helpers, even if the patients want them. In such a relationship, patients tend to keep secret much about themselves. Patients are more easily congruent in a relationship in which realness is valued and demonstrated in visible actions.

Empathy—getting at how the other perceives the world in the here and now—is also a cornerstone of the advocacy model of helping. To establish mutual goals and to determine which of those require the advocate to act in another's behalf necessitates an evaluative process that involves empathy. Although it is not quite so easy as the statement implies, one cannot help learning to be a good empathizer if one takes on an advocacy attitude.

In summary, we believe an advocacy model to be an effective avenue by which the definition of humanistic helping can be actualized at the level of direct patient contact. When such a framework is utilized from the beginning of patient contact, it incorporates the values placed on a professional problem-solving process; scientific know-how; and the subjective, personalized experience of patient and helper. Such a model also puts these values into perspective through a process of defining and evaluating with the patient—verbally or in writing or both—what can be expected. The kind of evaluation demanded by an advocacy model ensures that the totality of the patient's experience is utilized.

An advocacy framework is not only useful in initial evaluation but is also most effective when utilized as a frame of reference for both patient and advocate throughout their helping relationship. Overall, an advocacy model ensures that patient rights are protected on an ongoing basis.

Advocacy in Action:
A New Style Within the System

The advocacy model for implementing the humanistic helping goal also passes the difficult test of utility as it is applied to interdisciplinary team function and administrative operations. Ideally, the payoffs are higher for a group when the humanistic advocacy helping goal is held by all disciplines within any setting as a superordinate goal.

Superordinate goal, a term coined by Sherif and Sherif,[12] has the unique quality of being a commonly desired goal that cannot be ignored by group members and the attainment of which is beyond the resources and efforts of one subgroup alone. To the extent that any multidisciplinary group chooses to accept the humanistic advocacy helping goal as a superordinate one for their particular system, the Sherifs' work suggests the possibility of less intergroup tension and increased cohesive action toward ensuring humanism throughout their system. As the Sherifs state, "When groups in a state of tension interact with one another toward superordinate goals much desired by all, which cannot be attained by the energies and resources of one group, they tend to cooperate. In a series of activities involving superordinate goals, intergroup conflict and unfavorable stereotypes do become markedly reduced."[13]

When using a humanistic helping goal implemented through an advocacy model, increased evaluative thought can be given to such chronic problems as overlapping functions in team approaches to patient care and the sorting out of who is best able to help which patients with what. The distance often perceived between helping and administration can be shortened. A particularly poignant interview with a health-care agency director exemplifies all these issues. Although he speaks from the reference point of a mental-health center, the points that the director makes are applicable to any setting.

CASE IN POINT

Mental-health centers have several characteristics that are difficult to wrestle with. In our center we found that our initial requests for service have not always corresponded with what we originally saw ourselves here for. We have had to face the fact that old health problems come in new guises these days. Although some new health problems are expressed in traditional physical disease "costumes," some people are experiencing bona fide physiological disease symptoms that have become masked by confounding emotions and social slippage in the family. Some of our requests are referrals from medical clinics in which the persons were found to have no physical disease basis for the feelings that they were experiencing. These people don't always want to be here, even though they voluntarily seek us out.

Naturally we need a multidisciplinary staff, and we have a highly competent crew. All have their own unique contributions, which may not have a thing to do with their particular professions, however. It's not uncommon for a nurse to be a better group therapist than a psychologist or psychiatrist or a psychiatrist able to do a better family assessment and more willing to go right into the home than a social worker. Certain of our paraprofessional aides are highly skilled in the areas that some of our pros see themselves as having spent years to learn. Sometimes it's a draw as to who has the skills for a particular situation, and it has to be talked out.

We also have had to talk a great deal about being "territorial"—that is, who "owns" a patient or who is trying to be everything with the patient in a highly complex situation in which it requires more heads than one. Also I believe that we have had to avoid the staff trying to break down its functions around physiological things and emotional things—a sure way to break the patient up in pieces or at least leave the patient maybe feeling that way.

We have found the advocacy model helpful in shifting attitudes. A lot of edgy staff issues began to dissolve when we could begin to check our function against something other than disciplinary bias and traditional boundaries. Our biases in how we look at patients are real when you consider that each discipline has pretty much had its own way of looking at problems and what to do about them for a long time. It's hard to rise above and look at your work differently when you have been professionally raised a certain way, especially if you don't have a readily available way of looking at something any different than what you had confidence in.

Taking a position that we are advocates has also forced us to evaluate each presenting request for help more carefully before leaping into some vague "treatment" or unspoken assurance that we and we alone will do all the delivering to everyone that comes in the front door. Some people simply are not in the right place when they come; we have needed to help them get to the best place. We have found ourselves in the middle of some doozies, in which staff were way in over their heads and couldn't either call out for help with the case or level with patients that their situation called for more than we could offer.

We are reaching a point at which there is mutual trust between staff as to how patients are generally being responded to. I hope that to both patients and staff we seem more together. I think that we are doing a better job of avoiding patients' getting a different story from everybody that they talk to; yet I don't think we're giving out canned "group-think" jargon.[14] An advocacy attitude can prevent that: you are for the other in getting the best job done together, and that seems to come through. You can bet that some of our routines have smacked us in the face in going through this process, however. It is easy to lose track of what and who you exist for.

As an administrator I personally like an advocacy view of helping, since it allows "us guys at the top" a way to define that we are still helping. A lot of my activities seemed to the staff—and sometimes to myself—a lot of busywork. I sat down and evaluated everything I did in terms of when it was absolutely necessary for me to act in behalf of the staff and thereby in behalf of patients. When I could translate my functions like that, I knew more clearly what I had to do and what the staff had the power or authority to carry out—like saying "What did they need me for that they cannot do themselves to keep a sound operation going in advocating directly for patients?" I found that there were some decisions I did not have to personally make; some I did. I also began to realize that I was pretty damned important in advocating for staff and patients at levels that they did not have access to. Personally I no longer feel that lingering apology for not being in there slugging clinically. I can define myself around "making-it-possible" functions, and that makes me feel more productive.

As this example dramatizes, an advocacy frame of reference shared by health-care workers does more than just influence the way that persons think. New, visibly observed actions gradually emerge. In the preceding case in point, this mental-health center became not only increasingly efficient but also humanistically productive at the same time. New internal procedural systems emerged that helped the staff to develop an advocacy position with patients at the one-to-one level.[15]

Advocacy in Action:
Concern Beyond Agency Walls

An advocacy model can be utilized within all health-care settings and in response to any persons or their representatives who seek help therein. It is a framework of thinking that health-care workers carry within themselves. It is a guide to action that is adaptable to the special characteristics of patients and their particular needs for care.

Whether in an emergency room, obstetrical unit, outpatient clinic, or other setting, the advocacy model can apply. As helpers adopt advocacy attitudes and function, they become more aware of themselves and the effects of their behavior as it interrelates with that of patients. Advocates become activists in that they attempt to do something about the awareness that they increasingly develop concerning what affects people positively or negatively. As in the previous case in point, an entire agency became more aware of the impact of their own notions and procedures on those of others—patients and peers.

Health-care advocates also quickly become aware that there are many factors operating beyond their own particular behavior and the agency's walls that affect their helping processes within the setting. These factors that influence people's behavior before they approach a particular source of help we refer to as *presetting influences*. There are several levels of presetting influences that the patients have experienced that may affect their here-and-now help-seeking behavior.

1. *The influence of the patient's frame of reference and character style in responding to health problems or maintenance of health.* As garbled, passive, demanding, or inappropriate to the setting as their requests might seem at the time, patients would not have put the energy into getting there if something in their preceding experience did not seriously threaten their feeling of being "right with the world" or "in tune with themselves." Health-care advocates realize that it is important to explore at what point patients or their representatives concluded that there was a health-care issue of enough concern involved to reach out for professional help.

   Health-care advocates also need to know what this presetting experience was like for patients or their families. This information is needed in the patients' terms if one is to gain valuable knowledge of such things as the patients' sensitivity to lifestyle disruption; their personalized perceptions of what a "problem" is; the meaning or causes that they attribute to their problems; their willingness to care about themselves; how much professional assistance they think they need or can accept in addition to existing resources; and what they have already done to attempt to alleviate their situation. Through the interpersonal process of determining these personalized presetting influences, the advocate gets a clear picture of a person's own special definition of help and whether the person is in the right spot for the help that is sought and needed. Such a process of exploration with patients also contributes to their feeling that their help seeking is taken seriously.[16]

2. *The influence of sociocultural systems factors over which the patient has no control that affect ease in seeking help as well as personal expectations.* The health-care field has evolved in such a way that there is increasing distance between services and where persons reside. They can no longer bring help directly into their own self-system. At a time of high personal stress and decision making about what to do, those seeking health care are faced with an ever-broadening array of specialty settings from which to choose. The time gap between felt need and receiving something that is personally responsive to their particular concerns is increasingly longer. Indeed, part of the time gap between recognition of the need to "do something" and receiving help is sometimes attributable to patients' need to deny what

they are experiencing or what it might mean, but the concern at this level of preset-ting influence is those factors that confound patients' ability to use services when denial and resistance to help are not the major issues.

Advocates emphasize the necessity of full public articulation of a community's array of health-care resources—for example, making services visible by easy access to (1) what each distinctly offers, (2) information on how they can be simply utilized, and (3) ways to check whether the resources are credible and provide what they say they do. Humanistic helpers advocate for the availability of information on health-care ser-vices in the community and not only in the patient's behalf. Advocates recognize that, the smoother anyone's course is in finding resources, the easier is their own helping role when patients eventually seek them out.

Ideally, methods must be devised that complement the ways which persons have used to finding assistance in the past and that they still seem to prefer. For example, for the majority of the population, word of mouth has long been the primary mode by which to find health-care resources.[17] In part, this is because people are leery of enter-ing relationships with strangers when needs are highly personal. There is a tendency to trust an evaluation made by a friend or relative about a place or person, rather than one that is read about or heard about through impersonal media. However, given a highly transitional culture and the increasing lack of "someone in the know" whom one trusts and who is readily available, persons often feel at a loss in the search for help. For many, the telephone book and the Better Business Bureau have come to replace the close relative or resourceful neighbor across the back fence.

Many health-care professionals and agencies are aware of the public's increasing reliance on the phone book and utilize it to make their services visible; but it is a grossly inadequate resource manual, since its information is sparse.[18] Listings, ex-pressed in terms foreign to the prospective consumer, are not easily located. Its useful-ness requires a high degree of ability to formulate what one's problem is before the fact, as well as an understanding of complex community organization.

Phone-referral centers supported by community voluntary agencies are on the right track in providing some kind of coordination of existing resources as well as personal contact; but, to the degree that their listings are incomplete and relevant data about listings limited, consumer and professional referral decisions are still difficult to make. Those who monitor the switchboard are often inadequately trained to respond empathetically to a broad variety of help seekers. Of little assistance are the profes-sional disciplines, who do not yet agree on how much information about resources should be made available publicly or what media may be ethically used.

Given this confounding situation, seekers of help may simply seek out their physi-cians. Although the physician may be the appropriate choice in many cases, this ave-nue cannot be totally relied on as the solution to the public need for education and the delivery-system dilemma. The physician may or may not have the time or skills to define the health-care problem with the patient succinctly or in depth; or, if a "family physician" concept is not part of an individual's or family's system because of inclina-tion, mobility, or finances, help may be sought from an emergency room or some agency whose title apparently fits what seems to be wrong—or the person may do nothing at all for awhile.

Health-care advocates, therefore, are aware that these factors may significantly contribute to the kind of behavior that they observe or are asked to respond to when they encounter patients initially. By the time that patients gain entry into a health-care setting, they may be angrily impatient, fearful of rebuff and therefore compliant, victims of worry and isolation, or simply worn out from a runaround. Following is an example of presetting circumstances found all too commonly in our series of interviews. As will be seen, however, this patient was most fortunate in being with a hospital staff who were eventually responsive to what had happened.

CASE IN POINT

Jeff had just turned 45 years old when he experienced his first episode of pericardial pain. He had been in a new community for about six months and did not have a primary physician. He explained that he had "never been sick in my life" and didn't think that he needed to have a regular physician. According to the way that he saw the system, even if he had had a regular physician, he probably would have been referred to a specialist.

Since the pain persisted for several days, he began to think about its "maybe being a coronary thing." Quickly he contacted a friend to ask who was the best cardiologist in town. He called for an appointment, described the symptoms, and expected an immediate time slot in view of what he considered a serious personal crisis; but he was given an appointment for December 10—three weeks from the day that he called. He asked the secretary if he could talk to the physician directly. He was told that this was not possible.

He knew that he had other choices, but none appealed to him. He feared walking into a strange, impersonal emergency room and saying "I think I have coronary symptoms." Neither did he want to go back to friends to get the names of other cardiologists—maybe to be put off again. The delaying events in getting an appointment also played into an aspect of his personal response, which was to "deny the whole thing was happening." He explained that he "simply let it go for a few days." Three days later he was hospitalized with a severe coronary occlusion.

When interviewed later in his course of hospitalization, Jeff was angry and fearful—angry at himself for not pushing when he thought that he needed earlier help and angry at "the system" for not being immediately responsive. He was fearful that he would die, a fear that was intensified by his feeling that the hospital staff might not take his ongoing complaints seriously. His trust capacity was low regarding the staff as well as his own integrity.

With Jeff's permission, a discussion was held with his ward physician and unit staff about his prehospitalization experience. This discussion resulted in a number of changes in his care. Immediately the physician and head nurse talked to Jeff in more personalized detail about what had happened leading up to his admission. Jeff was reassured by the physician that his initial judgments about his condition were accurate and, by all means, his ongoing appraisal of himself would be taken seriously. The head nurse explained that, if he ever felt "put off" by the staff, they would discuss it in detail. Jeff also wondered, "Would it help anyone else if that cardiologist knew what had happened?"

The ward physician did talk directly with the cardiologist from whom Jeff had earlier sought an appointment. Later, the ward physician talked to Jeff about the results of that conference. The ward physician believed that Jeff's feedback to the cardiologist had resulted in a different initial contact and screening system that would avoid delay or rebuff or both.

Utilizing advocacy principles contributed markedly to a change in Jeff's feeling state and observable behavior. When last interviewed, his fear of not knowing what tomorrow would bring was still with him; but it was substantially moderated by his knowing that he could depend on the staff to do all that was possible. He was no longer clenched with unexpressed anger. He was still somewhat miffed at himself for his own part in the delaying tactics but was "learning to forgive myself." He felt good about expressing anger at having been put off by the initial cardiologist and hoped that his feedback had helped others.

As stated earlier, an advocacy model of humanistic helping implies that actions are taken in behalf of patients when it has been determined that, *on their own,* they or their representatives cannot bring the needed resources to bear on the situation. This policy would seem to require that everything possible be done by health-care advocates to make certain that the system itself is not contributing to the patient's inability to utilize what is available. It is one matter if health-care resources are well defined and maximally usable but the help seeker has such liability of personal function as to need considerable assistance in finding the appropriate sources of help. It is another matter if the resources are so hidden, ill defined, or chaotically organized that none of the prospective patient's autonomous strengths make a dent in getting where he or she wants to be. An advocacy model, therefore, demands that health-care resources be geographically coordinated and visibly articulated so that they are accessible to use— that is, defined and made available to the public in such a manner that, when they are confronted with a feeling that help must be sought, they can utilize their own resources to the utmost in finding the appropriate setting.

Advocates are also activists in their concern beyond agency walls regarding the plight of preclinical and beginning health-care workers. They recognize that beginning helpers are often caught up in the same complexities as beginning patients. As reviewed earlier, by their own definition and motivation, preclinical health-care students want to help. The time gap for them also—between wanting to help and being able to help—is long. Desirous of work satisfaction, beginning health-care workers are also faced with an array of settings into which they may enter. Some of these may not quite fit with their values or their professional or social skills. Many health-care workers have reported to us that it is difficult to feel that one has chosen the appropriate setting in which to work after the student years of briefly swinging through clinical rotations. Many explained that it was not until after they took a job and made fairly long-term commitments that they came to understand the main thrust that their position would require. For some, the fit was fortuitous. For others, there was a lingering dissatisfaction with their choice and "learning to live with it." Commitments to a poor fit are bound to have repercussions on patients as well. Following are excerpts from an interview with a nursing instructor who was found to be highly sensitive to characteristics of students that tend to affect work satisfaction.

CASE IN POINT

I suppose you remember the old professional adjustment classes; weren't they something like how to wear your cap, joining the organization, together with a smattering of nursing history?

I always felt that these classes led to trying to "be the same," rather than appreciating individual differences.

. . . I'd define professional adjustment as finding the best place to work that fits with who I am. It seems like that is not such a major thing to expect to find in such a broad field. There certainly are more opportunities today for diversity. . . . But students need to be more appreciative of "who they are" before they can size up a job more accurately.

Some years back, it began to occur to me that some students have a more interpersonal, social style—others, a less open style. Some are people oriented; others are more thing oriented, I guess you'd say. One gal seemed to function beautifully in her psychiatric rotation, but in intensive care, she was like Lucy setting up her 5-cent psychiatric stand in the middle of a typhoid epidemic.

. . . I'm trying to approach this adjustment process from the standpoint of helping students to become aware and value aspects of themselves, *at the same time* looking at what specific expectations are called for in certain tasks. I have no hesitancy to explain to students that, when they begin looking for a job, simply stay away from those situations that you know aren't your cup of tea; but in the meantime they need to experience a variety of situations they can try on for size.

In summary, both helper and those seeking help need experiences to work out preconceptions realistically—either having them validated if they are accurate or learning to correct mistaken interpretations early. Both beginning helpers and the consumer public require experiences from which they can determine if they are in the right place for the kind of help that they desire to receive or to provide. An advocacy model of humanistic helping requires that these experiences be provided both patients and helpers before formal entry into the health-care system and in the form of initial and ongoing experiences after entry into specific health-care settings.

Advocacy in Action: Redefining Health-Care Settings

Education of the public and aspiring health-care advocates as to the major functions of health-care settings can be a first step in simplifying help seeking or help giving. Education would assist both groups in discerning whether they were in the most appropriate place for themselves and in clarifying some preliminary expectations. To be meaningful, however, this educational process requires some form of classification of health-care settings quite different from those presently utilized. Traditional labels used to describe health-care settings are not only less than adequate but also are frankly confusing. They contribute little to clarifying the critical characteristics of the helping process that one can expect to receive or be expected to provide. They furnish minimal guides to behavioral evaluation that may be necessary within the setting. Present labels describing health-care settings miss the meaning of humanistic helping.

To review the traditional classifications still being used in the health-care field as to their usefulness and how they fail to lend the clarity needed in today's health-care system dilemma, the following general, but by no means all-inclusive, classifications are discussed: (1) public-health/private-health services, (2) inpatient/outpatient services, (3) specialty/general services, (4) adult/child services, and (5) emergency/non-emergency services.

Public-health/private-health services   The public-health dimension of classification traditionally has concerned the philosophy and actions taken by health-care workers hired by municipal governments or voluntary agencies dedicated to broad community health practices. The historical focus of the public-health dimension has been the prevention and control of disease conditions that affect large numbers of population—for example, communicable disease as it might be transmitted by water, sewage, food, group contact, or other means. In recent years, health-maintenance programs, such as prenatal and postnatal care, follow-up after hospitalization, and family-health counseling have been an important focus. Public-health has also long been the forerunner in the development of community clinics and maintaining the family home as a site of service delivery.

Private-health services, on the other hand, have gradually evolved into being further removed from on-site family and community organization contact. Unfortunately, private- and public-health service coordination has been less than friendly in some circles. This lack of coordination has led to public confusion as to the private sector's concern for broad health issues, in contrast to the emphasis on treatment of the specific disease entities of those who can afford to pay. To many, the public health/private health dichotomy involves those who are poor versus those who are "better-off." Stereotypes still abound in this area concerning the qualitative difference in the kind of services provided, depending on whether they are "private."

Inpatient/outpatient services   Traditionally, when someone was physically ill enough to die or so perceptually confused as to be unable to function in everyday life, residence in an inpatient facility was required. More recently, with the availability of increasingly complex diagnostic procedures that require patients to come to the site of technology, inpatient admission has taken on a broader, less crisis-oriented flavor. Coupled with this phenomenon has been the advent of health insurance that covers hospitalization but not outpatient or family home services. To get one's money's worth, many diagnostic appraisals and other noncrisis health-care services are now obtained on an inpatient basis.

Today, *inpatient* no longer means only that one is so resourceless as to have to be housed or that death is imminent. Within both inpatient and outpatient settings, one finds the living among the dying, the clear-headed among the disorganized and emotionally distressed, the rich and the poor, and often those who need a lawyer more than a medicine man.

Specialty/general services   Categorical breakdown within hospital settings, outpatient clinics, or private practice also inadequately assists either patients or beginning health-care workers to evaluate the specific kind of helping process required or expected, but they do provide more clues. For example, subsystem breakdowns along specialty-service lines, such as medicine, surgery, psychiatry, and obstetrics/gynecology, serve to predict with a certain degree of regularity the presence or absence of certain disease conditions that can be expected "to be seen." To the hospitalized patient, the specialty label may serve to give a hint as to the medical diagnosis—a phenomenon so dramatically experienced by Nikolayevich when, after being told that he had no malignancy, he was admitted to Cancer ward 13.[19] For beginning health-care workers, specialty service labels serve to suggest not only the conditions that they may encounter but also the kinds of technological knowledge and equipment that they must be prepared to apply and manipulate safely.

Specialty labels also allow some clarification as to expectations. Consumers may not like specialties to have evolved to such an extent that one feels "piecemealed." Yet for many, the notion of seeing a specialist assures them they are "getting the best." Nonetheless, the seeker of help generally knows, for example, that, if a setting or private practitioner specializes in ear, nose, and throat, personnel within that setting will probably not be concerned with one's abdominal pain, one's intense marital conflict, or one's child's neurological learning disorder.

Adult/child services   Categorical breakdown according to chronological age also assists the consumer to make some form of gross discrimination in choosing the setting. Some problematic situations are more age specific than others. People have some assurance that someone who specializes in children's problems will be more receptive to kids and can be presumed to be more knowledgeable about the evaluation and treatment of pediatric problems.

However, once again such classification tells little about the kind of helping process that one can expect. Particularly, age classification leads to categorizing human beings in such a way that comprehensive understanding and appreciation of the continuity of the developmental process is lost. For example, there develops a lack of appreciation that many adult behaviors have their roots in childhood; that a child is concerned with adults because of striving to become one; and that aging is not stepping into another universe but is an integration of both childhood and adult experiences combined with a host of years of living. Health-care workers can also lose sight of such issues as family interrelatedness across age groups; stress reactions of persons of any age often reviving behaviors typical of earlier developmental levels; or children's need for parent participation in their growth and development process, which goes on even during illness.[20]

CASE IN POINT

The hazard of using age-specialization categories was clearly dramatized one day when a postdegree trainee was asked why she was reluctant to sit down with a father and mother to share important information about their child. The trainee, who was the primary care giver, commented, "I only know how to work with kids. I don't know anything about adults—particularly parents. Maybe someone else can talk with them."

Emergency/nonemergency services   From the public standpoint, the definition of emergency is variable. People personally respond to a variety of deviations in their life continuum as such. Many times, public definition does not coincide with professional definition. Recently emerging in the field are also terms that take on a jargon flavor and further cloud the issue (e.g., the concept "crisis intervention").[21] For many professionals, this term has come to mean simply short-term intervention, in contrast to measures that continue over a long period of time. As is shown in the following case in point, the public is sensitive to this confusion and often does not know how to handle it. Our furnace repairman, who came to our cabin at 2 A.M., provided an example.

CASE IN POINT

"Maybe you can straighten something out for me, Doc. The other night my daughter had some kind of a seizure and scared the hell out of me, but could I get a damn doctor to come to the house? Not on your life. Now to me this was a crisis. This was my kid! I didn't want to take her out in the cold to find some help in an emergency room after something like that. To me that would make her worse. Now your furnace goes wacky, and it's 38 below. That's a crisis, and I come to you. No questions, right?

"Now for the rest of it—so I go to the emergency room, and I wait an hour for a doc. The nurse was very nice, mind you, but they always have to wait for a doctor; so what are they for? While I'm waiting, I see this sign—Crisis Clinic; so I ask the nurse what *crisis* means, and it doesn't mean what I think it means already. She says that means when people need just a little bit of help to get out of a jam; so what's a crisis anymore? I'm in one, I think; she thinks crisis is just a little thing; the doctor thinks it's nothing 'cause he's not even there. Now you tell me what this world is coming to. Just wait till some doc calls up and his furnace is out and it's below zero."

We got the message.

The traditional category reserved for crisis—house call—is generally a thing of the past.[22] It now means emergency-room services. But these seem to be in helpless confusion. Perhaps one can study no better microcosm of life in answering the empirical question of what is askew in the delivery of health-care services in America. Having mushroomed into a chaotic entry point to health care for a substantial number of the urban population, emergency-room service has gradually come to imply needing to be "everything to everybody" twenty-four hours a day.

To clarify and sort out service components that might be more useful in meeting the needs of those that show up in emergency-room settings, certain subcategories are being tried out in large urban areas (e.g., adult walk-in services and child walk-in services). Although these more refined subcategories may help to alleviate the snake-pit confusion seen in most large emergency centers, a method by which to analyze health-care situations is required that tells more than whether someone is grown or able to walk.

New dimensions   A more useful way to analyze the major functions of health-care settings and the situations that one may encounter within these settings is to utilize three *process* dimensions: (1) life saving, (2) life sustaining, and (3) life enhancing. Although not totally independent categories, for the purposes of clarity, the three dimensions are defined as if they were exclusive. As we begin to apply these dimensions to real situations in later chapters, their interactive nature as they might be utilized in the same setting will become more apparent. Briefly, the definitions of the three dimensions are as follows:

1. *Life-saving dimension.* Major focus: the prevention of imminent death.
2. *Life-sustaining dimension.* Major focus: the maintenance of good health or the restoration of physical health to the highest degree possible.
3. *Life-enhancing dimension.* Major focus: the maintenance, restoration, or further development of perceiving relationships with the world such that one feels emotional well-being—socially productive and self-satisfied.

These new dimensions are referred to as *process oriented* because they are action terms and allow evaluation of settings and health-care advocates in terms of *what they do*. In utilizing these dimensions, health-care advocates can appraise the setting in which they work in terms of such issues as the following: What is the major focus of this setting? Are we engaged primarily in life saving, life sustaining, or life enhancing? In some settings or with certain patients, more than one of the action dimensions may be operative simultaneously; yet advocates can further appraise: Even though this setting's primary function is to provide life-sustaining services, how often must we be prepared for life-saving functions to take precedence? What kinds of life-enhancing experiences are necessary for any particular patient to be able to sustain physical life? These dimensions can be further used by advocates as a definition base for community education—for example, assisting consumers to reconceptualize their problems in more realistic terms or more clearly informing the public about what health-care workers actually do.

Overall, the value of these dimensions in a framework for analysis is that (1) one can discern the helping actions required of both the health-care advocate and the patient in saving, sustaining, or enhancing life experience and (2) health-care advocates can more clearly determine the degree of technological input required, contrasted with the social/emotional understanding necessary to be life saving, life sustaining, or life enhancing. In other words, staff in specific health-care settings can determine both the content of the knowledge that their primary function requires them to hold and the degree and quality of the interpersonal process required to accomplish the overall goal of humanistic helping.

Table 6-1 charts the three dimensions in more detail as utilized in a variety of health-care settings. In Chapters 7 through 9, each of these new dimensions will be discussed in depth.

Issues for Evaluative Thought

Several basic principles underlying the understanding of oneself and others have been stressed throughout the text in a variety of ways: (1) behavior is multidetermined; (2) it is an integrated product of interacting physical, psychosocial factors that are internal and external to a person; and (3) the situational context in which one finds oneself has considerable influence on how one thinks, feels, and acts at the time.

In view of these principles, we have emphasized that, in the health-care field, one must know a great deal about disease, drug, and traumatic processes and how these factors affect behavior. We have also indicated that health-care advocates serious about humanistically understanding and helping people must also look at themselves and the characteristics of the setting in which they encounter patients as a vital part of what may be influencing behavior. It is not possible to come to know patients or oneself in isolation from "context variables."

We have discussed the influence of technical science as it affects the situational context and the behavior of health-care workers. Other social/cultural transitions have affected both the life-style of persons in general and those in the health-care field and make bringing patients and helpers together on some common humanistic turf a difficult task. For example, one can look back a few decades and remember the system by which a family called a health-care worker, generally a physician, *into* their environment. A certain degree of comfort could be experienced in the face of stress when someone whom people chose for help could be brought into their familiar system. The family was naturally "captain of the team" by mere virtue of having choice in who was allowed to enter their private domain. Because of this social structure in help giving, personalized stress reactions could be evaluated by the helper within the context of any given family's life-style. Not so any longer.

With the exception of home visiting by public-health nurses, social caseworkers, or physicians in experimental group practice, the predominant delivery site of any professional health care at present is within the life space of professionals. The distance of health-care workers from the life space of patients can numb the helpers' recognition that persons perceive their life experience as a continuum and that health-care settings into which they periodically enter are but foreign way stations outside their mainstream. Most people would rather be about the business of experiencing life elsewhere than in clinics and hospitals. Patients who prefer the illness role and settings other than their home base have problems other than illness per se.

Table 6-1.

Framework for Analysis Within an Advocacy Helping Model

Humanistic Helping Goal: development of an interpersonal process between helpers and patients or their representatives that integrates technological knowledge and personal/social experience in an interdependent way so as to provide both parties with (1) a satisfying, self-actualizing experience and (2) movement toward life goals to which both helpers and patients are committed.

		Characteristics of Interpersonal Process		
Evaluative dimensions	*Definitions of evaluative dimensions*	*Technological input*	*Social/emotional understanding*	*Degree of patient participation*
I. Life-saving	I. Prevention of imminent death			
A. Primary	A. Unanticipated emergency in community	High	Low	Low
B. Secondary	B. Emergencies secondary to such states as disease and trauma	High	Moderate	Low
II. Life sustaining	II. Maintenance of health and prevention of disabling complications in living subsequent to bodily insult			
A. Primary	A. Maintenance of good health through prevention of disease, injury, and developmental deviations	Low	High	High
B. Secondary	B. Prevention of death or disabling complications in living from disease, illness, or developmental deviations	High	Moderate-high	Moderate-high
C. Tertiary	C. Prevention of disabling complications in dying (e.g., physical and emotional suffering)	Low-moderate	High	High

Table 6-1.
(*continued*)

Evaluative dimensions	Definitions of evaluative dimensions	Characteristics of Interpersonal Process		
		Technological input	Social/emotional understanding	Degree of patient participation
III. Life enhancing	III. Maintenance, restoration, or development of a person's relationship with the world such that one feels emotional well-being—socially productive and self-satisfied			
A. Primary	A. Prevention of disabling complications in interpersonal relationships from social/emotional problems	Low	High	High
B. Secondary	B. Prevention of interpersonal problems in living secondary to effects of disease, drugs, injury, or developmental deviation	High	High	High
C. Tertiary	C. Prevention of dehumanizing residential care giving through establishment of humanistic helping goals	Low	High	Moderate

For helpers, however, health-care settings, except for their own health needs, are sought out of positive, nonanxious motivation. The social system of their occupational work is an integrated part of their continuum of life. To many health-care workers, the site of employment has become their second home. Within these highly complex social systems called *health-care settings,* sensitivity can become dimmed as to how milieu design and social interaction of those whose "home" it is influences the behavior of "outsiders." For health-care workers who wish to develop increased awareness of how a variety of context variables might be affecting the behavior of both patients and themselves, following are presented some examples of sensitizing questions that a group might explore:

1. What are the possible effects of the place where help is sought in influencing the power that we perceive ourselves to have in contrast to that of the patients?
2. How can we introduce ourselves and respond to patients so that our system makes sense in their frame of reference?
3. How are we introducing patients into our system in a way that ensures from the outset that we are allowing and contributing to experiences that are satisfying and more actualizing of the person's potential than those that were undergone before help was sought?
4. How are we relating to patients in such a way as to allow them full expression of their problems, values and life goals?
5. How can we check ourselves to determine whether the patient's goals for help are the same ones in which we are investing our energies?
6. How do we provide interpretation, recommendations, and treatment that require a high degree of technical input in such a way that patients can grasp the full meaning and appreciate our concern for them as total beings?
7. What seem to be the critical factors in situations with patients that seem most satisfying to us as helpers? What factors seem to be operating in those situations that feel the most frustrating to us?
8. What are the collective helping skills that we have as a group that can be shared among ourselves? What skills do we need for which outside assistance is required to accomplish our superordinate goal of humanistic helping?

In using these examples, we idealistically proposed that a group of health-care workers could espouse a commonly held goal and be about the business of self-evaluation; but, as is true in many group situations, individuals may find that they are alone in harboring a humanistic goal and advocacy model of helping. The overall group in which one practices may be found to have no defined goal that contributes to cohesive purpose; or one may be aware that so few hold to the goal in the particular setting that breakdowns in humanism frequently occur. In such situations, the individual or a small subgroup of helpers can evaluate themselves in relation to the total group with such questions as the following:

1. Given that I or my subgroup alone hold this humanistic goal in high value, what is the potential for carrying out such a goal in relative isolation?
2. What is the potential for me or my subgroup to influence other members of the larger group, and how might this influence be accomplished?

For the beginning helper in a student position or in an early employment phase, the feasibility of carrying out a humanistic helping objective can be more clearly ascertained by asking oneself the following questions:

1. Is this larger group of which I am a part going to help me learn humanistic help-ing?
2. Can they acknowledge what I can acknowledge and articulate—my being a novice and needing to struggle from time to time—or does my group tend to deflect from questioning and group learning?

Answers to the foregoing may be encouraging or discouraging. Although the goal of humanistic helping is a needed one and worthy of being held in high value, it does not automatically exist everywhere. Settings in which such philosophy and goals exist must be found or developed by advocates who hold such goals if they are to feel pro-ductive and avoid professional burnout. Sometimes advocates gain enough status or assistance of others to influence a group in these newer directions, but some advocates who thoughtfully evaluate the settings in which they work and find that their energies to accomplish such a goal for themselves repeatedly do not have productive payoffs, may have to leave and seek employment elsewhere.[23,24]

For the beginning employment seeker who desires to work within a system (in contrast to independent private practice), such a goal can assist in making pertinent observations of health-care settings and asking of relevant interview questions that are tied to meaningful specifics. By becoming increasingly sensitive to the goals and values that one holds, it is less difficult to evaluate settings into which one is considering entry.

In Chapters 7 through 9, we integrate both the humanistic helping goal and the advocacy model of implementation into a detailed discussion of each of the new dimen-sions of health-care giving—life saving, life sustaining, and life enchancing. We hope that these chapters will provide beginning health-care workers a clearer picture of the requirements of various settings and will lead to more personalized choices of where to work that fit effectively with the kind of help that they are both interested in and prepared to provide.

REFERENCE NOTES

1. Eric Hoffer, *Reflections on the Human Condition* (New York: Harper & Row, 1973), p. 56.
2. George L. Engle, "Enduring Attributes of Medicine Relevant for the Education of the Physician," *Annals of Internal Medicine* 78 (1973): 587–93.
3. See "Emotional Factors in Illness and Disability," in *Physical Disability and Human Behavior*, ed. James W. McDaniel (Elmsford, N.Y.: Pergamon Press, 1969), chap. 3.
4. Ian R. McWhinney, "Beyond Diagnosis," *New England Journal of Medicine* 287 (24 August 1972): 384–87.
5. For anyone wanting to do in-depth reading about the development of clinical-judgment abilities and internal evaluation models, Harty's work is excellent. See Michael K. Harty, "Studies of Clinical Judgment: Part I," *Bulletin of the Menninger Clinic* 35 (1971): 335–52 and "Studies of Clinical Judgment: Part II," *Bulletin of the Menninger Clinic* 36 (1972): 279–301.
6. Alfred J. Kahn, Sheila B. Kamerman, and Brenda G. McGowan, *Child Advocacy Report on a National Baseline Study* (New York: Columbia University School of Social Work, 1972), p. 14.
7. Ibid., p. 39.
8. "Making the 'Double Diagnosis,' " *Urban Health* 3 (April 1981): 41.
9. Ibid., p. 43.
10. Ibid., p. 43.
11. For an in-depth review of these concepts, see Chapter 5.

12. Muzafer Sherif and Carolyn W. Sherif, *An Outline of Social Psychology* (New York: Harper & Bros., 1956).

13. Ibid., p. 330.

14. Janis describes "group think" as the "desperate drive for consensus at any cost that suppresses dissent among the mighty in the corridors of power." Irving L. Janis, "Group Think," *Psychology Today* 15, no. 11 (November 1971): 43–46, 74–76.

15. Advocacy-oriented frameworks in the form of "patient rights" are available for agencies and large systems to use—if they will. See the American Hospital Association's statement on "A Patient's Bill of Rights" (affirmed by the board of trustees, 17 November 1972). The full statement appears in *Hospitals* 47 (16 February 1973): 41.

16. A particularly relevant Harris Survey concerning the public's feelings about American health care and patient rights was released in May 1973. Their nationwide cross-section survey of 1513 households revealed that 41 percent of the group believed that hospital patients are sometimes neglected or even victims of malpractice; 11 percent were not sure; 97 percent thought that "no person should be experimented on by doctors without the patient's permission and a full explanation from the doctor"; 78 percent believed that "every patient should be told the full extent of his illness and dangers, as well as the help he might receive from certain kinds of treatment." Comparably, 74 percent agreed that "any patient should be able to refuse treatment or medication even if it is strongly recommended by a hospital"; 62 percent thought that patients ought to be able to tell a doctor not to prolong life, 10 percent were not sure, and 28 percent believed that it is wrong. Telling a doctor to end life showed a lesser allowance factor: only 37 percent thought that it should be allowed, with 10 percent not sure and 53 percent believing that it is wrong. Because these are group statistics, they cannot be automatically applied to everyone; but they can give the advocate a general notion of the public's frame of reference and a base from which to explore with their individual patients. Complete copies of this Harris Survey may be obtained from Louis Harris & Associates, Inc., 1270 Avenue of the Americas, New York, N.Y. 10020.

17. Word of mouth apparently is still a powerful advertising force. In survey work done in the Office of Child Development/University of Colorado Medical Center Child Care Demonstration Project (Jane Chapman, Ph.D., Project Director), how consumers heard about the new resources was tabulated. In spite of planned public-media advertising programs within the "community system" of the medical center, the majority of applicants for information, counseling coordination, and direct child-care services had heard about the resource through a friend or co-worker.

18. Nowhere within a phone book is there a separate dictionary and map of public and private health-care agencies. Yellow pages in many cities still do not categorize nurse practitioners, physicians, psychologists, or social workers according to specialty practice. Concerned health-care groups—professionals or consumers—could do something about that. Beyond skeletal information about services offered, information on quality of service is almost impossible for patients to obtain except by direct experience. Helping the public to be aware of standards by which they may evaluate a health-care setting at the time of initial entry becomes increasingly important. Advertising agencies to whom the public can complain must also be highly visible. For useful suggestions that a community might try, see "How to Find a Doctor for Yourself," *Consumer Reports* 39 (1974): 681–91.

19. Alexander Solzhenitsyn, *Cancer Ward* (New York: Bantam Books, 1969), p. 1.

20. For further reading concerning a family focus in providing health care for children and adults, see Nathan P. Ackerman, *Psychodynamics of the Family* (New York: Basic Books, 1958) and Howard J. Parad and Gerald Caplan, "A Framework for Studying Families in Crisis," in *Crisis Intervention: Selected Readings*, ed. Howard J. Parad (New York: Family Service Association of America, 1965). Although these references may be viewed as rather old in view of rapid transitions in family life, they are reflective of some of its enduring characteristics. See also Cyril Worby, "The Family Life Cycle: An Orienting Concept for the Family Practice Specialist," *Journal of Medical Education* 46 (1971): 198–203. Particularly excellent and easy to read is Virginia Satir's *Peoplemaking* (Palo Alto, Calif.: Science & Behavior Books, 1972). The most refreshing part of her book is that it is not interwoven with references and documentation. She comfortably expresses her formulations from many years of experience. Satir is of the gestalt/humanistic tradition and author of another fine text, *Conjoint Family Therapy* (Palo Alto, Calif.: Science & Behavior Books, 1967).

21. See Lee Ann Hoff, *People in Crisis* (Menlo Park, Calif.: Addison-Wesley, 1978). See also Lawrence G. Calhoun, James W. Selby, and Elizabeth King, *Dealing with Crisis* (Englewood Cliffs, N.J.: Prentice-Hall, 1976).

22. The physician's house call is becoming revived of late in the evolving Health Maintenance Organization (HMO) system of health-care delivery. In a local Denver HMO demonstration, house-call benefits may be elected as part of a subscriber's health-care package for a slightly higher fee.

23. A particularly good reference to read before considering terminating your employment is Alexander L. George, "Adaptation to Stress in Political Decision Making: The Individual, Small Group and Organizational Contexts," in *Coping and Adaptation*, eds. George V. Coelho, David A. Hamburg, and John E. Adams (New York: Basic Books, 1974), pp. 176–245. See also Marlene Kramer, *Reality Shock: Why Nurses Leave Nursing* (St. Louis: C. V. Mosby, 1974).

24. For a full text copy of a physician's letter of resignation in the face of value-system conflict, see Appendix B. This letter was mimeographed and publicly distributed to the physician's staff so that there would be no question as to his personal/professional reasons for leaving. Only names and places have been altered in editing the letter.

SUGGESTIONS FOR FURTHER EXPERIENCE

In Chapter 5, a basic survey of patients was suggested as a sensitization to the consumer's perception of help as it might differ from that of health-care workers. At this point, select one of your patients with whom you have been most involved in providing extensive diagnosis and treatment. Evaluate the degree to which you have been working within an advocacy model by answering the following questions:

1. How did the patient find your setting?
2. What problem was the patient concerned about when help was first sought?
3. What had the patient done about this problem before seeking help in your setting? How useful or detrimental were these actions in light of present circumstances?
4. What meaning did the patient attach to personal difficulties on first seeking help; that is, why did the patient think that this was happening? What did the patient think was happening "inside"? What did the patient think was "causing" the problem? How did the event of seeking help disrupt the patient's continuity of daily living?
5. What did the patient want you to do about these difficulties?
6. At the outset, what was your appraisal of the patient's problem and the patient's capacities to assume responsibility in the helping process?
7. What did you share with the patient at the beginning regarding your notions about the problem, the patient's strengths, and what you could be expected to do?
8. What kinds of formal standardized tests have been used to appraise the patient's difficulties further? List all measures used and give the reasons why they were selected. In your judgment, were all these needed to provide safe care? Has the patient been informed of the reasons for the evaluation measures utilized?
9. How much of the results of the evaluation has been shared with the patient? How did the patient respond to feedback? How did feedback to the patient affect the need for renegotiation as to the goals of help?
10. How much about the patient do you still think that you need to know to help this particular person effectively? How do you plan to go about obtaining what you believe that you still need to know?
11. How does the patient presently feel about the nature of the helping process?
12. How satisfied are you with the helping process occurring between you and the patient? To the degree that you feel dissatisfied with the progress of the helping process, within which sphere of variables do you perceive the difficulty to lie? Patient variables? Setting variables? Helper variables? Effects of technical treatments (drugs, radiation, or surgery)?
13. Overall, is the major focus of this helping relationship life saving, life sustaining, or life enhancing?
14. What kinds of jointly made plans have been developed for that point in the helping process when your input is no longer immediately available?
15. How much do you feel the patient has learned about taking respectful care of his or her "total being" in the future?

Applying the Advocacy Model to Health Care

Chapter 7

The Life-Saving Dimension of Health Care

In overall purpose, the health-care field exists because people are concerned with the saving of physical life and with qualitatively enhancing how people experience life in the sense of physical and emotional well-being. Even disease-prevention programs have life saving as their ultimate goal in that they provide avenues by which to increase longevity. However, the life-saving dimension as spoken to for evaluative purposes in this text is more specific: its major focus is the prevention of imminent death through emergency actions.

In evaluating settings in helping situations against a life-saving dimension, it is helpful to break down the concept of emergency into two categories: primary and secondary. This categorization is useful because emergency life-saving activities, since they occur in various settings, have somewhat different psychological factors operating as they affect both helpers and patients, even though the specific technical options required at the moment to save life may be identical.

Primary-Emergency Life-Saving Situations

A primary emergency is an unforeseen crisis situation that occurs in the community, as opposed to within a formalized health-care setting. There is no predicting when or where the event will occur. These are events in which common sense alone dictates that something about a person's physical condition requires that skill in keeping people alive be brought to the scene of the event. There is little rumination about whether help is necessary. Motivation to let someone else with expertise take over is high. Examples of primary-emergency events are accidents, assaults, drownings, suicide attempts, coronary occlusions, strokes, perforated peptic ulcers, epileptic seizures, diabetic comas, delirium tremens, and alcohol or other drug overdosages.

Primary-emergency life-saving care involves two distinct phases: *phase 1,* from the time that the original bodily insult occurs or is discovered until the person enters the hospital emergency department; and *phase 2,* from the time of entry into the emergency department to the time of entering a continuing-care unit elsewhere in the hospital. Therefore, from the time of the precipitating event to the time of nonemergency status, the patient's care is entrusted to three teams of personnel: ambulatory, emergency-room, and continuing-care-unit teams. A high potential thereby exists for a breakdown in the continuity of humanistic and technical helping unless the organizational procedures that operate in the patient's behalf during this time are defined.

In primary-emergency life-saving settings—whether in a community with an ambulatory team (phase 1) or within an emergency department (phase 2)—a number of characteristics hold constant. For the patient involved or those closely related, the event comes as a total surprise. Threat to the continuity of psychological and physical life is at its highest. Care givers who arrive on the scene are total strangers to the patient and bystanders. Most often the patient is found in an unconscious state. Unconsciousness may be due to the trauma, drug, or disease process as well as the interactive effects of the psychological reaction to the suddenness of the event.[1] If conscious, patients in a primary emergency are often perceptually confused or disoriented—psychologically struggling to derive meaning from what is occurring, for which they were totally unprepared. In other words, patients in such situations have little data available to them from which to interpret what has just happened.

Health-care advocates who are involved in primary life-saving situations also have little data available to them about the specific situation when they initially encounter the patient. Particularly, this is so for emergency medical technicians (EMTs), who are generally first on the scene out in the community.[2] To the degree possible, information from the patient, relatives, or bystanders is utilized. However, the patient's physical condition is the main point of reference, and, on the basis of minimal input, health-care advocates must be able to function appropriately. Psychologically, they must be geared to primary-emergency stress; that is, they must develop the ability to expect anything and effectively cope with a high degree of uncertainty. Ideally, they have the capacity to incorporate the suddenness of an emotionally stressing event immediately into their frame of reference in such a way as to allow a model of action-oriented behaviors to be rapidly available to them.

Secondary-Emergency
Life-Saving Situations

Secondary emergencies are those that occur exclusively within formalized life-sustaining health-care settings. In these situations is present a higher degree of expectation that life-saving events might occur secondary to an event that brought the patient to the setting in the first place. For example, secondary emergencies are experienced during childbirth and surgery, in postsurgical and medical intensive-care units, in units that receive patients who have experienced a primary emergency, and in settings in which are patients in terminal phases of disease (e.g., those with carcinoma, heart disease, and renal failure). As will be seen, many of these settings must also carry out unique life-enhancing functions in great measure.

Life-sustaining settings that must be prepared for secondary life-saving functions have many characteristics in common with primary-emergency situations. As in the case of a primary-emergency advocate, helpers in life-sustaining settings must have similar knowledge of what to do technically in a life-saving crisis situation. They also must be prepared organizationally and psychologically for emergency situations that may occur at any time within their setting. However, there are some significant differences in experiencing a primary emergency "out in the field" in contrast to an emergency that is secondary to an existing condition within the hospital. For example, when a secondary life-saving event occurs, helpers have the advantage of a somewhat more organized environment and the opportunity of putting their life-saving competencies together with more specific preknowledge about the patient's physiological and social/emotional status. Helpers often have the further advantage of being able to anticipate a crisis by virtue of 24-hour surveillance of the patient's behavior. Emotionally, however, health-care advocates working through secondary-emergency situations with patients may find these experiences more stressful. Patients whom one has come to know personally may not be more difficult to relate to mechanistically during the crisis. What is more difficult is the deeper personal investment that one has in the outcome of a helping action for both the patient and oneself. No one likes to lose a patient to death during an emergency. It can, however, be more stressful to experience a human loss in secondary-emergency situations when one has come to know the other and that person has come to have personal meaning. Only if one has full knowledge that the patient does not have an investment in sustaining life does it hurt less to be present at its loss.

Psychologically, secondary-emergency life-saving situations are somewhat different for the patient and family. By virtue of a patient's already being within a hospital setting, these situations are not experienced by the patient or relatives as completely shocking or unexpected. Indeed, both patients who are acutely ill and those who are "on the mend" do protect themselves from the anxiety of complications that might occur. Sometimes, such defenses as complete denial of the seriousness of one's situation are apparent; at other times, optimism about the outcome is based on the reality of the patient's steady progress. Should serious emergency complications arise, patients, family, and health-care advocates must alter their perceptions. Nonetheless, for no one is the situation such that the event is totally unanticipated, as is the case out in the community, where primary emergencies occur. The patient and the family within the secondary-emergency situation have the benefit of recognizing that both equipment and personnel that they know are accessible in the immediate environment. This recognition, if the patient has experienced a competent, humanistic staff, contributes to trust and lowered anxiety both preceding and during a secondary emergency. Confusion and disorientation experienced by patients in secondary-emergency life-saving situations may therefore be less attributable to the difficulty in ordering perceptions because of a strange environment. Health-care advocates may experience less difficulty in reassuring and reorienting the patient to reality than they would in primary-emergency settings.

In both primary- and secondary-emergency life-saving situations, the overriding goal is the prevention of immediate death. This goal is highly dependent on technical prowess and timing—the capacity to mobilize knowledge of physiology, drugs, mechanical procedures, and equipment with organized speed. An emergency is no time to discuss the politics of using one emergency room over another or to end up going to the one farther from the point of the initial event. Neither is this the time in a hospital unit to search for needed equipment and damn central supply.

In both kinds of life-saving situations, the degree of participation that can be expected of or allowed the patient in directing the helping process is minimal if the saving of life is to occur. During the central aspects of the life-saving process, a verbal interpersonal relationship with the patient or relative is minimized. Interpersonal relationships between co-workers during the crisis aspect tend to be more mechanistic and focused on communicating about what to do; relationships during this time are rarely social. Among the staff, high degrees of trust that each quickly knows what to do when is crucial. Relating to the patient, the patient's family, and each other in a fully explanatory fashion traditionally comes after the crisis phase of the emergency—not during the specific life-saving process.

CASE IN POINT

Kay and her fiancé arrived at her home late New Year's Eve with bags of groceries in preparation for the next day's festivities, which included their engagement announcement. Kay's two adolescent children were at a neighborhood party down the road. Upon entering the house, Kay and her fiancé were surprised by Kay's ex-husband, who shot Kay's fiancé, Kay, and then himself. When the children arrived home, they found many police and ambulance personnel, who had been summoned by Kay before she lapsed into unconsciousness. One of the police attempted to inform and comfort the children, yet he did not yet know exactly what had occurred in terms of who did what to whom. Neither could he tell them if their mother would survive.

The children explained the next day that, while they had now received more explanations about their mother's condition—she was the only survivor—they still were in the dark about police suspicions that their mother might have shot both the men. They were bewildered by the prospect of "arrangements" and contacting distant relatives. The children were unused to crimes of violence except on TV, and they were still in shock from what they had seen in the bloody kitchen. They were appalled that they, as the "family," had to take responsibility for cleaning it all up, believing the police also "did those kinds of things."

It helped these adolescent children to learn their mother would probably survive and that it appeared she had not done the shooting, even though they had to face the shock that their father had done so. Helping them to get as many facts straight as possible enabled them to visit their mother, who would waft in and out of consciousness. It was also helpful for the ward staff to know the circumstances so that, in the children's absence, they could gradually help Kay clarify reality, shocking and painful as it was for her to have to incorporate.

Kay's return to consciousness and gradual recall was fairly typical for victims of such massive physical and emotional assault. At first, she would smile and warmly greet familiar family faces, at times begin to socialize, but then, within minutes, a wave of painful horror would spread across her face and eyes as she would remember and cry, "Oh, no, it really did happen." The family was comforted and less anxious because of the support and guidance of the unit staff, who were extremely sensitive and knowledgable in responding to Kay. If Kay asked about any aspect of the tragedy, a staff member would pull up a chair and sit next to her, touching her gently to give her added support. The staff never avoided answering what she wanted to know in order to fill in her gaps, but neither did they push her to accept more facts than her readiness indicated. By gradually learning the facts without overstressing her fragile physical and emotional state, Kay was, within 48 hours, able to provide more information to the police and to help the children make some of their immediately pressing decisions.

For the goal of humanistic helping to be fully realized in life-saving settings and situations, a division of labor may be required between (1) those health-care advocates whose primary function is characterized by swift, organized, technologically based mechanistic actions and (2) those who, during and after the crisis aspects of the emergency, provide patients and their representatives with "support"—that is, clarifying explanations of the patient's status, what must be done, or why certain behaviors of helpers take precedence over others. Following is a case in point in which an "explanatory advocate" would have been most useful.

CASE IN POINT

Mrs. M had been visiting her daughter Beth in Chicago and was flying back to California when she became unconscious on the plane. An emergency landing was made, and Mrs. M was taken by ambulance to a large city-hospital emergency room. Beth was immediately called long distance from the airport, and she arrived on the next flight. She called us in the middle of the night for advice.

Beth explained that we did not know her personally but that she had found us through calling a relative of ours in Montana, who suggested that we might be able to help out if she needed anything. What Beth seemed to need was some support in terms of information so that she could feel more trustful of the care that her mother was receiving in a setting that was strange to both of them. Beth explained that her mother had experienced "a stroke in the brain" and that she, Beth, was trying to decide about giving permission for the neurosurgery that was planned. Beth believed that good care obviously had been given her mother since, so far, she was still alive; but Beth wondered if the hospital that her mother was in was the best.

Some of the things that Beth had seen and experienced since arriving "kind of bothered" her: the emergency room where she went to make the initial contact was "swamped with all kinds of people that you practically had to walk over," and the "staff seemed overworked"; she thought that she had had to wait an awfully long time to find out what unit her mother was then in; she wanted to talk with the neurosurgeon personally, but so far he had not been available. She thought that she needed to know from someone whether the neurosurgeon had a good reputation and whether what she saw in the emergency room was any indication of the kind of circumstances that existed throughout the hospital.

Clearly Beth needed an explanatory health-care advocate on the premises from whom she could get some straightforward answers. When we arrived at the hospital, with which we were familiar, we were able to find health-care workers who could answer her questions, and Beth was reassured.

This case was not a matter of health-care workers' not having the information that Beth required; it was only that such information giving was not systematized in any way so that it could be utilized by her to reduce anxiety and to make responsible decisions.

As this situation demonstrates, in life-saving situations, the specific point at which a broader integration of humanistic concepts can be employed is the time at which it has been determined whether a life has been saved. If the person has survived, this is the point in helping at which life-sustaining functions come into the picture—that is, when the patient leaves the emergency department and is transferred to a continuing-care unit or regains status as a recuperating member of the unit in which the life-saving crisis occurred. At this juncture, the patient or the family or both require less of the total helping process to be assumed by the health-care advocate. More participant goal setting can begin or be reinitiated.

Summary Evaluation Guide

The life-saving dimension by which settings can be evaluated includes a primary- and a secondary-emergency focus. Health-care personnel and settings whose major thrust is life saving in primary-emergency situations are (1) those mobile teams that go to the site of the crisis out in the community during phase 1 of an emergency and (2) emergency departments of hospitals that are prepared to accept the patient in phase 2 of the primary emergency situation. Health-care settings whose major focus may be life sustaining or life enhancing also require preparatory equipment and skills for life saving situations; emergencies that take place within these health-care settings are considered secondary emergencies.

Beginning health-care advocates considering work in either phase 1 or 2 of primary life saving must evaluate whether what the setting requires fits them (i.e., their personal style together with their knowledge and skills). For example, such settings require staffs who can mobilize a high degree of technologically based knowledge with organized speed. To facilitate this behavior, personnel must be able to design settings that are more than just amply equipped; they must be compulsively organized for efficiency and dependability. Health-care advocates working within such settings must also be able to derive a sense of productivity and work satisfaction from stressful situations that (1) provide little personalized data about patients, (2) allow low-intensity, short-term interpersonal contacts with patients, (3) require a high degree of mechanistic, action-oriented behavior, (4) demand group effort that emphasizes a high degree of reliance on teammates to be efficient and dependable, and (5) contain a high potential for sudden death when a patient and family are least prepared.

Primary-emergency settings are not for everyone. Some health-care advocates prefer settings in which their function is not primarily dictated by emergency actions and the mechanistic behaviors that they require. Some health-care advocates need more data available to them before they feel comfortable enough to function competently in emergency situations. In other words, some persons do not "think so well on their feet," but, given more input about a situation, they function exceedingly well in secondary life-saving situations. Some health-care advocates, in spite of the stress involved in working through secondary emergencies with patients whom they have come to know, prefer longer relationships with patients; and some health-care advocates simply do not like primary emergency situations because they cannot psychologically cope with the traumatic physical appearance that is often encountered in patients in these settings.

Whether they choose to work in primary life-saving settings or in those in which emergencies occur occasionally, health-care advocates acknowledge that, in all life-saving situations, the following points are relevant:

1. In specific life-saving situations with patients or relatives, a health-care advocate recognizes the necessity for the patient's temporarily minimized role. In these situations, health-care advocates assume that the major goal—to prevent death—is shared by all, and they take total responsibility for acting in the patient's behalf only until that goal is accomplished.
2. Within life-saving settings, health-care workers advocate in behalf of patients with the system's administration to ensure that equipment and prepared staff are available to provide what their knowledge tells them is available to save lives.
3. At the broadest level of function in the consumer's behalf, the health-care advocate recognizes the need for an organized community plan concerned with coordinating phase 2 of primary-emergency care with phase 1 care—for example, utilization of other mobile emergency teams, such as fire departments, police, and private ambulance services. The health-care advocate recognizes that the minute saved by an effective community emergency plan saves lives; advocates cooperate with such a community plan. They insist on such a plan in behalf of patients if one does not exist. If the plan is not working, they express their concern openly.

As mentioned in the first point, the health-care advocate in life-saving settings must have the ability to evaluate when, in any given emergency situation, it is critical to begin implementation of a helper/patient interaction that includes increasing interpersonal process and consideration of social/emotional variables. This evaluation is the means by which the overall goal of humanistic helping has a higher probability of being accomplished. Following are the occasions in life-saving settings when the patient and/or family can be appropriately included in the helping process:

1. *When the patient is conscious.* Orienting responses to the patient during the crisis aspect of the emergency can help to clarify reality and lower anxiety. Behavior that is more cooperative and less disorganized is facilitating to the life-saving actions of the health-care advocate. A lowered level of anxiety on the part of the patient allows more coping energy in response to the physiological insult.
2. *When the goal of immediate prevention of death has been accomplished.* Explanatory interchange and realistic future-oriented goal setting can begin with patients and relatives. For example, patients and their relatives need to know at what point the patient's condition will show that the patient is "going to make it" and what they may now do to facilitate that process. This kind of communication contributes to trust and renewed hopefulness, both of which are essential to the patient's beginning to mobilize self-help processes, primitive or passive though they may be.
3. *When the patient is transferred from the care-giving responsibility of the primary-emergency team.* Orienting, explanatory interchange between the primary-emergency team and the health-care advocates of the continuing-care unit ensures continuity of the patient's physical and emotional safety. These coordinating interchanges between the staffs of different units avoid patients' being asked many questions about their condition at a time when such questions heighten, rather than diminish, external stress. The staff of continuing-care units are also less stressed to the degree that they have solid information about patients as a base from which to begin working.
4. *When the goal of immediate prevention of death has failed to be accomplished.* In no other situation of health care is professional helping often so abruptly terminated as when death of a patient occurs; yet, at no other time is ongoing help to family and relatives more important. Some persons have family resources to pick up on for the needed help that begins at this point. Others do not.

CASE IN POINT

Ada and her husband, John, were 55 years old. Their life together had been viewed by them as "idyllic." Childless, they liked being with each other most of the time; they had no financial problems, a lovely home, and two flourishing careers. John had never experienced a serious illness. Ada, however, had begun to experience some "female problems" that left her at times irritable and fatigued. Always interested in philosophy and new knowledge, Ada became intrigued with many Eastern and Western religious viewpoints that emphasized "mind over body" processes. Her reading seemed to help her periodic depressive responses to aging and its minor physical disruptions. Generally, she was enthusiastic about her newfound philosophy and found pleasure in talking about it.

One weekend, her husband complained of not feeling well. Ada's response was not worried; she encouraged him to think positively and get on top of the negative feelings. Complaints later in the day also did not seem to Ada to require special attention for John. That evening, however, her husband's symptoms became so severe that she realized that she must take him to the emergency room. When John and Ada arrived in the ambulance, he was pronounced dead on arrival.

Ada was in shock but, according to her recollection, "able to function." She remembers mechanically moving "like a robot" through the process of calling the funeral home and finding someone to drive her home. She vaguely remembers being asked at the emergency room if her children could be called, but she and John had no children.

On getting close to home, she became overwhelmed with the fear of staying alone; so she stayed with a friend until after the funeral. However, she could not go home after the funeral either. Beseiged by guilt at not responding immediately to her husband and fearful that imposing her philosophy had denied him care, Ada became sleepless and ruminative. She could not return to her work and believed herself incapable to handle her husband's business affairs.

When initially encountered in a help-seeking situation, Ada kept saying that she wished that someone could have helped her sooner. She thought that, as soon as her husband was dead, no one seemed to know what else to do. She wondered if she were selfish to think that someone besides her friends should have followed up on her; by the time that she sought help, Ada was preoccupied with whether she was "going crazy."

Shock, anger, grief, and guilt are common reactions experienced by a dead patient's relatives and friends, regardless of the circumstances. After a sudden, unanticipated death, these feelings can be even more intensely experienced.[3] When a patient dies in a primary-emergency situation, as in the preceding case, the family or others deeply involved with the patient are faced with suddenly having to make sense out of what has just happened. With no preparation, they must work hard internally to put the external event together with their frame of reference about life, death, and the particular meaning of the person who no longer lives.

Health-care advocates working in these situations allow the subjective, deep feelings of relatives and friends to be expressed. They listen carefully to presetting experiences that may be markedly influencing the response to the death of the patient. Because guilt about what "might have been done sooner" is often an aftermath of a primary-emergency death, health-care advocates can help reduce the intensity of guilt by giving realistic explanations of what apparently has happened and what they the helpers did to try to save life, even though they too failed. Following is a situation in which a simple explanation stemmed a fast-rising sense of guilt.

CASE IN POINT

Laura received a phone call from her friend Etta, who was sobbing because she had just learned that her only daughter was filing for a divorce. Even though Etta lived across town, Laura was immediately willing to go to her so that she could talk about Etta's problem with her in person. One-half hour later, when Laura arrived at Etta's home, no one answered the unlocked door. Concerned, Laura entered and found Etta slumped over in a chair. She was deeply cyanotic and not breathing. Laura immediately called for an ambulance.

At the hospital, Laura commented, "Maybe if I had gotten there sooner, she would still be alive." The physician countered her taking of responsibility by explaining that Etta had experienced a massive heart attack that undoubtedly had occurred immediately after hanging up the phone. He assured Laura that she had done the best that she could in responding to her friend's request to come and give support, but that, even if she had been there instantly, Etta's death probably could not have been prevented.

Laura continued to take her friend's death hard and openly grieved about her loss and the ironic fateful circumstances; yet, she did not have to wonder about her sense of responsibility in addition. She had received some basic information with which she could clarify reality.

Acting in behalf of relatives and close friends to put them in touch with resources that will assist them to carry out their grieving and their pragmatic responsibilities is also acknowledged by health-care advocates as contributing to the life enhancement of those who still live. Ideally, the advocate explores what kind of assistance is perceived by them as their need at that time and helps them to order the many priorities that a sudden death precipitates.

Health-care advocates also acknowledge that both they and their co-workers respond humanly to the loss of any life. Humanistic health-care personnel allow the experiencing and expression of their own feelings and those of their associates in finding ways to accommodate the loss for themselves philosophically, not simply in the light of how it might have been avoided through improved equipment or helping practices. Following is a case in point comprising a nurse's reflection on the process of coming to terms with her feelings about life and death.

CASE IN POINT

Things are gradually changing for the better in hospitals, I believe. People seem to be able to be more open with their feelings. I can recall when the message was clear that we "shouldn't show emotion." After my first patient died, I went into a broom closet to cry and was told to "grow up and get back onto the floor."

Then there were the polio epidemics that I remember so well; we were short of staff, there were not enough iron lungs, and patients were coming into the emergency room like the dike had broken—beautiful, healthy-looking people lying there—and at times we were helpless. My own cousin was admitted one night—a straping 6-footer with a wife and four children—but nothing we did helped. It seemed we didn't have time to feel, and we kept ourselves going on Dexedrine. We also had to fight the fear of our catching polio; at that time, gamma globulin was short, and it was reserved for pregnant women only. I remember a group of us talking one night about what we meant to humanity if we couldn't receive it.

For two months, I didn't shed a tear; I don't think there were any of us on that team that did. There was nothing built into the whole operation that said it was okay or allowed time off to bawl. Sometimes I think we substituted anger at things for grief about people and our helplessness.

After the major peak of the epidemic was over, we were gradually given leave. I remember sitting there watching a *Playhouse 90* TV drama, and someone died in the show. Suddenly, all my feelings came back, and I cried for what seemed like hours. I remembered patients and families whom I could not feel for or with at the time that the losses were so great. I felt better after that letting-go experience, however. I have never allowed myself or others to deny my gut-level reactions since that time. It helps remind me I am part of the human race."

REFERENCE NOTES

1. Review Hans Selye's "The Evolution of the Stress Concept," *American Scientist* 61 (1973): 692–99. Pay particular attention to his comments concerning adaptation and individual differences in the face of identical stressor potency. An easily read article nicely summarizing his major work.

2. A particularly outstanding text and a must as required reading for this chapter is James M. Mannon, *Emergency Encounters* (Port Washington, N.Y.: Kennikat Press, 1981). This is a well-done sociological study of an urban ambulance service, with particular emphasis on the personhood of emergency medical technicians and the stresses with which they learn to cope. The case studies and descriptive observational data are vivid and useful for beginners to review before field experience.

3. The "sudden-death" phenomenon is important for all health-care workers to be aware of within any dimension of care with respect to patients and close relatives. The finest article that we have encountered on this subject is George L. Engel, "Sudden and Rapid Death During Psychological Stress," *Annals of Internal Medicine* 74 (1971): 771–82. A comprehensive bibliography of 89 references follows the article. Engel classifies eight categories of life settings in which this phenomenon can occur: "(1) on the impact of the collapse or death of a close person; (2) during acute grief; (3) on threat of loss of a close person; (4) during mourning or on an anniversary; (5) on loss of status or self-esteem; (6) personal danger or threat of injury; (7) after the danger is over; (8) reunion, triumph, or happy ending. Common to all is that they involve events impossible for the victims to ignore and to which their response is overwhelming excitation or giving up, or both" (p. 771).

SUGGESTIONS FOR FURTHER EXPERIENCE

The life-saving dimension of care giving is one that the collective variety of health-care disciplines rarely can experience in common, partly because the techniques and responsibility for life saving are taught primarily in medicine and nursing. Therefore, the other disciplines can feel shut out by the mystique of this function, as does the general public. This situation also results in a type of existential experience and responsibility taking that may not be shared across disciplines.

Many students in medicine and nursing have related increasingly, however, that they too—with decreasing clinical practice time—lack the experiential comfort of knowing what is fully involved in primary and secondary life saving. Particularly is this so with respect to professional and student experiences in coping at the front lines where primary emergencies occur. Increasingly, medic-aide levels of personnel—for example, employees of private ambulance companies, city hospitals, or police and fire departments—go to the site of primary emergencies in the community. This appraisal is not to disparage the quality of care given at the scene—although our many interviews suggest a closer look. What is just as important is the increasing distance between patient and professional appreciation of real life events when students stay behind the moat. We are also concerned that the health-care disciplines whose members are not specifically given the public responsibility of life saving—but presume to understand human beings in the full gamut of their lives—are being educationally "protected." Not only can this lead to distance from the reality of an aspect of the human condition, but it can also lead to a lack of understanding of why their life-saving-oriented peers sometimes act as they do.

We suggest that students in any of the health-care disciplines, including medicine and nursing, who personally feel the need for beginning or additional experience consider doing the following:

1. Sit in the waiting lounge of a large city emergency room on a weekend night. Observe and talk with people about why they are there. Make mental notes of staff activities and evaluate these against the dimensions of technical, mechanical, and interpersonal functions.

2. Make arrangements to interview staff in life-saving settings (for example, emergency room and intensive care) about their experiences, their attitudes, and what they believe would assist them in providing better care. Ask them how they manage to incorporate humanistic activities into their patient care and simultaneously deal with their own stress levels.

3. Arrange with the police and fire departments to talk with or go with them on emergency calls. How do life-saving situations feel to them? Do they think that there is an adequate community

plan that assists them in coordinating their efforts? Read Arthur S. Freese, "Trauma: The Neglected Epidemic," *Saturday Review*, 13 May 1972, pp. 58–62.

4. With your instructor's cooperation, consider a home visit follow-up project concerning patients and families who have experienced and survived recent life-saving situations. Evaluate with patients or families or both their feelings about their experiences. Share your findings with emergency-room or unit staff, since they might appreciate feedback. Home visits are particularly helpful to one in becoming increasingly sensitive to the fact that life-sustaining and life-enhancing needs persist past discharge from the hospital.

Chapter 8

The Life-Sustaining Dimension of Health Care

The life-sustaining dimension of health care is a major focus in the greatest variety of health-care settings. It is concerned with the maintenance of health and the prevention of disabling complications and death after the impact of bodily insult. Characteristics of this dimension are similar to a relatively new aspect of health-care delivery emphasized within the framework of the Health Maintenance Organization (HMO) concept.[1] The key definition of care for the HMO is "those services aimed at preventing the onset of illness or disability, at the maintenance of good health, and at the continuing evaluation and management of early complaints, symptoms, problems, and the chronic intractable aspects of disease."

In contrast to settings in which a person's functioning is so impaired as to require emergency life-saving actions, life-sustaining settings and helping situations are concerned with a group analogous to what Garfield[2] describes as the "well," the "worried well," the "early sick," and the "sick." For the evaluative purposes put forth in this text, life-sustaining settings and situations can be defined from primary, secondary, and tertiary viewpoints. Although an oversimplification, one can roughly compare *primary* life-sustaining functions as pertaining to Garfield's "well" and "worried well" groups. *Secondary* life-sustaining functions are more applicable to those whom he describes as the "early sick" and the "sick." *Tertiary* functions are those unique life-sustaining functions that apply when death is inevitable and a terminal phase of life has been entered. The tertiary viewpoint acknowledges that dying is a special way of living.

More succinctly defined, the three aspects of the life-sustaining dimension include the following:

1. *Primary life-sustaining functions.* To accomplish the maintenance of good health through the prevention of disease, injury, or developmental deviation.
2. *Secondary life-sustaining functions.* To prevent eventual death or disabling complications in living from disease, injury, or developmental deviation.
3. *Tertiary life-sustaining functions.* To prevent the disabling complications of dying (e.g., physical and emotional suffering).

Within all levels of these helping functions, understanding the interaction of physiological, psychological, and sociocultural variables as they affect behavior is more complex than in life-saving situations. For example, the effects of illness, injury, and treatment measures influence a patient's usual life-style. Coping mechanisms that often cloud the feeling of being oneself come into play. A variety of ways of expressing anxiety are prominent and vary individually. Some feelings may be inner directed, with anger at oneself or vague notions of guilt. Other feelings may be directed outwardly toward other persons, God, or "fate," resulting in angry blame and impatience. The helper must possess a sensitive knowledge about the effects of chemotherapy—an intervention causing high susceptibility to alteration of mood and feeling like a stranger to oneself. Also, one's personal style and social interaction patterns often affect the particular form that disease takes. Intensity of symptoms is well known to vary with psychosocial interactive factors.[3,4]

In all three categories of the life-sustaining dimension, the degree of patient and family participation in goal setting is high in contrast to emergency situations. Often, total family involvement in defining concerns and determining helping actions is required—for example, with parents when the patient is a child; when the disease process, injury, or developmental disorder has seriously impaired the patient's judgment or communication ability; or when a patient approaches death and is unable to express wants and needs. Occasions that require ethical decisions are prevalent to a high degree in life-sustaining situations—for example, assuming parental rights in the face of evidence of neglect or abuse of a child; using methods of maintaining life beyond those requested by a patient or family; terminating fetal life; utilizing technology to maintain the life of a severely defective newborn; sustaining life with organ transplants; and protecting patients from uninformed research involvement. In life-sustaining settings there is no "protection" from complex patient or family influence, which may be willingly given up by them in temporary emergency life-saving situations. For health-care advocates, no routine set of mechanical tools or procedures is available to carry out the humanistic helping goal.

Although one must be sensitive to individual exceptions, patients encountered in situations other than life saving are generally not consciously stressed about death when they initially enter a health-care setting. Unless obsessed by fears about safety and death or of suicidal intent, most persons seeking help are concerned with becoming or staying well. Stress experienced on initial contact and over the course of care is highly dependent on (1) the feeling of trust that patients initially feel in the helper to assist them to get or stay well; (2) the threat that new information about themselves poses to their unique frame of reference, life-style, or capacity to survive; and (3) the kinds of psychological defenses that they are utilizing to protect themselves from experiencing real or imagined threat. Even if patients have sought out many helpers concerning a chronic fatal condition, each new contact initially offers an opportunity for new insights or perhaps the long-awaited breakthrough.

Patients entering settings with a primary and secondary life-sustaining emphasis seek services in a conscious state and under their own power, so to speak; yet, staff sensitivity must be high as to whether a person is in the right place for the most appropriate help. This sensitivity must be implemented within the context of (1) what such concepts as sick, well, and help mean to each patient and helper and (2) recognition that health-care resources are poorly advertised out in the community. Sensitivity must be high to the fact that drugs and the disease process that the patient may be experiencing influence perceptions, emotions, and the ability to communicate. Health-care advocates working in these settings are therefore prepared for patient concerns to be variably expressed. Some will be vague, some specific, some expressed in biological language, and others in more psychological terms; but, verbally and nonverbally, they will be expressed.

Health-care advocates working in these settings are sensitive to the impact of their own health-culture language and concerned that the language terms that they are using be similar to those of the patient to allow the full communication that these situations demand. Asking patients to define what they mean by their individual and colloquial terms is important in trying to genuinely understand them. This definition of terms can be done in direct and indirect ways. For example, several years ago, when we were working in a storefront drug clinic serving all ethnic and economic groups, new patients were asked to write down for the first week how they felt every morning on arising. This request was made to learn what patients were experiencing, as expressed in the language most familiar to them. Terms glibly used by the health-care disciplines were rarely found (e.g., anxious, depressed, disoriented, obsessed, and aphasic). Moods often were described in color terms, such as *black, gray all over, kinda rosy today, pea yellow-green.* Commonly, descriptions that suggested views of mind/body disconnection were found—for example, "like I had died all over except in my brain," "no cramps in my muscles but so messed up in my head," "my mouth had the slurs," and "I had to tell my arms what to do." Anxiety states were described in somatic terms, such as "having the nerves," "the shakes in my stomach," and "my heart beating fast all over my body." Many patients talked of "being behind drugs"; yet, this same phrase did not mean the same thing to all. For some, the phrase meant that they had gone back on drugs, similar to "falling off the wagon"; for others, it was a way to describe what it felt like to have no control, with all willpower succumbed to the power of the drug and what they had to do to get it. In contrast to "soft" drug users, those with a history of "hard" drug usage (opium derivatives) consistently spoke of withdrawal symptoms as "being sick," and "well" as a state of being either on their preferred drug or at some point in treatment at which they no longer felt a physical craving for the drug. To determine symptoms of actual physical disease process within this subcultural framework of sick and well was difficult until one knew the language of the patient.

Before entry into life-sustaining settings, patients have made a preliminary personal decision to seek help. Sometimes it is a self-made decision, but help seeking also occurs because of outside pressure—for example, a spouse's insistence, a school's request for evaluation of a child, a grown child's concern for an aging parent, or pressure by the court on a drug user. Also, many help seekers have used other helpers along the way regarding their central focus of concern. Some of these others may have been professionals; some may have been neighbors, family, or quacks.[5] Some persons, like Ada in Chapter 7, have utilized various mind-over-matter approaches or religious faith healing.[6] The incidence of self-treatment with a wide variety of nonprescription medications over chronic periods of time is high in our national culture. These medications are often perceived as such an ordinary part of life that the patient forgets to mention them.

Health-care advocates in life-sustaining settings are more than just curious in wanting to know about the patient's process of deciding to come for care and the various ways that the patient has tried to reach a desirable state of well-being. Advocates recognize the need to have a high degree of understanding of "illness behavior"; they recognize that it is a psychosocial process that goes on with people even before they seek assistance and often after they are "under someone's care."[7] Advocates understand the influence that such behaviors will have on motivation to change, the ability to work out mutual goals, and the willingness to follow through.

CASE IN POINT

Mr. and Mrs. C were initially seen at the neighborhood health clinic. Because they spoke English poorly, they were accompanied by an interpreter whom they trusted from their church. They wanted a physical examination for their 9-year-old son. The prime movers in their obtaining help were public school personnel, who had insisted on an evaluation for their son, because he was failing in his academic work and was constantly fighting—particularly with children far younger than he, whom he frequently injured.

The parents agreed with the school that they had a problem, but it was obviously more serious as experienced at home and in the neighborhood than even the school was aware. Tearfully the parents explained that their son had "always been a bad boy," yelling obscenities at them, hitting his sister, often refusing to eat, stealing, and setting fires. They said that they had "tried everything to help." The health-care advocate explored with the parents what kinds of things they had tried. *Everything to help* was defined by them as yelling back at him, beating him, locking him in his room and sometimes out of the house, denying him food after he refused to eat, hanging him by his feet from a basement pipe and setting a small fire below his head to "teach him."

In no way did the parents recognize the severity of their responses to their son's behavior and the part that it played in the problem. Neither did they seem aware of the similarity of their own behavior to that of their son. When asked what they thought was responsible for their son's problems, they both said that he had "something in his brain that should be fixed by the doctor." When further asked how they had come to see the cause in this way, they explained that he had always been a difficult child, being "an early baby who almost died." More specifically, they believed that a serious fall and head injury at the age of 2½ years had perhaps caused it.

A complete evaluation by the medical center interdisciplinary team yielded no indication of neurological disorder such as the parents had hoped to find. The child's academic difficulties were found to be a product of his struggles with bilingual reading and writing skills. He had received no assistance from home, where the parents spoke only their native language. They made no effort to learn English and had relied for many years on their young children to intercede socially and economically when English was required. Church school twice a week was taught in the family's native language and only further removed him from the emphasis and practice on English skills that he sorely needed to master productive interchange with his peers and teachers. His public school had failed to analyze his repeated reading and writing errors for the simple confusions occurring between English and his native language. The special education that he had been receiving for "perceptual difficulties" naturally resulted in missing his central academic difficulty, and his frustration was further piqued.

The parents were upset at the evaluation's yielding no evidence of brain injury. Such a conclusion disrupted their frame of reference concerning the cause, effect, and cure for their child's problem. Let the school staff do what they could, but things were really no better at home, they explained. Their secondary approach was to utilize their own notions even further: the father would take the son back to the old country for a month's visit. The parents thought that the trip would prove to the child that they really loved him, and, with fond recall, they expressed how the climate, the food, and the clean water would help the problem with which we had failed.

This was a difficult point for the primary helper. Substantial shifts in perceiving and responding to the child were necessary if he were to remain safely at home. Home visits and the regular helping sessions for both the child and parents seemed to validate the report that the parents were no longer physically abusing the child, yet the total situation was still a powder keg in that, should the child "blow up" at a critical point of family pressure, the parents were still vulnerable to old patterns of response.

Staff discussions concerning what the parents were still saying yielded the conclusion that the parents were still unable to shift their long-held beliefs about their son, even though what they were willing to try was more beneficent. They were somewhat closer to recognizing environmental influences. The staff agreed to support the parents' plan with the condition that both parents and their son continue in counseling after the therapeutic vacation.

After the return from Europe, the parents perceived their son as again having the same difficulties. They requested that something "quite serious" be done. They wanted the boy taken from home because they could not live with him any longer. They wanted him in a "special school." The child also had been enthusiastic about his parents' idea and stated, "Maybe there will be a playground and toys and lots of cops around the place to keep bad grown-ups from getting the kids." Insistently, the parents held to this third approach to help. The advocate did not resist. With the assistance of the clinic staff, a local residential program was found. The parents explained to others that, because of school problems, their son needed this kind of program. They work long extra hours to pay part of the monthly fee. The child agrees with his parents' perceptions of its having been a school problem. He has flourished physically, socially, and psychologically. He has caught up in academic subjects. He maintains his native language skills through occasional weekend visits with his family, and when he wishes, through staff at the residential center. His home visits are often precarious; however, both the child and parents terminate them when pressure builds. Neither the parents nor the child ever wish to talk about his remaining home permanently.

As can be seen in this case, the clinical diagnostic method designed to determine the presence or absence of biological disease or developmental disorder—of high value as part of a comprehensive appraisal—is inadequate as the only central reference point from which to evaluate.[8] Critical interacting psychosocial variables are missed if this method is used alone. Considerable personal information is eventually necessary if advocates are to evaluate accurately and relevantly.

Therefore, staffs in life-sustaining settings must be prepared to develop artful, individually oriented interpersonal relationships with patients from the beginning of contact. The patience to listen before acting is an essential staff characteristic. Developing quicker ways to understand the patient's frame of reference concerning problems, philosophy of life, and views of help is often more critical than the speed with which clinical diagnosis and technological products are brought into the situation. Coming to know the patient in this way also allows the advocate to formulate more accurately how much reality feedback certain patients can tolerate about their circumstances and the ways in which this feedback might most effectively be communicated.

The preceding case also demonstrates a point made in the previous chapter—that, in some situations, a health-care advocate may have to utilize functions that reflect more than one dimension of care. In the particular case of Mr. and Mrs. C and their son, the ongoing evaluation and helping process involved a high degree of primary life-sustaining care, in that deterring physical abuse of a child prevents injury; but to accomplish this end effectively required a high degree of what is referred to as the life-enhancing dimension of humanistic helping. As will be seen in more detail in Chapter 9, settings or situations whose major focus is on problems in living are referred to as *life enhancing*. Advocates in any primary and secondary life-sustaining settings have to be able to discern when the patient's major difficulty is concerned with self-perceptions and relationships to the world that have no correlation with a physical disease process. Patients such as Mr. and Mrs. C and their son have serious problems in living. Had they been dismissed from care after the finding of no neurological disorder, they would have received no help for their problems in living with each other and the larger society. Even if a neurological disorder had been found, the parents might have continued to view their son as "bad." Both parents and child would still have required long-term assistance in how to give up old behavior patterns and assume more growth-enhancing ways of experiencing one another.

Once the full ramifications of a problem are discerned, the patient's health-care advocates must determine whether they have the necessary expertise or are comfortable with providing the kind of help needed. If the advocates within the setting are unable to provide the necessary help, then the helping function is to see that the patient is provided with an appropriate resource; that is, should Mr. and Mrs. C's primary advocates have been unable to effect an ongoing helping process concerning their life-enhancing needs, several avenues might have been utilized—for example, making a helping setting whose major focus was life enhancement available to them or bringing in someone with the needed skills from the first setting's health-care team. It is not the intent of the advocates of humanistic helping to insist on each helper's having all the in-depth skills that a situation requires. Rather, the intent is to insist on the application of sensitive evaluative skills, with needed resources being brought into the situation to ensure relevant continuity of care.

In reality, few health-care settings neatly fit the categories of primary and secondary life-sustaining. That is why health-care advocates in our present delivery system cannot rely alone on what a setting does but must intimately focus on the characteristics of the patients who enter the settings. Let us explore a few settings whose major focus more clearly fits the definitions, as well as some factors that require advocates to function discriminately and multipurposely.

Primary Life-Sustaining Settings

Settings with primary life-sustaining functions are those that offer health checkups and information that can be utilized by the patient to maintain already present good health. A traditional example of this level of care is the public-health well-baby clinic. Within such a community-based clinic, one finds mothers bringing presumably well babies for health appraisal, not for treatment of acute symptoms. Through continuity of observation of the growing child and educative family input through the mother, early detection of potential problems is more likely.[9] It is hoped that shared health information will be utilized broadly at home, thus increasing the probability of practices that contribute to overall good family health. For example, counseling concerning such matters as immunizations, nutrition, birth control, and childrearing is often available in such settings.

Analogous settings for adults are being developed in some communities. These are referred to as multiphasic screening clinics. In such settings, adults can obtain "read-outs" on their state of health and what might be done to maintain or correct that status.

The primary life-sustaining function of health appraisal is usually an outpatient service. However, while specialized settings concerned only with prevention and maintenance of health may provide excellent helping services, when symptoms of a confining disease process are found or the person or family is found to have serious social/emotional problems, the continuity of care-giving frequently breaks down. For example, a mother might obtain information from one setting suggesting that her infant has a serious disorder but be required to seek out yet another setting because of the limitations of a well clinic. If she becomes pregnant, she may have to go to a prenatal clinic. If her husband and she are experiencing marital difficulties, yet another setting may be required. When patients must go from setting to setting, the incidence of information gaps is high, and demands are great on patients to reestablish trust and familiarity with caregivers. In recognition of the need for people to experience an integrated view of care with an integrated view of self, many general and teaching hospitals are developing family-health-care outpatient centers that have an underlying holistic and continuity-of-care philosophy.[10] This system's development also takes into account the increased utilization of inpatient settings to appraise the well or worried well because of the technical equipment available, as well as because of the limits of health insurance. With the addition of home-based continuity of care, the newer models of care ideally provide a central body of helpers for family members' wellness and sickness, whether care is life saving, life sustaining, or life enhancing, and in whatever setting is required for any one family situation.

Secondary Life-Sustaining Settings

Workers in secondary life-sustaining settings are concerned with persons who already have or are presumed to have some form of disease, injury, or developmental disability. These persons may be treated on an outpatient or inpatient basis. Again, the influence of the question of which setting health insurance most adequately funds is a clouding issue. Also utilized as a criterion is the severity of a person's disease process, which may require the surveillance of 24-hour care.

Ideally, the decision as to where the most effective secondary life-sustaining care can be provided is not dependent simply on the availability of technical equipment or on economics. Hopefully, it includes as much emphasis on what is socially and psychologically most fitting to the individual patient. Certain decisions cannot be measured in dollars and cents. When health-care advocates allow patients to weigh the alternatives when hospitalization versus outpatient care is at issue for diagnosis or treatment, some interesting data about what makes that person's life meaningful emerge. "Difficult" hospitalized patients are often a result of insensitive appraisal of the patient's readiness for or acceptance of inpatient care. Consider in the following case what the long-term negative effects might have been for "Grannie Mae" had her wishes not been heeded and if she had experienced inpatient social isolation from those facets of her life she held dear.

CASE IN POINT

Grannie Mae got on a city transit one morning and found her way to the walk-in clinic of a local hospital. The secretary recalled her vividly, since "she seemed so fragile, and I couldn't imagine how she got here on her own steam. She was peppy though. She insisted I call her Grannie Mae because her boyfriend did, and she didn't have any time for that 'Mrs.' stuff, as her husband was long gone."

Grannie Mae explained to the physician, whom she referred to as a "young twerp," that she felt weaker than usual, had occasional dizzy spells, and wanted to get "all fixed up." The physician explained after a preliminary check that her blood pressure was fairly high and suggested that she consider going into the hospital for a few days for a thorough physical examination. He asked her what she thought. Grannie Mae's response was an immediate, absolute no. Didn't he realize that she had two cats, a dog, her plants, and a gentleman friend living downstairs whom she had to watch out for? She suggested that she could come and go for any tests that she needed.

Because of her frail appearance and age, the physician and nurse both commented on the inconvenience to her of coming frequently to the clinic. "Don't you know," she explained, "coming here on that new bus thing is the first time I've had an excuse to go anywhere in three years? I always wondered what that metro thing was really like to ride on, and it's fun."

The staff did not insist. Grannie Mae faithfully kept her appointments and seemed to thrive on the experience.

In secondary life-sustaining situations in which one finds the early sick and the sick, the advocate therefore recognizes that part of a patient's reaction to disease, injury, or developmental deviation is interactively involved with self-concept, social productivity, and the capacity to relate effectively to family, peers, and caregivers. In no other dimension of care is it so important to evaluate with the patient both initially and on an ongoing basis the patient's personalized view of self and the larger dimensions of life as they interact with technological treatment measures.

CASE IN POINT

A disheveled 50-year-old Mrs. B was admitted to the psychiatric service, clutching a photograph taken of herself approximately 20 years before. She was inattentive to any attempt of the admitting staff to interview her. Repeatedly she asked the staff whether they knew who she *really* was and how famous she once was. Each of the staff and patients was pressured by her to look at the photograph. She insisted that they recognize that under her "mask" she was a famous movie star. Any hint of disagreement or withdrawal from her demands led to an unintelligible tirade and threats to call her attorney.

An interview with her husband clarified several aspects of her life relevant to her current behavior. The picture was of her, and indeed he believed her to have been a beautiful woman—a characteristic in which they both had taken pride. However, approximately five years before, she had been discovered to have widespread carcinoma of her reproductive system. Medication utilized as part of her treatment had led to severely masculinizing side effects. He remembered that neither of them had been apprised of this possibility. When the physical changes, including voice quality, began to appear, he felt his wife's concerns were dismissed by caregivers in light of the positive effect that the treatment was having on the carcinoma.

He believed that, after a serious suicide attempt a year before, his wife had become more obsessed with thoughts of her former beauty and her present appearance. When she began insisting that she was really a movie star and became abusive when he did not agree, he decided that he should take her to the psychiatric hospital.

Suicidal patients, in spite of the low value that they may seem to place on their existence, have their own way of expressing the basic need to live. This need is complex and requires careful, empathetic listening, in that their desires are intricately interwoven with existential conflict resolved by hopelessness and helplessness. It is important to take suicidal expressions seriously, whether they are directly or indirectly verbalized—and not just because a person "might mean it, do it, and make the staff feel bad." The expressions of suicidal intent are genuinely a part of that person's frame of reference at the time. They deserve serious humanistic consideration in understanding that person's view of coping. Whether one means to do it is not an irrelevant issue, but it also signifies that the person is seriously hurting inside and is sending a signal that says "Help!"[11]

Following is another case in which a patient's total concept of self was defined in an illness mode.

CASE IN POINT

Lee was admitted to an inpatient medical unit with complaints of severe headaches, dizziness, and occasional aphasia. During the initial history taking and physical examination, the physician became particularly sensitive to Lee's preoccupation with telling about his many illnesses and close calls since early childhood. Lee was curious about what his present symptoms meant but not with the anxiety that might be expected in view of how incapacitating they were.

The nurses became even more aware of Lee's need to talk incessantly about his past illnesses, "as if he were proud of them." They also observed that he seemed to have none of the frustration that patients often experience in the face of aphasic difficulties. The nurse assigned to his care related that he had shared the information that he had always wanted to be a physician and hoped that he could learn more about "this hospital business" this time. She made an offhand, but astute, comment: "It is as if there is no personality to this man aside from a long medical record."

In a preliminary staff meeting concerning Lee's presenting problems and early findings, the consensus was that Lee's symptoms pointed to a possible brain tumor. Beginning concern was raised for Lee's identification of himself around illness—never health. The question arose as to what to tell Lee. Previous conversations and observations were utilized with him in a conference that assisted the staff to learn more in depth about his life-style and frame of reference, perhaps giving more clues as to what and how to tell him.

Following are excerpts from a subsequent conference between Lee, the physician, and the nurse of his unit team:

Dr. A: Miss M tells me you have always wanted to be a doctor. . . .

Lee: That's right. Things didn't work out so well with all my sickness, but I've always read up on medical things. Had to keep up with my own ills, you know.

Dr. A: Then you must know a lot about what's going on with you now.

Lee: Thought you'd never ask. Frankly, I think I could have a tumor or maybe a small stroke.

Miss M: Lee, you seem so calm about what are both serious conditions. I'd like to understand that better.

Lee: Oh, I'm used to lots of things happening. I won't give you any trouble. Dr. A, when do we do the pneumoencephalogram?

In the remainder of the conference, they outlined for Lee what procedures would be useful in fully determining what was causing his symptoms, including his suggestion of a pneumoencephalogram. They also explained what the possibilities might be. Lee was un-abashed. He seemed almost enthusiastic about what he could learn. What a brain tumor might mean seemed to have no impact on him.

Although Lee's demeanor made explaining the facts and enlisting his cooperation easy, the staff was concerned. Not only did the brain tumor contribute to a mood of nonchalance,[12] but apparently Lee derived a sense of self from his history of multiple illnesses, with which he was obsessed. The present situation only seemed to embellish his "reason for being." The staff knew that they had a difficult task ahead in the treatment and rehabilitation phases. He did have a chance to recover, but the staff's problem lay ahead: Did Lee want to? Could he without "giving up" an even more chronic illness mode?

Persons who are obsessed by thoughts of safety and the state of their health are difficult for the staff in life-sustaining settings to deal with. In the acute phase, such persons are miserable and spend enormous amounts of energy organizing their inner reality and outer world to ward off flooding, paralyzing anxiety. Externally observed behavior is of a highly compulsive nature, taking a variety of forms. Depending on the individual, incessantly talking about one's condition, meticulous cleanliness and hand-washing, withdrawal from associating with others, inability to leave a circumscribed space, and obtaining many medical diagnoses, medications, and treatment schedules are often observed. These patients should not be confused with the lonely and fearful who utilize health-care settings to fill an existential void and to obtain someone to be concerned about them. Neither should they be confused with those who may have a disease process that has so affected them that they sense quite accurately that they are in the throes of a critical process. Obsessed patients with highly organized compelling thought and motoric behavior patterns require a health-care advocate who has consid-erable skill with these kinds of chronic, deep-seated difficulties.[13]

As the preceding cases also strongly suggest, health-care advocates are sensitive to determining if any helping process is contributing to a more self-actualizing experience than that which the patient experienced in isolation prior to seeking help. In other words, is the helping process assisting the patient to learn effective coping strategies in living with the perceived or actual threat to a preferred life-style? As the health-care advocate comes to learn: explore, explain, and ask when in doubt. If one finds that ongoing specialized help in the form of life-enhancing counseling seems necessary, the advocate facilitates a referral early on in the life-sustaining process.

Overall, the evaluative usefulness of the different categories of primary and sec-ondary life sustaining is most effective in helping advocates to sort out the many pa-tients whom they see with variably expressed concerns. This differentiation is not to be interpreted as a dehumanizing kind of categorizing or as a method by which health-care workers can quickly dispose of the well to get on with the "real business" of the sick. It is a way to assist helpers in recognizing that they have a responsibility to evaluate clearly what patients express—to respond differentially, neither treating everyone as diseased nor conversely treating those who do not fit a disease model as "crocks."[14]

In life-sustaining settings, it is particularly important for health-care workers to appreciate that, for most people, the "mind" and "body" are consciously experienced as an organized whole. Therefore, any view of psychobiological disorders—those highly related to social/emotional stressors—must be evaluated within the holistic (integrated whole) context. Patients do not have psychobiological, or psychosomatic, disorders in their heads, so to speak. It is dehumanizing to express or imply that the patient's problem is somehow imaginary. Through thorough educative feedback about the interrelationship of factors influencing their disease or pain process, patients can more effectively participate in their own helping process. They can put their energies into understanding and cooperating with useful treatments and life-style changes rather than defending against believing that they are "nuts" or the implication that they are consciously doing it to themselves.

Contrasting primary and secondary life-sustaining functions is also a way to discriminate more consciously that a different view of human behavior is required if the goal is for persons to maintain the good health that they have versus mobilizing their participation when a threat in the form of an actual disease process is present. It is difficult to find the key in motivating people to practice early detection methods without alarming them unnecessarily about eventual trouble. Contrast this difficulty in motivation with the automatic motivation that seems to occur when "something" has already happened or the threat of imminent death is present. Prevention motivation requires attaching concern to something or someone of personalized value. For example, contrast the response to many years of public education about routine breast examination with the sharp increase of diagnostic help seeking after the discovery of malignant tumors by Betty Ford and Happy Rockefeller in 1974. Knowledge concerning breast self-examination and follow-up procedures has been around for a long time. Obviously, the high degree of personal identification with these women was a major motivating force in use of the knowledge at that particular time.

Following is a case in point that gives an example of what health-care advocates face in designing effective prevention and health-maintenance programs.

CASE IN POINT

Carl, age 39, is a free-lance carpet layer. He has a wife and three children by his second marriage. His first wife and two children are in California, where he "tries" to send as much money for child support as he can. He does not have health insurance because "I don't work for any one company." He does not contract independently for health insurance, since "There's not enough money left at the end of the month." Following are excerpts from his interview with us regarding his attitudes about health care:

Q: What do you think about health care in America?

A: Not much. It's too expensive.

Q: If it was cheaper or even free, would you use services more than you do?

A: Not me personally. I figure it's for the wife and kids. I make the bread and can't afford to be sick. The TV tells me I smoke too much, and my wife thinks I'm too thin. She keeps harping about seeing a doctor, but I feel okay; so why should I go and have them tell me that something's wrong. I'll just keep going until I feel something is wrong; we all get it someday.

In the meantime I'll keep working; what I don't know don't hurt me. For the kids it's different; I want them to have the best.

Carl sees himself as being primarily of monetary value to the family, and he takes the chance of extending his productive time as long as possible. He does not make logical future-oriented connections between maintaining health and the ability to work that the statistics show. He uses his own personal logic, which is fatalistic. As he said when asked about the kind of person that he saw himself as being, "I always play the long shots—win some, lose some."

Changing Carl's attitude and behavior concerning prevention of health difficulties would be difficult. An idealistic, preaching health-care worker would have an unproductive experience in motivating him through "do and don't" health education. He himself says that he already disregards the public media and admonitions of his wife. He perceives them as always telling him what he ought to do and withdraws from any person or force that he identifies that way. Carl will probably show up for health care when something concrete overtakes him on his way to work one morning.

Following is an interview excerpt regarding what kind of patient Carl thought he would be if he ever had to be hospitalized for a serious illness:

A: It's hard to say—probably a real bastard. It'd be hard thinking that life had caught up to me. I don't know—maybe I'd fight like hell to get out of there and get back to work. Maybe I'd hit a real downer. I've had a couple of those in my life.

Q: Do you ever think about becoming ill like that?

A: Nah.

Dying and Tertiary Life-Sustaining Functions

In life-saving settings, the major function is emergency action to prevent death, but efforts often fail. It is a difficult time for the family and health-care advocates, but the experience of death is somewhat different in these circumstances than the experience of death that is lived through in life-sustaining settings. To review, the patient and family in primary life-saving situations have quickly entered the life space of a health-care team; and, when death occurs, the family often quickly leaves the field of professional helping concern. In life-sustaining settings, the issue of dying and approaching death is often lived with for a considerable period of time by the patient and the persons for whom the patient holds deep meaning.

Death is always a point in the patient's life and in health-care practice at which many existential questions about living and dying surface and press for answers. In settings in which death occurs quickly and unexpectedly, these issues merge after the fact, and the immediate caregivers are relieved of working them through within a relatively short period of time. In such situations, it is easier to hide behind the shroud of technology and the lesser emotional challenge of brief contact. In settings in which dying is a chronic experience and the point of exact death unpredictable, existential concerns must be lived through with the patient, family, and co-workers. To avoid the existential threat of dying and death, the staff have to work harder and longer. Our concern is that health-care workers' avoidance of the dying and failure to respond to the patient's and family's desires, existential anxiety, and struggles to derive meaning at this point in life lead to the patient's and family's emotional suffering (e.g., helplessness, hopelessness, and finally giving up).[15]

The relief of physical suffering during the terminal phases of illness is a traditional, well-practiced function in health-care settings. However, many helpers are novices in the prevention of emotional suffering while a person is living through a terminal process. Neither have the professions been perceptive in viewing this point in life as having potential for the personal growth of the patient and family, as well as for that of the health-care advocates themselves. Too often, the social/emotional experiences of the dying patient have been left to the family alone or to representatives of the patient's religious beliefs. However, what of those who have no family present or those whose family seem unable to assist the patient in working through the deeply personal feelings of the experience? What of the many who have no well-organized religious belief to help them through or those who find that their belief assists them only with explaining experience after death rather than the experiential aspects of living while one is dying?[16] What of the understanding of dying and death that health-care workers need beyond the catalog of life-saving technical procedures?

To become functionally concerned with the social/emotional existential aspects of death and dying, one must learn more about the experience, but it is a difficult phenomenon to get close to, since it is an experience fraught with avoidance, fear, and isolation.

Historically, death has always been viewed as something that happens to everybody some day; thus, humanity has developed personalized rituals and beliefs to account for that time. Persons have thoughts of death in their everyday life more often than one might suppose; yet they also keep a rationalizing distance from its reality to ward off its unknown aspects, to protect life spirit in the here and now, and to enjoy future-oriented capacities without morbidity. In recent years, however, those in this culture seem more vulnerable to the depersonalization of death, for example, associating it with the failure of science or believing that it happens only to the aged, who are increasingly isolated socially.

Increased personal distance from the fact of death and the experience of dying is in part a product of cultural changes in the past few generations. Scientific technology has pushed the statistics of death further into the chronological years.[17] These factors contribute to death and dying becoming the most highly personalized experience for which persons are increasingly less well prepared during the course of early development. For example, advances in health care and life saving have contributed to a quality of living in which childhood is no longer riddled with such experiences as loss of a parent through death in childbirth and the loss of siblings and close relatives to epidemics of communicable diseases. As reliance on technological failure to explain death increases, philosophical existential discussions with children can be avoided or their necessity overlooked. When 20th-century death does occur, the increased use of hospitals and nursing homes as sites of dying and the use of the mortuary as a place to carry out rituals of respect and grief have also denied the growing child a home- and family-based experience with these realities. Ever increasing geographical distances between close relatives contribute to the likelihood that a family may come together only after death has occurred, not during the dying experience, from which they might learn.

The most vivid reflection of the depersonalization of death in our culture comes in the observation that, simultaneous with the foregoing factors, death surrounds growth and development in the form of impersonal television victims of violence and the fuzzy knowledge that thousands have died in a number of recent wars somewhere in the outer reaches of the world. Not only do such cultural factors influence the depersonalization of death, but they also lead to the dehumanization of life as well.

However, cultural circumstances alone do not make the understanding of dying and death difficult. The individual, subjective nature of the phenomenon makes it a life experience impossible for another to know or identify with in its fullest. It happens only once and cannot be practiced. Neither does one have the preparation of knowing in what time, form, or place it will ultimately occur for oneself or others. The closest primary experience, therefore, is as an onlooker, as one suddenly left behind, or as a participant only insofar as one stays with and listens to what the dying are trying to communicate.

The personal meaning that a dying person holds for one also influences the ability to learn about the experience. Subjective feelings that accompany the loss of someone close cloud the imagination of what the other might have experienced at such a time; the focus is on oneself and one's grief. Even when the knowledge of someone meaningful having a terminal condition becomes reality, often shock and reluctance to believe reduce the ability to relate humanely to the person in life-enhancing and learning ways.

Evolution of the "health-care culture"—always a reflection of the larger social culture in which it is embedded—has contributed to the denial of the personalized meaning of dying and death. Until recently, professional education programs for health-care workers stressed primarily technical life-saving and life-sustaining procedures (e.g., the use of pain-killing drugs, machines, chemicals, and dramatic surgery to maintain physical function). In the face of death, health-care workers have been well educated in legal and ethical procedures concerning pronouncement of death and the care of the body after expiration. However, these educational approaches alone only further a dehumanized attitude about death and dying—denying health-care workers a guided personalized experience for their own growth, as well as perpetuating the interpersonal distance between patient and helper at a time when closeness is most needed.

Through the courageous efforts of humanistic researchers, such as Dr. Elisabeth Kübler-Ross, the concerns of the dying and documentation of the subjective experiences of death as they are lived through by patients, families, and helpers have been made more public.[18] Her work has stimulated further personal/cultural research, which finds that, in spite of the sophisticated technological advances in contemporary society, how people desire to experience death now is generally how people found it most helpful generations ago. A particularly appropriate study to this point was carried out by Bryer, who surveyed the stable, multigenerational Amish community. In this society, she found the following conditions as most helpful in coping with death:

> (a) the continued presence of the family, both during the course of the illness and at the moment of death; (b) open communication about the process of dying and its impact on the family; (c) the maintenance of a normal life-style by the family during the course of the illness; (d) commitment to as much independence of the dying person as possible; (e) the opportunity to plan and organize one's own death; (f) continued support for the bereaved for at least a year following the funeral, with long-term support given to those who do not remarry.[19]

Caring for the dying patient and the family in ways that integrate humanistic values is becoming part of the curriculum within medical and nursing schools and social work programs.[20] Valuable first-person accounts of those who have closely experienced death with a dying friend or spouse are being written. In some parts of the country, special hospice settings that focus specifically on the humanistic care of the terminally ill are being developed.[21] With this public support for the humanistic needs of the patient and family, many persons are choosing to experience dying once again within their home and family circle.[22] Deferring to health-care workers to make decisions alone about dying and death is gradually being abandoned in favor of shared responsibility with those to whom it is happening.[23]

Health-Care Advocacy at the Time of Dying

Except as experienced in emergency life-saving situations, the process of dying creeps up on the person to whom it is happening. Long before the patient or family knows or acknowledges knowing, advocates in secondary life-sustaining settings know when the terminal phase of disease or trauma has begun or has a high probability of ensuing. Telltale physiological clues that cannot be denied are available to advocates. These clues give caregivers preparation time to contemplate added technological measures that might yet be helpful. Such clues also provide advocates with beginning psychological preparation for the loss of the stranger whom they know and in whom they have an emotional investment.

Yet stress is high for health-care workers during that period when they know what the probable course of the patient's life will be and the patient and family have yet to know the reality. For the patient, this period of time can be what Bernstein and Dana[24] refer to as a time of *closed or suspected awareness*. Closed awareness is described by them as contributing to a "conspiracy of silence and avoidance among hospital personnel, the physician, and family members. The patient's environment is controlled by means of duplicity, social games, and contrivance." As to suspected awareness, Bernstein and Dana describe what can occur:

The patient is continually engaged in a contest for information with the hospital staff. Staff members attempt to control their contacts with the patient, so that information is not inadvertently made available. Distance is maintained and relationships are impersonal. Questions are met with evasion, vagueness, expressionless features, and the inevitable "Ask your doctor." The hospital personnel are unable to be human in their relationships with patients by these implicit or explicit rules against providing information.[25]

When whether "to tell" looms as the major question, humanistic helpers recognize that the answer is not simple. No clear-cut humanistic rule exists for telling patients they are dying. From our own experiences with dying patients and their families, together with the overwhelming research findings, we favor open awareness between helpers and patients for the supportive energies that mutual expression of feelings frees up. Because of the opportunity that awareness provides patients to choose to do their last-minute business of living in more open fashion—to withdraw peacefully or to make important life changes—we are loath to deny anyone this opportunity. We also believe that people ultimately do better with realness, a process that Ruffin believes to be critical at any point in the health-care process, particularly at the time of dying:

> I believe the most important aspect of the subject is honesty. It is not only our duty and obligation to report to the patient our honest evaluation of his health, but truth is the factor necessary for the development of a relationship that will help carry the individual through a crisis, such as grief or death. We are all most comfortable when we can be our true selves—without fear of being unacceptable; to be otherwise is phony and necessitates living a lie which results in anxiety. . . . [26]

If there is any general principle to use in telling, it can be derived from a humanistic viewpoint, as found in Kübler-Ross's statement that the question should not be "Do I tell my patient?" but rather "How do I share this knowledge with my patient?"[27]

Yet, we do make exceptions. These are exceptions to be struggled with, challenging the nagging thought that perhaps ultimately all of us are vulnerable to wanting for others what we want for ourselves. One exception we will all make sometime, somewhere, with someone yet to be known: supporting the denial defenses of those who are dying and perceive themselves to be ultimately alone. For patients for whom there is simply no one willing to help them work through the experience in their own way, we question the further isolation and despair that open awareness with no support can reinforce. Another situation that requires individual consideration from an open awareness viewpoint is that of family members' feeling that they themselves cannot bear to acknowledge the pain of their loved one's awareness and holding to their frame of reference, which they ask or insist that helpers follow. An ethical humanistic struggle is involved in this circumstance, and at times concealment must be allowed.[28] In our experience, only by coming to know the patient and family members' depth of relationship and how they have shared "knowing experiences" in the past can one sensitively decide. A controversial, yet deeply moving, description of such a circumstance is put forth by Werkman[29] in a poignant book written in tribute to the courageous dying of his young wife.

CASE IN POINT

In a letter to his wife's siblings, Dr. Werkman struggled to explain the nature of Alexandria's disease and the symptom cycle that it involved. He explained to them that, except for a miracle, the leukemia would allow her a survival time of only a year or two. With hopefulness, however, he attempted to console them with the knowledge that, with drugs, she might feel perfect in a few weeks and remain so for a number of months. These reasons for not openly telling his wife were further explained, giving insight into the depths with which he too shared the experience: "That is why I haven't told her what she has, nor have her doctors. They feel strongly that it only adds to the burden of the illness when she is feeling pretty well. Also, when it first happened, I realized in talking with her that she wanted hope, not doom. I would have wanted the same, and I still do. I don't feel at all that this is deception, but rather a decent humanity. When she really wants to know, her doctors will tell her. I might add that they are very warm and fine people as well as excellent physicians."

Obviously there is no definitive rule for what a patient should be told. Neither is there any rule as to specifically when. Those who know each other develop a sense of timing—do humanistic helpers who have come to know their patients in more than mechanistic ways need a rule of thumb to answer their questions? And as to what or how information about dying and death is shared, if, from the onset of contact and evaluation, one has established an open, humanistic, and advocating relationship, these questions need not suddenly be at issue. If one sincerely comes to know one's patients' perceptions about living and their personal, cultural values as they affect wellness and sickness and can separate them from one's own, only small cobwebs of ignorance remain as dying becomes reality for others.

Yet a thorny issue remains for health-care advocates with respect to the question of who shares information and provides ongoing support to the patient. In settings in which closed or suspected awareness is the prevailing atmosphere, the informational system between the milieu staff and the patient may be impaired because of the mandates of the primary caregiver—usually a physician. Even if the physician, in fact, has not disallowed open communication with the patient, a generalized feeling among some health-care workers and families is that, if the physician does not fulfill this obligation, no one does.[30] Although, traditionally, the majority of physicians are known to be against relating honest information about a fatal illness,[31] one cannot help but wonder if alternative health-care workers do not use the traditional hierachical status and obligation, or perceived mandates, of the physician as a hiding place from the open communication that they themselves wish to avoid.

An advocacy model can be applied at the level of solving the dilemma of closed systems that are perceived as being maintained by the physician. The framework provides several alternatives. First, an advocacy model requires evaluative realness on the part of those who perceive themselves closed out from patients. Health-care advocates must determine whether they are using the physician as a way to avoid their own feelings. If not, risk taking in the face of old habits and established policies can occur. For example, one can listen to patients and be sensitive to the awareness or need for awareness that they may be struggling to share. So often health-care workers become caught up in unconscious closed-system patterns that the importance of spending time listening to patients has gone by the wayside. Questions do not need to be sharply avoided in a closed system simply because one does not believe oneself permitted to provide information. Questions can still be answered. For example, no law prohibits sharing the realness of the situation with the patient; that is, the patient can be apprised of one's limits to share; but one can still offer needed support. One can offer to advocate for asking patients by straightforwardly sharing patient concerns with those who do hold the information that they seek. Following is an example of a nurse's advocacy in the face of a mandate that patients definitely not be told their diagnosis or condition. As this case suggests, the nature of the physician in traditional settings must be understood and worked with in behalf of the patient as long as the doctor controls the situation—both as to helping potential and the truth.

CASE IN POINT

In our particular unit, Dr. K's patients were not to have their diagnosis or condition discussed with them. He believed that life should be pleasant for them, and he medicated heavily with opiates. As you know, medication may help with anxiety from pain, but not from wondering if one is dying. I thought that I could not counter his orders to talk to patients about these things, but increasingly neither could I avoid a patient's open questioning of me. Often right after Dr. K left after visiting his patients, I would be asked pointed questions that suggested that they really knew and were struggling to have someone verify their conclusions. I felt uneasy with my responses, which seemed to be such obvious detours; some of my reactions were just plain rude, I'm afraid. I found myself angry at myself and Dr. K. I believed that, if he would be straight with his patients, I could give more to them; but I had to find an open way to do it, since I was unwilling to "go underground" with the patients.

I decided to take the risk with my good relationship with Dr. K and to convey my feelings directly to him when such a situation came up again. Initially, he shrugged me off and muttered something about my being impertinent, but I persisted by explaining that I had written the entire dialogue that I had had that morning with Mr. T and put it in the nursing notes. Would he read it and give me some help in how to handle it the next time?

Dr. K surprised me by admitting that he couldn't bring himself to be as open as "maybe he should be." He asked how it would be easier for me the next time that I felt pressured by Mr. T's questions. I explained that I would feel better and believed that the patients would too if I could at least tell them that, although I couldn't give them the specific information that they needed right then, I would help them ask Dr. K in his presence. Dr. K agreed to try.

Following is a lengthy case in point that further illustrates the struggle to relate openly with a dying patient. In this situation, it was difficult to actualize closeness to the patient even when the physician gave the nurse full rein to do as she wished. It is also an example of the value of integrating technological life-sustaining functions with interpersonal process in such a way that a life-enhancing experience could occur for both the patient and, ultimately, the nurse. Consider the concepts with which this young nurse grappled concerning positive regard, congruence, and empathy—often difficult behaviors to carry out with the dying patient who is unpleasant or strenuous to care for.

CASE IN POINT

I remember struggling with some of Carl Rogers' early statements about the need for "unconditional positive regard" for patients. I would sit in class and think I understood, nodding amen! Then I would run back to the wards for evening shift to find I'd been assigned to Mr. G *again*. I felt like everything I had heard discussed in class went out the window. How could I feel positive about that old duffer?

He was a difficult patient to care for. Not only did he have carcinoma of the spine with metastases to the right hip, but he also had active tuberculosis (involving isolation procedures, Stryker frame, and lots of medication and treatments). Foul-smelling drainage came from an open ulcer on his back that resisted everything that we did. Also, he had a miserable personal way on top of it. Either he would not talk—just glower—or else he would use tough backwoods language to tell me how lousy his care was and where I could go with it.

Just as soon as I would finish with his care every few hours and be out of all that isolation garb, he would turn his light on. I'd stand in the door and ask what he wanted, so I didn't have to get into the gown, mask, and so on again; but, no, he would insist that I come in; *then* he would tell me something that he wanted that meant I had to go out into the ward again and do the whole procedure all over. I felt as if he had me dangling like a puppet.

I was not without some form of sympathy. I knew life was miserable for him—an unpleasant way to die—but I was miserable in my own way. Nothing that I did helped him, and I didn't like him. To compensate for that ugly thought, I tried to imagine how he might have been before all this happened. I imagined a nice guy whom something rotten had happened to, to explain his behavior. That wasn't working either; so I talked to my P.M. supervisor—a neat gal. She was willing to go with me the next day to talk with the day staff about how I felt and to ask for ideas on what we could do evenings.

I needed to know if those on the other shifts felt the same way that I did. They did. Nobody liked Mr. G, and nobody liked to go in and take care of him. His physician didn't like him much either and encouraged a "stiff upper" and said to "do anything you like with him because he isn't going to last much longer." I thought to myself, that's a fine thing to say when you don't have to go in there but once a day on rounds. I was also curious about what "anything" meant. He explained that it was anything that we could come up with that made life more pleasant for us nurses.

I said that I would feel more comfortable if I could just level with Mr. G about how difficult it was for us to take care of him. One of the holier-than-thous on the staff who never took care of him jumped on me for that, saying that I was putting my needs first and shouldn't do that; but I believed that, if he could just decide what he wanted, it would be easier to meet his needs. How could I if I didn't know what they were? I knew what mine were. I was discouraged in trying to guess his and always thinking that I was missing the mark.

As a group we didn't come up with any specific horrendous plan. I was disappointed with that. I still felt at odds with the thought of it all seeming insurmountable. Reflecting back, I believe that a large part of me was hoping that I would get support simply not to work with Mr. G anymore. Instead I was encouraged to stick with it and test out my feelings about it. It was like a freedom trap. I wasn't happy about not being allowed to avoid the situation, but I did get support to try anything. I now realize how wise the group was, at least in terms of what this approach eventually allowed me to learn.

"Unconsciously—I hadn't planned it—I went into Mr. G's room first that evening. I was surprised at his greeting comments: "You're early; you never come in until last." He was right. A few seconds later he growled, "You don't like to come in here, do ya?" I asked him how he knew, but he went into that quietness again. This time I was not going to ignore it or try to fill in the gaps with superficial chitchat. I dove in, saying "Mr. G, when you get silent like that, I get frustrated because I don't know what's going on or what to say."

Still silence for the longest time. Inside I gave up. Finally, he said, "All I see is people's eyes. Haven't seen a whole face up close since I came here—those masks, those screens—but I can read eyes now, and you don't like being in here, I can tell. You just pretend to be nice." I took another chance on my newfound honesty and told him that he was right. I went further to explain that there was something else about me that maybe he didn't know: that I thought that he was not easy to take care of and sometimes it was difficult to go in there. At that he became furious and accusatory. He told me that I didn't like to be there because he smelled and because he had consumption and I was afraid I would get it. Now about that I did not think he was so accurate. I was used to smells. Heavens, years ago I had learned to close off nose breathing reflexively so I didn't gag in worse situations than his; and it never occurred to me that I would ever get TB, since I had had the BCG and I knew good isolation techniques. But how could I tell him any more of how I felt—like how derogating it felt always to be told how lousy I was and called assorted names and how angered I would get at his light's beeping on all the time?

Maybe I was going overboard on my needs, I thought; so instead I tried to put it into a "we" kind of thing and said, "Mr. G, you and I don't really see eye to eye. I want to give you what you want, but you always seem to ask for things when I am out of the room and never when I'm with you. Can't we make some kind of deal, so I'll know what you want when I can give it?" My God, there was that long silence again, and again I waited him out. Very quietly he finally said, "But then you won't come in here."

Suddenly it dawned: if he related all that he wanted me to do when I went in for his treatments and P.M. care, he was afraid that he would be isolated from any interpersonal contact the rest of the evening. I took a chance on my insight and asked, "Are you telling me that one of the things that you want is company?" He started to cry and tried to hold it back with sobs; then he began swearing about his being such a damn fool for crying like a baby. He said that he thought that he was going nuts, being strapped in like a dog with no roommate and his family up north and his dying in misery. He went on to explain angrily that he seemed to see one of us only when we had something that we thought was good for him, but he wanted me to know for damn sure that everything that we did hurt him and didn't help. It hurt when we turned him on the frame and always scared him "with you little punks trying to do it." The drugs made him nauseous; dressing the wound on his back was excruciating. He really analyzed our problem well when he said, "Now, if I call you in here when *I* want something, then I know that you aren't going to bring pain in with you."

The next day he was curious about what I had meant about making a deal with him. I said that I wasn't sure but that I thought that it should have something to do with making life more enjoyable for both of us. He lapsed into silence again. After our open communication of the day before I was apprehensive that maybe we would lose the gains that we had made, but this man had a cycle that I was beginning to understand. It was hard for him to "be close." Whenever he was not angry and demanding he seemed not to know how to express his feelings. I was willing to bet that, afraid to cry because of how it would look, he also covered his inability to put grief and suffering into words with silence. I decided to leave that insight alone and not push him. I thought that I had pushed him a lot already in the previous two days. Maybe after awhile he would trust me enough to share more openly.

I also thought that I could not leave him hanging about what I meant by a deal. Just off the top of my head I came up with something that might be reasonable. I offered to make an agreement with him about those times that I did not have to be in the room to do his treatments and change his position. Since I knew my limits, I believed that I had better not let him name what he wanted and then knock him down with my reality. I said that I was thinking about a plan in which every day before I came onto my shift he would think of all the things that he wanted me to do for him while I was in the room. I would do them. Then I would spend ten minutes each hour sitting in the doorway where he could see me; we could shoot the bull, or I could read to him, or I could write letters for him. I explained that, during all the time that it took me to get in and out of the isolation garb, I could be sitting in the doorway and spending time with him. I did think that I had to add that, if during those ten minutes an urgent request came up for me to do something on the unit, I might have to leave. Could we try it? He agreed.

It is hard to describe what this did for him and me. I became more organized, believe it or not. I'd find myself mapping out my duties and other patient contacts to be sure that I would have those ten minutes. He also became more organized; like he would have a list of things ready for me each night. He began to think of things for me to read when we ran out of "bull." He had anchors now to something besides raw time, which must have dragged endlessly.

Our plan affected the rest of the staff as well as the other patients. Those ten minutes became "old G's time," and nobody dared to bother me during that time, it developed. One evening when a new patient came in, I heard another one explaining what I was doing in the doorway. The old patient kindly admonished the other to "leave her alone unless you're dying." Mr. G became part of the social group in another way too. You know how the men joke about their sexual feelings when they have been sick and hospitalized a long time. Every once in a while some of the other men would jest through the door "How do you manage that trick, you old goat?" I saw a sense of humor in Mr. G in response to jokes like that that I had never seen before. Increasingly, we saw other patients doing the doorway socializing with him. I never had had other patients that I was working with ask about him before, but that became common.

It is probably obvious that Mr. G and I became close, but he never talked openly of his feelings about dying again until the last day. He simply said that evening when I came on duty, "I'm going to die tonight." I cried briefly and made an awkward comment about that not being on his list of what he wanted tonight. He smiled wanely and said, "I know, but I do."

I asked him if he wanted his family called, and he said no, not until he had gone: they couldn't get there in time, and he didn't want them to feel bad about that. He wanted me to call in the physician, so he could tell him not to do anything except to let somebody be with him. I sat down by him after that, and he soon fell asleep. In about two hours—I forget—he simply died.

I had never watched a simple death like that before. I was always doing things. I loved that old man. He really made me look at myself. I'm not religious, but my experience with him made me realize why people have wanted a life hereafter. I would like to think that I could see him again.

As the preceding case in point also emphasizes, on becoming close and opening the door to those who are dying, one learns more about oneself and what the experience means to the patients. Persons in any walk of life learn when they step out from behind denial and fear. Some patients learn how to do this for the first time at the point of feeling the reality of dying. For example, some patients initially face the approach of death with immobilizing fear of the unknown and of isolation, emotions that are sometimes rooted in long-held fears from childhood; but with open closeness, the patient can potentially make self-satisfying shifts.

CASE IN POINT

During an acceptance phase of her dying, a 60-year-old widow reflected, "I never experienced release of a lifelong fear of the dark and being alone until I began to die. I spent a lot of time talking about those old fears. My doctor helped me understand that I can survive that. I used to challenge him that I could not—definitely not. One night I woke up and simply did not feel afraid in that room anymore. I'm just not afraid, as I always used to be. If I should just happen to live, I will never be the same."

For other patients, the circumstance of the finality of dying provides a need and opportunity for pulling things together with others that their previous life circumstances and defensive demeanors seemed to preclude. Following is a case in point in which a 70-year-old man felt actualized after a lifetime of feeling misunderstood and always at unsatisfying odds with his family.

CASE IN POINT

"I'm glad I'm dying and still have my senses. There have been many things for me to settle and make right with my folk. I used to fear getting just struck down and leaving things up in the air. Does it sound funny to say that I feel kind of good about my ending? The beginning and the middle were not so hot."

From the young as well, when unburdened by the emotional pressures of disbelief and tragedy-laden attitudes of family and staff, one can learn much about dying. Often the young child can be a remarkable teacher of how life and death are ultimately experienced by each in a uniquely personal way. With candor and yet with all the richness of the integration of childhood, Marty talked about his life as a dying youngster.

CASE IN POINT

I'm missing the kids in school and what they are probably doing in science right now. I have this molecule model I'm working on here, and I have to get it done real soon. I just wish mother would stop bugging me whenever I say that I've got to get it done. I really do.

Oh, I miss my dog and my little brother because being stuck in this place I can't tease him. He's really going to miss me because I always used to tease him all the time. Say, have you seen that movie about Big Foot? Do you think that they will ever find one up here in the woods? I sure wish I had been able to see that movie—well, maybe some day. When you go back over to school, will you give this picture of Big Foot to Roddy Jay? I always promised.

As all the cases in point suggest, advocates working in tertiary life-sustaining settings require understanding of a wide variety of emotions that patients, family, and they themselves will express during a dying experience. In understanding patients, health-care advocates recognize that the emotions of those who are dying may be reflective of distinct life-defending phases, as they incorporate and cope with the inevitable fact of death. The advocate becomes sensitive to the well-documented stages of denial and isolation, anger, bargaining, depression, and acceptance.[32] Advocates commit themselves to experiencing these phases *with* a patient in flexibly discriminative ways, allowing emotions to occur but not insisting that they must. They humanistically integrate technical skills within the context of patient and family wishes with the knowledge that they assist in maintaining the one thing that persists throughout the stages of dying—hope. Hope may seem like a tenacious denial of the ultimate, but it always has been a spark in the human life-force, and the dying are human to the end.

Summary Evaluation Guide

The overall focus of the life-sustaining dimension of care is the maintenance of health and the prevention of disabling complications and death after the impact of bodily insult. Appropriate, effective functioning within this level of care requires a high degree of competence concerning society's present scientific physiological and technological knowledge with respect to (1) prevention of developmental disability, physical disease, and trauma, (2) recognition of its presence as early as possible, and (3) appropriate, accurate treatment and remediation. Yet, because of the interrelated nature of human functioning and people's perceptions of themselves as total beings, this dimension of care also requires high degrees of understanding of and utilization of social/psychological processes. Therefore central to all functions of the life-sustaining dimension is the integration of technologically based knowledge, equipment, and diagnostic clinical methods with a high degree of feeling-based understanding as to how one's personalized frame of reference influences health, illness, life, and death.

Because of the chaotic, multifunctional nature of many health-care settings from which patients seek help, we have proposed several levels of life-sustaining function around which health-care advocates might more discriminatively evaluate their patient's needs and the helper's actions. To delineate more accurately the appropriate care of any given patient, the advocacy model of humanistic helping emphasizes that, on initial contact, the following entry experiences be provided the patient.

ENTRY EXPERIENCE: *Establishment of the problems and goals of help as perceived by patients (or their representatives)*

Relevant questions:

1. Is my level of communication with this person such that I am getting the clearest picture of what is meant to be expressed?

2. Is this person expressing problems in physical, psychological, or socially based terms?

3. Does a physiological process appear to be interfering with the patient's ability to articulate problems and wants?

4. May social-context variables be interfering? That is, how has this person been responded to by others before seeing me within the present setting? In other settings? Am I seeing this person in a place that allows quiet and privacy for feelings to be struggled with? Do I have the time available to explore this person's view of self and life situation adequately?

5. How may internal psychological stress be interfering? That is, how does this person's preoccupation with the problem interfere with ability to come up with goals for help? How might it affect a previously felt and observed productive style? Are present coping styles—conservation/withdrawal or fight/survival—habitual or are they a response to the immediate threat?

6. How clear a picture do I have of this person's value system, self-concept, and the importance placed on remaining or becoming healty? Do I have an adequate view of this individual's belief system as it may affect a casual view of problems, what can be done about them, and who will be trusted to help?

7. Am I adequately determining this person's strengths at the same time that I am grappling to understand the person's limitations and definition of the problem?

ENTRY EXPERIENCE: *Determination if the setting in which help is sought is the most appropriate site for the desired or required help to occur*

Relevant questions:

1. Do those in the present setting have the evaluative capacity to explore fully all the relevant ramifications of this problem as the person involved sees it?

2. Am I or are others within the present setting willing to make another helping source easily available if another should appear to be more beneficial?

3. How do the concerns and wants of this person clash with my value system? Am I able to sort out our feelings from each other and continue to assist, or are my own feelings immobilizing of my best function?

4. Am I prepared to allow others within the present setting to assist me if this person's situation exhausts my particular skills in understanding or bringing the needed help to bear?

5. Is my relationship with this person such that I can openly explain why this may not be the right place or the appropriate helper without sounding rejecting? That is, have I conveyed this information in such a way that transfer of care giving can be perceived to be the best therapeutic choice?

ENTRY EXPERIENCE: *Articulation of the overall philosophy of the health-care setting and health-care advocate in such a manner that expectations of the patient on an initial and ongoing basis are realistic—neither overestimations nor underestimations of the amount or quality of help that is to be forthcoming*

Relevant questions:

1. Have I effectively shared with this person what is my understanding of the problems and what is expected as help?
2. Am I prepared to incorporate the patient's corrections or agreements into the formal helping plan and follow-through process?
3. Have I adequately and in understandable terms shared with this person what else I perceive to be related to the problem or concern that might be explored? Do I present my ideas in such a way that the patient can distinguish between hunches and fact?
4. Have I clarified the extent to which the person wishes to know about findings along the course of help, and am I prepared to stand by these wishes?
5. Have I established how much about the problem, new findings, and treatment this person wishes to be shared with the family?
6. Does this person need assistance in formulating information to be able to communicate it to others in a preferred way?
7. Overall, is there anything that I have promised or allowed the patient to believe might be forthcoming in the helping process about which there is considerable doubt that either I or those in the setting can deliver?

The preceding guide to entry experiences also has high utility in evaluating the helping process on an ongoing basis. Health-care advocates recognize that, although initial evaluation is a solid baseline process from which to begin, ongoing help requires evaluative checkpoints along the way.

As is undoubtedly clear at this juncture, the interplay between the health-care advocate's frame of reference and that of the patient is of vital import. This interplay is what determines whether the help is helpful and is what makes for the reality of the life-enhancing function threading throughout both life-saving and life-sustaining situations. Focusing on the mere existence of life does little to forward humanism if the essence of who one is loses or gains no meaning in the life-saving or life-maintaining process. It is as the aging woman announces to the unseen figure of Death in Eve Merriam's "A Conversation Against Death":

> And what did I want for my life to be?
> I wanted then
> the same thing as I want now:
> everything![33]

REFERENCE NOTES

1. HMOs have evolved rapidly and in various forms. These organizations, based on four principles, constitute (a) an organized system of health care that accepts the responsibility to provide, or otherwise assure the delivery of, (b) an agreed-on set of comprehensive health-maintenance and treatment services for (c) a voluntarily enrolled group of persons in a geographic area and (d) are reimbursed through a prenegotiated and fixed periodic payment made by, or on behalf of, each

person or family unit enrolled in the plan. See U.S. Department of Health, Education, and Welfare, Health Services and Mental Health Administration, *Health Maintenance Organizations: The Concept and Structure*, DHEW Publication no. 0-426-030 (Washington, D.C.: U. S. Government Printing Office, 1971). See also chapter 6, "A Note on the Concept of 'Health Maintenance Organizations,'" in *Public Expectations and Health Care*, ed. David Mechanic (New York: Wiley, 1972), pp. 102–11; and Ernest W. Saward and Merwyn R. Greenlick, "Health Policy and the HMO," *Milbank Memorial Fund Quarterly* 50 (1972): 147–76.

2. Sidney R. Garfield, "The Delivery of Medical Care," *Scientific American* 222 (1970): 15–23.

3. For a fine annotated bibliography concerning the interrelatedness of physical illness and self-concept, see Vickie A. Lambert and Clinton E. Lambert, *The Impact of Physical Illness and Related Mental Health Concepts* (Englewood Cliffs, N.J.: Prentice-Hall, 1979). Other suggested required readings for this chapter are John E. Adams and Erich Lindemann, "Coping with Long-Term Disability," in *Coping and Adaptation*, eds. George V. Coelho, David A. Hamburg, and John E. Adams (New York: Basic Books, 1974), pp. 127–38; Alan S. De Wolfe, Robert P. Barrell, and Jonathan W. Cummings, "Patient Variables in Emotional Response to Hospitalization for Physical Illness," *Journal of Consulting Psychology* 30 (1966): 68–72; Lawrence E. Hinkle, Jr., and Harold G. Wolff, "The Nature of Man's Adaptation to His Total Environment and Relation of This to Illness," *Archives of Internal Medicine* 99 (March 1957): 442–60; Helen P. Klein and Oscar A. Parsons, "Self-Descriptions of Patients with Coronary Disease," *Perceptual and Motor Skills* 26 (1968): 1099–1107; S. H. Schmale, "Giving Up as a Final Common Pathway to Changes in Health," *Advances in Psychosomatic Medicine* 8 (1972): 20–40; and Eberhard H. Uhlenhuth and Eugene S. Paykel, "Symptom Intensity and Life Events," *Archives of General Psychiatry* 28 (1973): 473–77.

4. Biofeedback procedures have been useful in providing much support for an integrated view of behavior. This approach has also provided useful ways for patients to participate in altering the responsiveness of their own neural mechanisms. See Barbara Brown, *New Mind, New Body: Biofeedback; New Directions for the Mind* (New York: Harper & Row, 1974).

5. James Harvey Young, "The Persistance of Medical Quackery in America," *American Scientist* 60 (1972): 318–26.

6. Harold Sherman, *Your Power to Heal* (New York: Harper & Row, 1972); Hans Holzer, *Beyond Medicine* (Chicago: Henry Regnery, 1974); Andrew Neher, *The Psychology of Transcendence* (Englewood Cliffs, N.J.: Prentice-Hall, 1980). For an appreciation of healing as an integration with worship and philosophy of life, see Robert L. Bergman, "Navajo Medicine and Psycho-analysis," *Human Behavior*, July 1973, pp. 8–15.

7. Mechanic discusses illness behavior from several standpoints: (1) as a culturally and socially learned response, (2) as a coping response to situational difficulties, and (3) as an attempt to seek secondary advantage. See chapter 12, "Response Factors in Illness: The Study of Illness Behavior," in David Mechanic, *Public Expectations and Health Care* (New York: Wiley, 1962), pp. 203–22.

8. If it seems that we are harping on the medical clinical diagnostic model, we are, but not just because physicians use it. Many, if not most, of the health-care disciplines use modifications of this process, in part to ape the medical field in the struggle for "professionalism" and in part because the model is an effective adjunct to comprehensive evaluation. Our point is to caution against over-reliance on it and denial of its limitations. See Ian Renwick McWhinney, "Beyond Diagnosis: An Approach to the Integration of Behavioral Science and Clinical Medicine," *New England Journal of Medicine* 287 (24 August 1972): 384–87. An excellent text that emphasizes the holistic approach in initial evaluation is Mathy D. Mezey, Louise H. Rauckhort, and Shirlee A. Stokes, *Health Assessment of the Older Individual* (New York: Springer, 1980).

9. A limitation of agency primary life-sustaining settings is the decreased opportunity to observe naturalistic mother/child interactions at home. Home visits by the public-health nurse or social worker associated with a family-oriented clinic are useful for more accurate observations and the general comfort of the parent. For those interested in honing their skills in evaluating and working with the mother and child, see Alfred L. Baldwin and Clara P. Baldwin, "The Study of Mother-Child Interaction," *American Scientist* 61 (1973): 714–21.

10. "Holistic health" has had a difficult time gaining professional and public acceptance in some parts of the country. It seems to us that this lack of acceptance is due in part to the term *holistic* being applied to certain clinics and food stores that evolved in the late 1960s and 1970s and which, in many cases, were frankly unsafe. In our area, there have been "holistic health food stores" that simultaneously sold self-healing products, literature ranging from diet manuals to astrology, and drug paraphernalia. In the fall of 1981, the Denver headlines extolled an investigation of a large "holistic" clinic in which clientele were treated by a "communications psychologist" with colonic irrigations and health foods. Clients with previously undiagnosed carcinoma and other serious diseases are now testifying and pressing charges. Obviously, the term *holistic* is a misnomer for such a clinic, as it seems that their focus is primarily the digestive system. What we are pressing for is that the already existing body of health-care professionals listen to what people say they want in terms of holism and provide it safely. For a text concerning continuity of care, see Sally R. Beatty, *The Hospital and the Community* (New York: Grune & Stratton, 1980).

11. Innumerable references are available concerning suicide. For a brief, but comprehensive, overview of earlier formulations, see Edwin S. Shneidman, "Preventing Suicide," *American Journal of Nursing* 65 (May 1965): 111–16. For ethnic differences, review Andreas M. Pederson, George A. Award, and Alan R. Kindler, "Epidemiological Differences Between White and Nonwhite Suicide Attempters," *Mental Health Digest* 5 (December 1973): 27–29. Two books to review are Alfred Alvarez, *The Savage God* (New York: Random House, 1972), and Jacques Choron, *Suicide* (New York: Scribner's, 1973). Alvarez not only writes about his own experience with attempted suicide but also presents many personalized examples. Choron is more objective in his presentation. Any of the back issues of the *Bulletin of Suicidology* (published by the National Institute of Mental Health, U.S. Department of Health, Education, and Welfare, now discontinued) are valuable to review.

12. For a valuable article concerning the affective responses (emotional mood) often observed in patients with organic brain disease, review Edwin A. Weinstein and Robert L. Kahn, "Personality Factors in Denial of Illness," *Archives of Neurology and Psychiatry* 69 (1953): 355–67. This is a particularly helpful article for boning up diagnostically when a patient's denial of illness seems to have little relationship to dynamic defensive mechanisms or the patient's usual coping style.

13. See chapter 2, "Obsessive-Compulsive Style," in David Shapiro, *Neurotic Styles* (New York: Basic Books, 1965), pp. 23–53.

14. See Robert E. Reynolds and Thomas W. Bice, "Attitudes of Medical Interns Towards Patients and Health Professionals," *Journal of Health and Social Behavior* 12 (December 1971): 307–11; and H. J. Skully, "Classes of Patients as I See Them," *Canadian Medical Association Journal* 105 (21 August 1971): 361–63.

15. Particularly review Schmale, "Giving Up," p. 23. *Helplessness* is defined by him as the feeling of being deprived, let down, or left out that is perceived as coming from a change in relationship about which the person feels powerless to do anything. *Hopelessness* is defined by Schmale as a feeling of frustration, despair, and futility perceived as coming from a loss of satisfaction for which the individual assumes complete and final responsibility and believes that nothing more can be done to reverse the failure. *Giving up* was found by Schmale to be present to some degree prior to the onset of disease and problems in living of all categories.

   An exploratory study by Nash found that 90 percent of the terminally ill he studied gave responses reflecting a sense of powerlessness, lack of control, unrelatedness, and an overwhelming sense of loss. See M. L. Nash, "Dignity of Person in the Final Phase of Life: An Exploratory Study," *Omega* 8 (1977): 71–80.

16. The Christian religion has placed great emphasis on an afterlife and the rewards and punishments therein—depending on thought, word, and action behaviors. Anxiety and guilt concerning life's experiences can become intensified as a patient who holds such beliefs nears the time when beliefs may be actualized. For some, religious beliefs about "the other side" hold great comfort and diminish fear; for others, the opposite may be true. Even though patients may initially profess to have broken away from their earlier religious beliefs, they may, during the dying process, need to experience the rituals of their former faiths. As one patient explained, "I want last rites to cover all my

bets." Some individuals have spent considerable energy throughout their adult lives defending a "fallen away" or avowed agnostic position. It may be difficult, as dying becomes a reality, for some to admit deeply subjective needs to reevaluate their position to ensure forgiveness and a less punitive threat of the unknown. Health-care advocates are sensitive to where dying patients—and their families—stand in relation to religious beliefs and what they need to do about them.

17. See Bernice L. Neugarten, "Social Implications of a Prolonged Life-Span," *Gerontologist* (Winter 1972): 438–440.

18. Elisabeth Kübler-Ross, *On Death and Dying* (New York: Macmillan, 1969).

19. Kathleen B. Bryer, "The Amish Way of Death," *American Psychologist* 34, no. 3 (March 1979): 255–61. An excellent overview and bibliography is included in this article.

20. An excellent conference review on this subject is Austin H. Kutscher and Michael R. Goldberg, eds., *Caring for the Dying Patient and His Family: A Model for Medical Education* (New York: Health Sciences, 1973).

21. Bryer, "The Amish Way of Death," p. 260.

22. The data from the cross-age and cross-ethnic study carried out by Kalish show that most respondents would rather die at home if they had a choice. See the summary of Kalish and Reynold's work in Antoinette A. Gattozz, "Death and Bereavement: A Cross-Ethnic Study of Attitudes and Behavior," in *Mental Health Program Reports*, 6, ed. Julius Segal and Muriel R. Reich. DHEW Publication no. HSM 73-9139. (Washington, D.C.: National Institute of Mental Health, 1973). We suggest that the entire paperback be obtained because of its comprehensive excellence. Write to Superintendent of Documents, U. S. Government Printing Office, Washington, D.C. 20402 (Stock no. 1724-00326).

23. The finest article we have reviewed on this subject is Raymond S. Duff and A. G. M. Campbell, "On Deciding the Care of Severely Handicapped or Dying Persons: With Particular Reference to Infants," *Pediatrics* 57, no. 4 (April 1976): 487–93. The title of this article is a misnomer in that it may deflect the reader from its full implications and widespread application. See also Marvin Kohl, "On Death, Dying, and the Karen Ann Quinlan Case," *The Humanist*, 36, no. 1 (January/February 1976): 16. In this same issue, review Joseph Margolis and Clorinda Margolis, "On Being Allowed to Die," pp. 17–19.

24. Lewis Bernstein and Richard H. Dana, *Interviewing and the Health Professions* (New York: Appleton-Century-Crofts, 1970), p. 151.

25. Ibid.

26. Kutscher and Goldberg, *Caring for the Dying Patient*, p. 48.

27. Kübler-Ross, *On Death and Dying*, p. 36.

28. When reflection is needed in the face of the exceptional struggle, we suggest reading a small, but thoughtfully rich, book: Clark E. Moustakas, *Loneliness and Love* (Englewood Cliffs, N.J.: Prentice-Hall, 1972). Particularly relevant is chapter 7, "Honesty Versus Truth," pp. 105–114.

29. Sidney L. Werkman, *Only a Little Time: A Memoir of My Wife* (Boston: Little, Brown, 1972), p. 72. Werkman is a sensitive clinician, teacher, and author of other works for the beginning health-care worker in psychiatry. This book is a first-person account of his experience with death and dying. It is excellent in developing a greater appreciation of another's inner reality and the importance of empathy.

30. Kalish's study supports all the many others that reveal that the majority of people say that they would want to be told if they had a fatal illness. A physician, family member, or minister or priest were named, in that order, as to who should tell. See Gattozz, "Death and Bereavement," p. 56.

31. Bernstein and Dana summarize the studies concerning physician resistance to open communication with patients in *Interviewing and The Health Professions*, p. 153.

32. Kübler-Ross (*On Death and Dying*) describes these stages in detail. It is important to keep in mind in reviewing her work that she found "most" dying patients to experience these stages. The humanistic advocate acknowledges that not all people may experience these phases or in the order that they are described, just as, in earlier growth and development, there are discernible phases, but each child or adult experiences them uniquely. One does not insist that a phase of development occur according to the book.

33. Eve Merriam, "A Conversation Against Death," *Ms.*, September 1972, pp. 81–83.

ADDITIONAL REFERENCES

Following are some of our favorite teaching references when helping students to appreciate the complex emotions surrounding death and dying.

Sharon Golub and Marvin Resnikoff, "Attitudes Toward Death: A Comparison of Nursing Students and Graduate Nurses," *Nursing Research* 20 (1971): 503–8.

John H. Kennell, Howard Slyter, and Marshall H. Klaus, "The Mourning Response of Parents to the Death of a Newborn Infant," *New England Journal of Medicine* 283 (13 August 1970): 344–49.

Paul C. Rosenblatt, Douglas A. Jackson, and Rose P. Walsh, "Coping with Anger and Aggression in Mourning," *Omega* 3 (November 1972): 271–83.

Bernard Schoenberg et al., eds., *Anticipatory Grief* (New York: Columbia University Press, 1974). This is one of the finest compilations of the recent literature; it is a must for all beginning helpers.

Avery D. Weisman, *On Dying and Denying* (New York: Behavioral Publications, 1972).

J. C. Quint, *The Nurse and the Dying Patient* (New York: Macmillan, 1967).

Chapter 9

The Life-Enhancing Dimension of Health Care

One of the goals of this text has been to sensitize health-care advocates to the multiple factors to be considered in better understanding the persons they wish to help, as well as themselves. We have stressed that (1) human beings are a vital composite of inter-relating biological, psychological, and social forces; (2) an individual's particular nature emerges from the complex interaction of specific genetic endowment, life circumstances of the distant and immediate past, and the present situation; (3) one's collective life experience is interwoven into a highly personalized frame of reference concerning the meaning attached to oneself and to the world around one; and (4) people are simultaneously conscious and unconscious beings and yet generally experience themselves as an integrated whole.

We have asked health-care advocates to look at these many factors that may be affecting any patient's behavior before making concrete snap judgments about patient identity and what the problem seems to be. We have also asked health-care advocates to look within themselves to consider how what they think, feel, believe, and act may be related to what there is about the patient that they do not understand. A major purpose in asking advocates to come to understand patients in this way is simply this: *health-care workers in any setting have the tendency to ascribe too quickly to a patho-*

logical category any behavior with which they are uncomfortable and that they do not understand immediately. This kind of categorizing is perhaps one of the strongest deterrents to a humanistic atmosphere within health-care settings. Such a view also too quickly brings closure to what could be an exciting venture with patients and co-workers in solving the mystery of what they do not understand about each other.

One of the major messages of this text has been a generalizable life-enhancing theme—that by reexamining the health-care culture and incorporating more humanistic goals into its various subsystems, life for patients, students, and staff might become more understandable and self-satisfying. In this chapter, we are going to talk more about that particular theme in more specific terms. Our particular emphasis is a life-enhancing function in certain helping situations and settings whose major focus presumes to be social/emotional based in order to help patients experience their lives as somewhat better than before help seeking. Health-care settings whose major focus is life enhancement are those whose primary functions are the maintenance, restoration, or development of people's relationship with the world in such a way that they feel emotional well-being—socially productive and self-satisfied.

Patients who are met within such settings are generally those who according to their own perception or that of society have difficulty in relating effectively to others in their immediate or larger environment. A basic concern of those who seek help willingly or unwillingly is how they or someone else is behaving. For some, this concern is because their own or someone else's external or overt behavior is distressing. Common behavioral manifestations that motivate help seeking are extreme withdrawal, acute and chronic depressive responses to traumatic events and significant losses, hyperactivity, explosive anger, or behavior that is chronically inappropriate in terms of time-honored social norms.

The primary concern of yet others may be their internal experience or covert behavior; that is, their thoughts and feelings create consciously felt anxiety. Distress concerning internal behavioral experience may be expressed in a variety of ways—for example, anxiety expressed in reactions of muscle and soft tissue organs as well as in thoughts and emotional states. To some persons, their thoughts and feelings seem unrelated or offensive to their stated beliefs or way of life. Others may have come to view their present way of life as incompatible with their notions of self and what they have always wanted to do, as seen in certain phases of burnout or mid-life identity crises.

Problems in Living: Disease or Dilemma?

Traditionally, health care concerned with "those emotional things" was thought of as occurring only in guidance clinics, psychiatric units, and mental hospitals. Today, such an attitude is recognized as stereotypic and denying of full-bodied understanding and helpful health services to all patients, regardless of setting. Relegating social/emotional understanding only to interventions with a "patient" population also denies the humanity of health-care workers and the knowledge that it might bring to them in learning to grow as individuals and effective group members.

Within this area of health care, there is no agreement on what to call persons who seek help in settings primarily concerned with the life-enhancing function—for example, "patient," "client," the "disturbed," or the "mentally ill." Neither is there any consensus as to who is best prepared to work with persons with minor to major difficulties in relating to themselves and others: Is it to be those with special psychiatric, psychological, or mental-health training, or can it be anyone who comes out of a general health-care curriculum? Should it be a physician, nurse, psychologist, or social worker? What of the paraprofessional?[1] The question has also been raised: Does the care of those with social/emotional-based problems of living belong within the province of the health-care disciplines at all?

Underlying the surface conflicts as to what, who, and where are two interrelated controversies:

1. What is "normal" and what is "abnormal" behavior?[2]
2. Is disease involved at all in the problems in living that involve perceptions of self and others and social relationships?[3]

For centuries, the question of what is abnormal behavior has been a thorny problem. At present, in spite of the medical profession's attempts to categorize people with detailed diagnostic DSM III labels[4] and the psychologists' batteries of standardized tests, it is cultural anthropologists who keep reminding people that definitions of normal and abnormal behavior are not universal. Internationally, as well as regionally within nations, what is taboo in one culture may be normal in another. Depending on the attitudes and beliefs of any culture's given social-control structure, there may exist an "in" group, and woe be to those who deviate. In the history of Western civilization, and to varying degrees in the present, those who do not conform have been called "crazy," "mad," "heretics," "sinful," "hippies," and, more recently, "punks."

The United States has an appalling history of how deviants have been treated, in spite of the humanistic, freedom-giving themes within its constitutional base. The early 1900s found the country becoming dotted with brick and mortar structures to house those who behaved in ways that frightened or otherwise were in the way of the family or community. Away from the eyes of the "normal" (the desired goal of the social community), these asylums for the "insane" became pits of the severest form of degradation.

In the middle of the 20th century, humanistically oriented groups that showed growing concern for this nationwide system of "concentration-camp" facilities began to form. A new term was coined: *mental illness*. The vogue of this terminology had positive effects, but it has also deterred full understanding of both the problems and the effective interventions. Positively, for example, the relabeling of the banished behavioral deviant as *mentally ill* helped in calling attention to the plight of institutional persons and the need for "treatment." The sympathy engendered by this terminology heightened the public's and helping profession's concern, as manifested in the form of dollars and specialty helpers. It also gave the public other terms for the deviant besides *crazy, mad, insane,* or *witch.* Simultaneously, however, efforts to make mental illness akin to physical illness to increase the public's ability to get close to the problem has led to oversimplification of the problem and overemphasis on technological approaches to "cures," (e.g., electroshock, insulin-shock therapy, and massive drug treatment).

Inappropriate or excessive use of the term *mental illness* and the medical disease model to which all forms of behavioral deviation have gained rank, sorely overlooks the social concomitants of this health problem. For example, such a model has increased society's tendency to label any behavior considered unusual as "illness." This belief denies the public the sensitization and understanding of the interrelationship of social, economic, and psychological factors that are a part of persons' becoming or feeling caught in "behavioral traps." Such a view also denies the public the understanding that the culture in which their children grow and develop influences many of the problems later expressed. An illness model also allows society at large to defer the problem to someone else (e.g., the health professions). The illness model, therefore, is vulnerable to being a defense mechanism against social institutions' doing anything about contributing factors or helping processes.

The disease model also holds a defensive trap that ultimately does not work in the individual's favor. It becomes too easy for the patient to say to the health-care professions: "I have an illness; you do the curing; you have all the answers." With physical disease and trauma, a temporarily useful coping mechanism may be to set the affliction aside from one's view of self and fight to overcome its biological effects; but, for those whose essential problems in life are how they view themselves and relate to others, how often is there identifiable disease or injury to isolate, to fight, or to acknowledge as a part of oneself?

The health professions themselves have contributed to society's and the individual's denial of the social/emotional concomitants of the problems and where responsibility taking broadly lies. "Illness" as a new way to view behavioral deviants came along at a time when the field of medicine was beginning to swell with scientific breakthroughs. It appeared at one time that the contributions of new discoveries might be the magic solution. Particularly, great hope was placed in the chemotherapies and biological causation. Society at large, desirous of "letting John do it," has been more than willing for the medical sciences to take over; but, simultaneously, social side effects of our technological culture have soared, and people struggle with them as bona fide social/emotional difficulties—not as disease that can be expunged. For example, increasing distance from close, meaningful relationships is reflected in such phenomena as unsatisfactory marriages, runaway children by the thousands, child abuse, and increasing ingestion, by young and old alike, of agents to alter mood and blur the effects of external realities.

Sending recalcitrant Tommie "off to the doctor" or getting Mary off her bitchiness kick with a "complete physical" and "maybe some medication" does not always get at the focus of ultimate concern. Helping Henry to cope with interpersonal work circumstances by immediately responding to his request to "give me something to keep me from being uptight" may not be ultimately helping Henry. Also, the staffs of hospitals for the care of persons who apparently cannot live in the greater society well know that medication and mechanical treatments alone have never been all that is involved. To the extent that any segment of the health-care-worker force responds to patients and their families with medications, mechanical treatment devices, and hopes for a technical science breakthrough alone, we believe that the health-care field is perpetuating a narrow perspective and less than adequate care.

There are, however, several elements of the health-care system that have long been aware of the sociopsychological implications of what are termed *emotional problems,* particularly among the psychiatric and public-health subsystems of medicine, public-health and psychiatric nursing, clinical psychology, and psychiatric social work. Those who joined with and have remained committed to the 1960s community mental-health movement are most significantly aware of (1) the interrelating contributory factors of social and economic circumstances as they affect development of problems and (2) the efforts that need to be continually made in moving society at large to help out in both attitude shift and priorities for the tax dollar as they affect humanistic quality in social institutions.

This community-oriented group of mental-health workers have also become increasingly sensitive to the necessity for focus on the interpersonal process and the various forms that this process must take in helping, both at the level of prevention of later difficulties and in intervention when a call for help is made. This group is also sensitive, however, to the proclivity for other health-care disciplines surrounding their "subspecialty," as well as the general public, to "let them do it." When one holds to a view that the most appropriate care occurs within the community because that is where the reality of the problem and the helping process lie, it is not an easy task. Attitudes change slowly. Mental-health workers with a community interpersonal approach deny society's wish to keep "those who bother" out of public view. Such an approach, as it becomes stronger within the health-care field, also denies many health-care workers the complacence of believing that they are accomplishing something by writing a prescription. In the mental-health movement, obtaining cooperation to look at things differently or more complexly is often hard to come by, even after 20 years of concerted effort.

Our view of the area of concern referred to as emotional or behavior problems is not a simple one. We believe that a number of phenomena occur within this broad area and that it is inappropriate (at times unsafe) to relegate any one discipline to being responsible for those persons whose behavior is frightening or mystifying or who "don't seem to have anything really wrong with them." We also do not believe that there is any one way to understand the person who often displays behavior that cannot readily be interpreted.

As repeatedly mentioned or implied throughout the text, all behavior has meaning, is multidetermined, and requires multiple approaches to understanding any particular human being. For example, in Chapter 8, health-care advocates were sensitized to the influence of presetting events and behaviors that might well be influencing the nature of the patient's complaint and methods of coping with it. As the review of suggested references for that chapter reveals, often stressful events of a social/emotional, highly interpersonal nature precede the onset of physical illness and influence the form of disease experienced by the individual. In view of these phenomena, health-care advocates in life-sustaining settings were reminded to explore carefully with patients what might be precipitating or simultaneously occurring factors, including interpersonal difficulties.

Repeatedly, we have also cautioned health-care advocates to "listen" for early complaints to be expressed in either biological or psychological terms. This sensitivity is equally important for health-care advocates working in the life-enhancing settings, such as counseling centers, guidance clinics, and mental-health centers; that is, patients who seek help with problems in living have a high probability of simultaneously being vulnerable to the onset of some form of physical disease. As Holmes and Rahe's[5] work suggests, particular attention should be focused on those persons who seek assistance after the death of a spouse, divorce, marital separation, jail term, death of a close family member, or previous personal injury or severe illness. Thus, health-care advocates working in primary life-enhancing situations must also be prepared for emotions in response to the recent event or cluster of events to be sometimes expressed in physical disease terms, even though the patient's central focus of concern is not disease related. Often, the onset of physical disease during the life-enhancing helping process signals the degree of stress that the social/emotional problems may be stimulating.

Just as the interpersonal process is the critical core of any helping process, in life-enhancing situations, it cannot be overemphasized; that is, there is a necessity for an interpersonal process of great depth that allows advocates to get close to, understand, and humanistically relate to patients, regardless of other adjunctive therapeutics that may be required. We encourage this interpersonal process to be richly integrated with an advocacy attitude to (1) counter the social myths about mental illness, (2) diminish stereotyped notions of patient incompetency, and (3) place more appropriate responsibility on patients, families, and society at large. For example, an advocacy position recognizes that, when help is sought, whether concerning minor or major interpersonal or intrapersonal disruption, and when the patient, family, or related social institutions do not feel adequate to make the responsible choices, then the primary goal of the helping process is to assist any or all of them to do so.

Open and realistic awareness between the patient and the advocate regarding the mystique and stereotypes surrounding emotional problems and mental illness is just as important in life-enhancing situations as open awareness in life-saving and life-sustaining experiences. As a first step to being more authentic with patients at the time that help is sought in life-enhancing settings (or any other setting in which patients may happen to end up), helpers themselves need to evaluate how they feel about persons with these kinds of problems and what they believe should be done about them.

Although necessary, it is difficult for health-care workers in all settings to be more discriminative in evaluating and responding to persons whose expressed feelings and overt behaviors do not fit with classic biological disease categories or traditional social norms. To clear away some of the confusing morass in this complex field, we have found it useful to break down the life-enhancing dimension into categories of function. The categories subsumed under the major focus of this dimension take into consideration (1) that individuals experience varying degrees of interpersonal and intrapersonal disruption and (2) that, etiologically, there are different factors that contribute to a person's perceptions and their overt behavioral style, some of which are secondary to physical disease and drug influence and some of which are non–disease related. Some of the latter stem from earlier, but undetected, developmental deviations of neural or biochemical function. Others derive from the effects of cultural disruption. The three viewpoints from which the life-enhancing dimension of helping can be more definitively evaluated are primary, secondary, and tertiary aspects of care:

1. *Primary life-enhancing functions.* To prevent disabling complications in perceptions of self and interpersonal relationships stemming from social/emotional problems.
2. *Secondary life-enhancing functions.* To prevent difficulties in self-perception and interpersonal problems in living secondary to the effects of disease, drugs, injury, or developmental deviation.
3. *Tertiary life-enhancing functions.* To prevent dehumanizing residential caregiving through the establishment of humanistic helping goals.

Primary Life-Enhancing Functions

Early needs for help   Throughout the health-care system, there are opportunities for function concerning life-enhancement issues. For example, there are times when a patient simply wants to clarify information to be able to understand something better or when a parent wishes to discuss how to do something more effective with the children so that their healthy growth and development may be ensured. Primary life-sustaining situations are replete with opportunities for this kind of life-enhancing function, which is based on the stress-reduction power of knowledge.

Health-care advocates also observe that, increasingly, individuals seek out health-care settings for what seems like the opportunity to "simply rap." Specifically, this kind of help seeking is seen in community-based mental-health centers; but, as any experienced health-care advocate knows, it is a common phenomenon in any health-care setting. Public-health nurses have long been aware of both the need and value of the home visit as the opportunity for a harried mother to "let down" and talk out loud about her dilemma as she perceives it. University health-center counselors know the value of simply being available for students to come in and try out ideas on someone else.

Common to this level of help seeking is the request of people for someone with whom they can struggle with philosophical existential questions that have become highly personalized for them. Following are some of the issues that health-care advocates frequently encounter that are entirely unrelated to a disease process, but that the person perceives as a highly personal dilemma nonetheless:

"How can I find more satisfaction in my job when I feel like such a drone?"
"How can I feel like the person that I believe myself to really be if I am tied down with four kids?"
"How can I have a better marriage than that which I witnessed my parents having?"

"How can I live more at one with my minority peers when I feel angry both at them
and the honky?"

"How am I going to be able to cope with the fact that I am getting old?"

"How can I best act on what I have always wanted to do?"

Each generation has its own set of questions about existence and its meaning, and
all societies have had their unique systems for assisting their people with problems in
living—the oracle, the priest, the guru, or the prophet. Although religious groups still
utilize their pastor, priest, or rabbi, many of these traditional functions have been
rapidly supplanted in our Western culture by the counselor or the psychotherapist.
This group is perhaps the least underemployed in the country and that people want
these services is reflected in the increasing numbers of health-insurance plans that
provide for mental-health consultations. That people are concerned about living more
actualized, better lives is also reflected in the wave of popularity of books concerning
such subjects as how to live more happily, how to achieve more satisfying expressions
of sexual feelings, and alternative life-styles.[6,7]

In life-enhancing settings, health-care advocates have to be particularly sensitive
to themes in the patient's complaints that are reflective of responses to living in a mass
society. Seeman defines six forms of alienation that can occur in response to the sense
of community that is lost in the face of technical efficiency, geographical mobility, and
mass culture.[8] He speaks of the feelings of (1) *powerlessness,* in which one has little
expectancy that one's own efforts can be influential in gaining personal or social rewards; (2) *meaninglessness,* in which one has little expectancy of being able to predict
the outcome of social events; (3) *normlessness,* or not being bound by conventional
standards and implying a high expectancy that socially unapproved means must be
used to accomplish goals; (4) *value isolation,* causing rejection of the values highly
esteemed by others; (5) *self-estrangement,* or engaging in activities that are not valued
or rewarding in themselves; and (6) *social isolation,* or low expectation for social acceptance—for example, as expressed in the feelings of minority groups concerning loneliness and exclusion. Again, expressions of these feelings in response to our rapid
cultural shifts do not constitute disease, but that does not mean that health-care advocates do not have to grapple with these feelings in their patients as well as in themselves. Health-care advocates stay in tune with their contemporary culture to help
patients define problems more accurately, as well as to help with more creative solutions. As will be reviewed in the following chapter, the above characteristics are high
contributors to the syndromes of existential burnout and job-related stress reactions.

Within the group of persons asking the existential questions, it is generally the
case that, with the opportunity to talk out some of the issues, people go about their
business of daily living trying out new modes of thought and action on their own; or
they may join one of a number of actualizing groups that are unrelated to health-care
settings per se.[9] Their anxiety is of the expected developmental quality that precedes
or immediately follows the experience of risk taking and change—for example, as one
encounters new life experiences or considers a new way that seems to fit with a particular view of oneself.

Subtle expressions as clues to more complex problems   Within the group ask-ing these "how" questions may also be those who are indirectly referring to more serious interpersonal circumstances than their initial question implies. For example, beneath what seems like an offhand question about childrearing or the need to talk about life in general may lie a mother's need to talk about a pattern of child abuse in the family.[10] Many life circumstances that people are enmeshed in are to them touchy and embarrassing, and their cries for help are indirect. In addition to child abuse and neglect, we have found the following situations also to remain undercover for some time during initial or subsequent interviews: recent abortion, adult battering, alcohol-ism, concealed felonies (e.g., embezzlement, drug dealing), heavy drug use, homosex-uality, extramarital affairs, and unwanted pregnancy. Therefore, as reiterated in the previous chapters, taking time at the point at which a person first enters a health setting to determine fully the most accurate picture of what the patient is actually talking about is not only humanistic but is also a measure of safe helping practice. A general principle prevails: *listen to the person in front of you, listen to your professional hunches, and tactfully explore with the patient as trust grows.*

Some persons seek help in life-sustaining and life-enhancing settings when al-ready involved in what seem to them overwhelming circumstances to which they read-ily admit. Anxiety is high, and their usual coping styles seem to them ineffective. Again, in keeping with the advocacy model of humanistic helping, the advocate starts with getting a full picture of the problem and the proposed solutions as the patient sees them. However, as this "knowing" process ensues, the perceptive health-care advocate may sense that other factors are involved. Following is a case in point that exemplifies such a situation. On initial contact, the young patient was open about the problem as she saw it. She wanted assistance to carry out the solution that she had thought out on her own.

CASE IN POINT

When 18-year-old Lois came to the health center, she was three months pregnant and unmar-ried. The father of the child, Tom, had left the neighborhood immediately on hearing of her pregnancy. Marriage was out of the question, and she definitely did not want to keep the child. She thought that she knew little about abortion but would be in favor of it "if I am not too far along."[11] If abortion was not possible, she wanted help to be able to give up the baby immedi-ately after birth. Her parents knew about it and were not chastising. She felt remorse about the situation as it affected them, however, since she had been expected to help out in the family.

Her wants and desires were straightforward. However, Lois seemed emotionally shat-tered by her present circumstances. Through bits and pieces of an often digressing conversa-tion, she spoke of the close relationship that she had had with Tom. It was puzzling that she felt no anger or resentment toward him. In fact, she often took a defensive role for him when there was nothing in the advocate's exploring that seemed to call for it.

Without denying Lois her options, the advocate believed that a deeper exploration of this determination not to keep the child was warranted. The helper was aware through her pre-vious experience that considerable covert ambivalent feelings are experienced by women concerning either abortion or relinquishment of a child. Lois was asked to come back the next day for an appointment when more time could be allowed her. A thorough developmental history concerning the health and parenting patterns of both Lois's and Tom's family seemed an appropriate place to begin. Lois agreed that she would like to talk about this.

During the course of the following session, Lois revealed that both she and Tom saw themselves as "inner-city kids" whose only stability was their friendship while they were growing up in the same neighborhood for 18 years. Early childhood comparison of their each having a "goofy" brother was part of their friendship bond. Friendship eventually felt to them like being in love. The interview also revealed more significant reasons why Lois wanted not to have a child: she and Tom were convinced that any offspring that they might ever have would be retarded like their brothers.

Reassurance through using general statistics about retardation would have been to no avail in countering Lois's insistence on not having a child. However, individualized facts specifically related to Tom and Lois's situation just might be. It was explored with Lois as to whether she and Tom would consider her pregnancy differently if they had no history of retardation in the family. Her response was an immediate "Of course, then it would be different. You can understand that, can't you?" She was asked if it had ever occurred to her that maybe the kind of retardation present in their families was not inheritable. She had never considered it. In fact, she knew nothing about the concept of retardation except for the meaning it held for her in the form of embarrassment, extra work around the house, and fears of her own offspring's being the same way Lois was asked if she wanted to find out more about what had contributed to the retardation of her and Tom's siblings in order to know more about what they really might or might not be up against. Did she think that Tom would want to know? She thought that he might and would try to find him to ask.

Tom was not immediately found, but, with permission from Lois, her parents were contacted for a family conference to determine if they would cooperate in evaluating how her little brother's retardation might have occurred. They agreed, and it was found from the parents' report and supporting hospital records that, during delivery, a severe anoxia of the infant had occurred, leading to serious cerebral dysfunction. With the news that Lois's little brother did not have a condition that was inheritable, Tom readily agreed to talk with his parents about a similar evaluation of his young brother. Little Davie was found to be a child with Down's syndrome who had been born when Tom's mother was 49 years of age—again a situation in which direct inheritability was not at issue for Tom and Lois.

These facts about a family constellation in which no other history of retardation was present served to reassure Tom and Lois about the probability of their having a normal child. It was explained that, of course, in any pregnancy and delivery, there is not a 100 percent guarantee, since any decision to have a child is the first step in the risk taking that parenthood involves. But, with good prenatal monitoring by the clinic and Lois's commitment to take good care of herself, the probability of a normal child was good. They accepted this level of reassurance, and, with the support of their families, they married.

As often as he could get off work, Tom would accompany Lois to the clinic during the pregnancy. He was the more apprehensive of the two and needed personal reassurance that everything was going along fine. He wanted to be present during labor and delivery to keep an eagle eye on things as much as to give Lois needed emotional support. A normal son was delivered, and Lois keeps well-child appointments. Periodically she openly admits to needing feedback that he is accomplishing his developmental milestones in a normal fashion.

In the preceding case history, there ensued a happier ending than might have been experienced. In part, the ending occurred because of the sensitive health-care advocate, who, although allowing Lois to explore her own options, at the same time followed her own curiosity and hints from her knowledgeable experience base. Had she not done this, Lois might have been supported in an alternative of abortion or relinquishment without ever understanding anything more about her reasons than when she came in the front door. Not only did the actions of the health-care advocate lead to a more enhancing resolution of the current set of circumstances, but the helping actions also introduced Tom and Lois to a completely new set of perceptions about their families, themselves, and their own future. This kind of help is preventive at the same time that it accomplishes the working through of an immediate problem.

This case also exemplifies the benefits of open awareness to facts as well as feelings. Too often in such situations as the foregoing, helping actions are focused so intently on the emotional support that a situation seems to require that the usefulness of factual knowledge as a helping tool is overlooked. Sometimes neglect of factual knowledge is a defense of the helper against a painful reality; that is, factual knowledge is overlooked or watered down because the helper has a difficult time sharing bad news and coping with the subsequent emotional support that such a reality may require on an ongoing basis. Particularly in situations requiring evaluation of children and feedback to parents facing probable developmental deviation of a child, the helping function is stressful for everyone. Yet, information sharing and counseling with prospective parents or parents of a defective child require a high degree of openness, honesty, and detailed educative explanations in understandable language. To deny parents factual knowledge denies them a reality within which they can work and choose to do something remedial with professional help. To do other than be honest only reinforces illusions of what parents would rather have or the helper would want for them in the best of all possible worlds. It is unkind to mask the reality for parents and send them off into daily living only to have them come to know at some later time when they no longer can deny the limits of their child's ability. In any health-care setting, factual feedback that is unpleasant to convey need not engender hopelessness and helplessness. When simultaneous reassurance is given that a humanistic helping process is available to help individuals work through crises that new knowledge brings to their awareness, then it is easier to share reality and experience its effects.

When a patient's goals cannot be supported   There are several cases in which the advocacy principle of helping the patient to accomplish personal goals does not fit with what the advocate can support, regardless of how life enhancing the patient perceives such goals to be. These cases are those which involve felonious activities or the willful taking of life.

An example of such cases occurs primarily in life-sustaining settings when the conflict about "mercy killing" arises from time to time. Although euthanasia is a complex philosophical issue, health-care workers in these settings have a number of guidelines to follow. As was seen in Chapter 8, although people believe that they have a right to tell helpers what not to do to prolong life, the majority of people think that it is wrong to ask a physician to terminate the life of a dying patient deliberately. Although this issue will be debated for years to come, health-care advocates ethically and legally cannot support euthanasia.[12]

Periodically, within life-enhancing settings, a health-care advocate will encounter a patient with a terminal disease who is coping with it by thoughts of suicide. Empathetically, one may understand the patient's perception of the situation and not condemn it; yet, in the commitment of saving life, the helper advocates for alternative ways to face dying and death. So also is it with patients in such deep existential pain about life's circumstances that they see suicide as a resolution to either despair or deep-seated vindictiveness against those whom they perceive as inflicting pain. Acknowledging the patients' ultimate choice, the health-care advocate sticks by the suicidal patients and fights with them for life alternatives to experiencing the human dilemma. The advocate cannot go to the grave with them and help them in.

In all settings, health-care advocates occasionally encounter patients whose general life-style is built around values and actions in the greater community that advocates find offensive to their own personal belief system. Some of these circumstances involve persons who are known to engage in criminal acts or who are reputed to have violated some of the basic tenets of humanity in sub rosa fashion. When such a patient enters a life-saving or certain of the life-sustaining settings, the advocate can share with the patient goals for "wellness" and prevention of imminent death as it relates to physical disease and injury. Defenses against wondering what that person will do with that health and life after leaving the clinic or hospital are available to insulate the helper. One may be able to fall back on the centuries-old commitment of the health-care professions to treat disease and injury and to save life regardless of who the patients are or what they have done.

Health-care workers in life-enhancing situations have a more difficult task concerning such patients, particularly when the patient asks for help in maintaining or enhancing a life-style that is contrary to the legal or moral underpinnings of the community. Following are two cases in point for contrast. Characterologically, the patients were similar and had life-styles that neither advocate could endorse. In both cases, the message concerns the goals for help that the patients set for themselves, the issue that allowed a differential response for the advocates involved.

CASE IN POINT

Frank's description of himself as unreliable was a characteristic that showed up early in our contacts. He missed the first two appointments, and, when he finally came, he was half an hour late. Physically he appeared well put together; he was fashionably groomed in expensive leather clothing. His medium-length hair was well styled and his face tanned. He had a cool, calm, matter-of-fact demeanor that lent him an aura of being somewhat older than his 25 years.

He stated that his main concern was that he might be "crazy." He based these fears on what his wife and peers told him—yet he insisted that he did not care what others thought about him. What he thought they might be reacting to was explored. He thought that they were saying that because of his "willingness to do anything for money" and the fact, to which he admitted, that he lied a lot. He did not know why, but he had begun to think a great deal about this lately. He wanted my reassurance that it was not crazy to do "anything," such as "contracting on people." It had never bothered him before. He wanted to keep on with what he was doing, but with none of the new feelings about it.

Frank's confusion about whether he was crazy seemed linked to what he fantasized that to be. He simply thought that it should be "like you don't know what you are doing." He believed that he was aware of what he was doing at all times, when he did things, and why— at least to the extent of his awareness that he was motivated to "make it big" through money. It had never occurred to Frank that his wife's and friends' knowledge of his being an un- abashed "hit man" had anything to do with what they were reacting to in calling him "crazy." He agreed that "just maybe" others would look at it that way. He said that he did not have "normal reactions," particularly when he was hurting other people; but he did not see this as crazy. It had just always been that way for him.

The question of how it had always been for him was asked. His calm demeanor disap- peared, and the first overt signs of anxiety were exhibited—for example, restless shifting of posture, commenting on his having to go back to work, smoothing his hair, clearing his throat frequently. He requested to leave to go to the toilet and then changed his mind and said that he really had to go back to work and he would talk about it the next time.

He did come the next time. He began where we had left off, which was surprising. What was the force motivating him to come back and to begin to talk about what had made him so anxious on the previous occasion? His response to my curiosity was calm and matter of fact. "I figured out if you're going to help me not be bothered by those feelings I'd better tell you what you want." He did not seem to register my explanation that I had asked about his past to help him get a better view of what he wanted to avoid repeating and some choices about where he wanted to go in the future. He saw no relationship of that to his present problem. He said that being a kid was "something left behind" but he would talk about it anyhow.

He had been "a waterfront kid with nothing." He was one of 11 children and saw his mother as a "squealer" who would tell on him to a punitive father. "The old man" used to hang him by his thumbs in the garage for his misbehavior. Nothing else that he had been through in life did he see as important. He was not interested in alternatives to his present life- style. All that he wanted was to make big money. If he could have three wishes, he would open a wig and hairpiece shop for men and women and a porno and shine shop and get into a "hustle" for which he first needed a few more grand. He didn't want anything to interfere with his work now because he needed to keep making lots of money for the really big hustle.

I explained to Frank that what he was asking was impossible for me to help him with. He needed to know that my personal and professional ethics did not allow me to cooperate with his wish to deny the emotions that he was beginning to feel concerning killing and inju- ring other people. I explained that I could agree with him only insofar as he expressed needing help, but I thought that we were miles apart on what the goal of that help should be. His reaction was a calm, matter-of-fact "So that's that; I guess I'll just forget about it." He did wonder if I would see his wife and calm "that ____ down about leaving all the time."

His wife, Mary, came reluctantly for only one visit. She explained that she did not think that coming to talk would do any good. She did want to leave Frank but could not "when it got down to it." She harbored an almost unquestioned belief that during her first marriage she had caused her first husband to "go bad." She believed that she had probably done the same thing to Frank, since she had viewed him as "straight" when she lived with him before marriage and now he was not. Therefore, in her view she could not leave him, but she did want him to be "put away," since she was afraid of him from time to time. Furthermore, his sporadic drug usage bothered her. She thought that it was a bad influence on their children. As to her feelings about Frank's being crazy, by contrast, she seemed to be less concerned than Frank. She thought that he was "just plain nuts" for doing those things. She saw his behavior as being like that of a little boy who always wanted his own way, regardless of who or what might interfere; and she had not hesitated to tell that to Frank periodically.

She reported that Frank was to appear in court within a few days to face sentencing for a collection of felony convictions. She was certain that he would be sent up for a "long, long time." She thought that he was uptight about it. She did not particularly care; becoming a cell widow was to her a positive resolution. She looked forward to going back to school during his anticipated imprisonment. She planned to wait for him maybe; it would depend. There was nothing that she thought that any of us could help her with.

A review of Frank's clinic record revealed that he had spent six months of the previous year in a county jail after a burglary conviction. He admitted to being arrested "40 or 50 times" in his life for various misdemeanors and felonies. He did have several felony charges against him at that time. None were for the illicit activities that he had admitted to during our interviews, those for which he wanted help to continue "without being bothered."

He stopped in the doorway of the office the day before he was to appear in court. He quipped, "At least wish me luck." I explained that it was going to take more than that. He smiled and said, "I know that."

In sociopathic fashion, Frank wanted to continue his life-style with no disruption from anyone or anything, not even from his internal feeling states. He wanted to use a publicly acknowledged helper to assist him in this process. The health-care advocate could not do this and could not refer him to anyone who would assist him with his specific goal. Obviously, feelings about his actions that he had repressed, suppressed, or otherwise set aside were beginning to break into awareness. He wanted to get rid of his feelings rather than to listen to what they might be telling him. He wanted to leave the past behind and precariously maintain a way of life that would, in his view, get him closer to the goal of making it big. Frank obviously found someone to help him in the way that he desired. Two weeks after the last contact with him at the clinic, he was seen driving down the boulevard in a sleek new car. Six months later, he was found dead at the edge of town, and who did it remains a mystery.

Frank's life-style can be deemed appalling. How he had been living at the time that he sought help could have, for the helper, been a factor in not wanting to continue to work with Frank, but this was not the issue. Many persons who come initially for help have been leading "appalling" lives beneath a cloak of social and economic propriety. The issue here is what the person set as his goal and what he expected the advocate to help him in achieving.

Contrast the case of Frank with that of Gilberto, who had lived within a similar social context—drugs, murder, extortion, heading up a prostitution ring, and all the usual trappings.

CASE IN POINT

Gilberto, age 29, was admitted to 4 West from the state penitentiary. The prison did not have a complete hospital for the inmates; so anyone who became critically or terminally ill was brought to the university hospital. Gilberto had a cirrhotic liver condition and bleeding esophageal varices. My understanding was that he had almost died of hemorrhage before they brought him down from the prison. We were all so concerned in keeping him alive that night that who he was or what he was in prison for did not even pass our minds. Looking at his record the next day revealed that he was in for life subsequent to a stabbing murder that had occurred two years before in a Green Bay bar.

Gilberto was in critical condition for some time, receiving many transfusions. Often he was too weakened to talk for any period of time. It became apparent that he probably was not going to make it. If we did not know, he at least thought that he did. He flatly said that he was not going to. He began to talk more about himself. He wanted to "put his life together." He wondered if anyone would be willing to listen and help him with that if they knew what he had been. Telling him that it did not matter what he had been did not satisfy him. He wanted to talk out loud about what he saw his life as being. I asked if he was daring me to like him in insisting on telling me. He thought that, yes, maybe he was testing me, but he wanted to look at it all again, and maybe I could learn something about "how not to be."

Methodically each day he would talk about his life. He started from the beginning, as if he were telling a story. First, he told of his life as a blond-haired Mexican child, who never seemed to fit with his peers in a small Texas border town. An adolescence of moth-and-the-flame activities between school and police authorities followed. Next came his rise to power within the gang; then he went into the drug business as a way to meet ever-increasing needs for status and money. At 22, he felt proud of being the youngest behind-the-scenes pusher in that part of the country; he had a covey of goons to carry out whatever violated his moral code. He himself was never a drug user until the age of 25, at which point his structural world began to crumble, what with poor decisions in keeping his organizations going, getting into the middle of the "mess" that he had always been able to stay out of, becoming broke, scrounging drugs, dirty needles, shooting up in gas-station rest rooms while running from the police, and being blackmailed and afraid. He had never directly murdered before the Green Bay incident, although he knew of at least five or six deaths for which he was responsible.

At the end of the story, he wanted to talk with a priest. He believed that he had some things sorted out at that point and could include in his confession everything that he wanted to say. He asked whether after that I could help him find something to do that would make him feel that he was worth something— "at least like someone who has helped other people."

The last two weeks of Gilberto's life he rolled gauze, made tongue blades, and folded four by fours for central supply. Several patients were brought to his bedside in wheelchairs to simply "rap" with each other. They were lonely and found pleasure in commiserating and joking with him. I told Gilberto that I had never talked before with anyone who had been in the drug business. I asked if he could give me a few hints on how I might help persons caught in the trap if I ever found myself in that kind of work. One of the things that I remember his saying was "Don't ever let anyone con you into helping them with anything you don't want to do."

Patients who do not cooperate   For all the advocate's efforts to develop a helping framework within which understanding between two persons can be maximized, some patients simply do not seem to cooperate. For a number of reasons, which may or may not be shared with the advocate, this lack of cooperation may be evidenced when the patient suddenly stops coming for help. In some cases, the patient may be discouraged with a certain form of help or the personal style of an advocate that to the patient seems "not how a helping person should be." Understanding would be ultimately an easier task if patients would express these feelings directly. However, many patients within health-care settings are in awe of the professional and reticent in being real. In many life-enhancing situations, patients who are struggling with a lowered self-concept and learned helplessness may be no better able to tell their advocates what they think and feel than they are able to communicate with those in the broader community whom they perceive as "keeping them down." Patients with retarded affect and poor verbal facility as a result of chronic depression[13] are particularly prone to unexpressed discouragement and resentment. Some patients who were coerced by others to seek help in the first place may simply decide on their own that they want none of that and disappear.

Particularly in life-enhancing situations, in which the goals are to develop a more actualized, self-satisfying life-style, health-care advocates must have their eyes wide open to the paradoxical nature of change. First, any attitude or habit of a significant nature is slow to change even when patients say they want to experience life differently and put much effort into the helping process. Second, anxiety accompanies both positive and negative changes in life-style. Patients who poorly understand that change is often slow or those who have a low tolerance for felt anxiety often wish to terminate forward progress when the stress of new gains seems to interfere with the way that they think they should be feeling. For some, the stress of new gains faces them with the necessity of giving up an immature life-style of need for instant gratification and low responsibility for what happens to themselves. At this point, such people who "seemed to be doing so well" sometimes return to old life-styles with even greater intensity. This phenomenon often is experienced in community-corrections settings concerned with adult and juvenile offenders. For an in-depth review of the dynamics occurring in these situations and how one can more effectively work with those who are developmentally immature, see Appendix C, Understanding Narcissism.

It is hoped that advocates can establish a relationship in which the specific reasons for resistance become available to both the helper and the patient. In the absence of facts, it is well to keep in mind a general concept: patients will choose to do what they perceive to be in their best interest at the time. Health-care advocates have to get used to the fact that they will encounter patients who will make choices about pursuing help with which the advocate will disagree. Ultimately these choices must be allowed as the only alternative that the advocate has is to insist on doing it the helper's way "for the patient's own good"—hardly a reflection of the autonomy that the advocate presumably is fostering.

To prevent and cope with uncooperative, or "backing off" behavior, the health-care advocate has available the tools of the advocacy model of humanistic helping. If the advocate has interpersonally involved the patient in a comprehensive evaluation, provided adequate, understandable feedback, and established mutually determined goals from a variety of choices realistically available, the helper has done the best that one can do. Although it is a difficult fact to acknowledge, some patients need their old way of doing things for whatever existential pain that it brings more than the anxiety that they perceive themselves having to experience to grow and change. Ultimately, one has to face that not everyone can be helped.

CASE IN POINT

Martin sought out assistance at the mental-health center after several brief blackouts at work and a recent history of insomnia. His complaints seemed directly related to the events surrounding his recent mutually agreed-on marital separation. However, a complete physical examination was carried out to ensure there being no organic basis for his symptoms. None was found.

Superficially, Martin expressed pleasure at his newfound freedom from Sheilah, whom he perceived as a dull, boring woman who was overly preoccupied with the children and "all those housewifey things." He was dating again and liked "burning the midnight oil," but he found his blackouts and sleeplessness interfering.

In discussing the goals that he would like to work for in the therapeutic sessions, Martin wanted to work through some of his difficulties in "starting life all over" and trying not to make the same mistakes that he made in his first marriage; yet, Martin never seemed to be able to explore the future that he said he wanted to experience. He became increasingly preoccupied with Sheilah and his inability to stay away from his former home; yet, he was resistant to going back and working out with Sheilah some of the problems that he thought that they had had.

In the middle of this seeming impasse, Martin showed up one day and announced that he was going back to Sheilah even though it would "be just like it used to be." He believed that was "better than nothing."

Behavior that frightens or mystifies   Many patients who voluntarily come or are brought by others to outpatient or inpatient life-enhancing settings behave in ways that health-care advocates find frightening or mystifying. Some advocates, particularly beginning students, have never seen human beings act in certain ways. Moreover, they feel at a loss when, in addition, they are expected to "do something" with the behavior presented. Understandably, stress can be high for the advocate in this kind of situation. Unless the beginning advocate has experienced highly stressed, disorganized behavior in a family member or friend or grew up in an inner-city area where broad latitude is given for deviant behaviors, most beginners have a fairly low comfort level with someone whose actions are different from those sanctioned by their own cultural norms.[14] Second, many patients are difficult to understand, no matter what one's experience base may be.

Particularly difficult are those patients who are experiencing what is referred to as *disorders of thought:* in formal diagnostic language, these kinds of disorders refer to psychotic reactions.[15] Patients may experience disordered thinking and inappropriate behavior stemming from unique perceptions for a host of reasons. As we shall see in the section on secondary life-enhancing function, psychotic and psychotic-like reactions can stem from cerebral insult in the form of injury, disease, or the effects of drugs. However, for many psychotic reactions, no organic causes can be determined by present methods. In such situations, these reactions are assumed to have evolved from a variety of social/emotional developmental circumstances from which a patient has come to derive meaning about the self and others in a highly disordered way.

A disordered thought process is expressed by patients in a variety of ways, all of which seem to have some highly unique, significantly personal meaning that makes sense only to the individual. Disorders in perception can be in the receptive as well as the expressive mode; for example, what the patient sees, hears, feels, or otherwise takes in is often misinterpreted. Expressively, the patient's disordered perceptions may be reflected verbally, in writing, through inappropriate social behavior, or all three. Language may suffer various distortions; for example, nouns, adjectives, and verbs are often interchanged and sentences disconnected. Occasionally, new words are simply made up. Patients may be, but often are not, receptive to feedback that their language does not make sense to others. Sometimes they become angry that the helper is not hearing or seeing the world as they do. Often patients put much energy into trying to get other persons "to see their way" and to appreciate how vital this is to their survival. Following is one of 17 letters written to police, lawyers, and various bank managers to plead for something to be done with a person whom Angela had perceived to have made her "do things."

CASE IN POINT

Dear Bank Manager

Save in main vault till police get it as evidence for prosecution of a criminal doctor, hypnotic sex perversion and mental disarrangement through mind changing drugs, 2 sets of recordings one true, one the mind changed for evil patient (myself). However no one assaulted me during marriage except him under his hypnosis—that's what I found out last week decided to kill me with a huge dose of candy coated, so he told me, but maybe under hypnosis I dug them out of the trash burner (45 of them) perhaps added 50 more (100 seems to be the number). This destroys the mind and it is too late now. I think this happened after midnight last Friday. I'm positive. This had to be the time for a "feeling" experience. I had them while under hypnosis.

Angela

Keep in main vault as vital evidence give to police only!

Angela had been hospitalized in a psychiatric unit of a general hospital after being brought to a mental-health clinic by her husband. She was brought for help after a week of sleeplessness, an inappropriate visit to the president of their local bank, and innumerable phone calls to the police concerning her perceived plight. This behavior seemed to be precipitated by her husband's finding out about a brief affair. The affair had in reality occurred, a fact that her husband learned about through her confessing to him remorsefully.

Her letters and lengthly verbalizations were intense and energy depleting, since she insisted that the one who had "done these evil things unto me must be captured and punished."

She did not think that she could rest until this task was accomplished. Food and liquid intake were dangerously low, since Angela was certain that she would succumb to hypnotic influences if she ingested anything from strangers. Medications were effectively utilized in reducing her life-threatening anxiety level, which bordered her on physical exhaustion. In addition, a critically needed interpersonal process was slowly initiated. Many hours were spent with Angela in sensitively leading her through the confusion of her reality. This process eventually enabled her to develop understanding and forgiving acceptance of her own role in her current circumstances.

Not all patients with disorders of thinking express themselves with behavior as verbose or hyperactive as did Angela. Some patients appear closed in with their preoccupying thoughts, visual images, or internal auditory experience; but mystifying they all seem when one is trying to translate and reach out to them for common meaning. Following is a letter, found in a wastebasket, that was written by a young man who periodically would go for days without uttering a word to his family. At the time that his family asked the public-health nurse to visit, Bernie was acting as if nothing existed in his visual field.

CASE IN POINT

Folks
June 1060/35¢
Astors are pretty flowers
Pres. Richard Nixon
Brides beautiful apt.
Hidden danger in Cincinati
How to be a girl. Glorious summer evening
and Bernie

Health-care advocates who encounter patients with disorders of thinking have a doubly difficult task. They must attempt to evaluate and offer help based on a patient's highly individualized frame of reference that often seems like a foreign language. Coupled with this helping task is the need for health-care advocates to cope with their own feelings of fear that the patient's "strangeness" or aggressive behavior may engender; yet, health-care advocates must come to appreciate that the patient also is fearful and trying to make sense out of internal and external reality, albeit through highly ineffective coping strategies. Even with this realization, frustration can be high for the advocate from what, on occasion, seem to be ineffective attempts to get through to those who seem unintelligible or suspicious.

Reactions of health-care workers in the face of patients' behaviors that mystify or frighten or both are commonly (1) to avoid the patients as much as possible or (2) to respond to them in gingerly ways that disallow closeness and the opportunity to find out what is going on in their inner reality. These response patterns with a group of 19 postdegree continuing-education nursing students were studied by J. Chapman for a six-week period of time.[16] It was found that there was a cluster of patient behaviors with which the student group and clinical-setting co-workers felt most uncomfortable; for example, behavior that was hostile/aggressive led to the highest degree of discomfort, followed by that which was manipulative, destructive, unresponsive, untruthful, nonverbal, impulsive, and demanding, in that order. In contrast, students preferred working with those patients who might be considered the picture of mental health—for example, those who were cooperative, intelligible, verbal, responsive, considerate, attentive, and helpful. Follow-up as to what specific emotions the group felt in response to their rated categories suggested that approach or avoidance depends on (1) whether helpers think that they themselves will get hurt, (2) whether they believe that they can "get through" and understand what the patients are talking about, and (3) whether the patients seem to have the ability to cooperate with the staff in the helping process—that is, whether they can act in their own behalf. Patients who were both hostile/aggressive and unintelligible posed the greatest threat and were subject to the strongest avoidance by helpers.

Patience and gradual trust building cannot be overemphasized in the attempt to accomplish the ultimate helping goal: that the patient reestablish accurately perceived links with reality and less self-negating coping strategies. Therefore, the advocate works (1) with the patient interpersonally in establishing a reality base that can be trusted by the patient at the same time that (2) the helper is working for the patient in catalyzing a social milieu in which educative, effective group relations may be experienced.[17] A humanistic advocacy model again can be a helpful guide in negotiating responsibility taking with the patient. Discriminatively, the advocate assumes responsibility when the patient's judgment is precarious; yet, the advocate is ever aware of maximizing the patient's participation in goal setting and determination of helpful experiences as quickly as possible. As one's experience grows with patients having disordered percepts, one comes to appreciate that such patients are rarely out of contact with reality 24 hours a day.

Family concern and need for involvement is high in these situations. Family members also experience fear, mystification, and frustration with respect to the patient's demeanor and responses to them. In the helping process family involvement is variable, depending on what the advocate believes is required to understand more fully the patient's circumstances and the possibility of the family members' becoming a positive, therapeutic force. Although one would like to believe that all family members will be eager to rally around and join helping forces, experienced health-care advocates are aware that considerable familial alienation may be already a hard reality by the time that the patient seeks or is brought for help. Nonetheless, the health-care advocate attempts to maintain ongoing involvement with the family if this appears to be in the patient's best interest. To the degree possible, the advocate is responsive to the patient's judgment in these matters. Open awareness with families is again emphasized to counteract the many social myths that surround these situations, to facilitate personalized understanding of the patient's dilemma, and to provide the family with insight into the realistic effort that they may need to put forth if they are willing to become therapeutic in life-enhancing ways. Of major importance in working with disturbed young people is to understand families, as Haley says, as "organizations with a hierarchy deserving of respect."[18]

Summary   Within primary life-enhancing situations, the focus is on those circumstances in which no disease per se is evident as a central or contributory concern in the patient's experienced problem. A central unifying thread in understanding these situations is that of anxiety that is variably expressed in response to social/emotional-based difficulties in interpersonal relationships. Interpersonal difficulties, if secondary to anything, are secondary to how the person has come to view the self and others, how those views are acted on, and the resultant unsatisfactory payoffs in the sense of personal and social well-being. As is characteristic of the primary life-enhancing level, the expression of these difficulties may vary from philosophical existential concerns and the desire for alternative life-styles to severely disruptive perceptual difficulties that require the reestablishment of concrete links to an inescapable reality. For persons in any of these circumstances, the goals are (1) to prevent disabling complications of a long-term nature stemming from the social/emotional difficulties to which patients are already responsive when they seek help and (2) to explore alternative coping strategies from which the patient may choose in seeking a more self-satisfying and socially productive way of life.

Secondary Life-Enhancing Functions

In secondary life-enhancing situations, there is a somewhat different focus than discussed above. The concern in these situations is for the social/emotional impact on patients and their families secondary to the experience of disease, injury, drugs, or developmental deviation. In contrast to primary life-enhancing situations, advocates in secondary situations must take into account these concrete organic factors and do something about them simultaneously with focusing on their effects on a person's highly personal frame of reference.

Patients requiring assistance with a secondary life-enhancing focus are most frequently found in life-sustaining settings. Several different sets of circumstances may be found to be directly contributing to the patient's behavioral difficulties:

1. A definitive form of brain disease, injury, or intoxication that interferes with perceptual or motor function or both
2. Development of behaviors that frighten, mystify, or frustrate the patient, family, and health-care advocates subsequent to initial evaluation of disease or trauma
3. Serious perceptual and comprehension disabilities stemming from congenital, prenatal, and early postnatal trauma or deprivation

Direct influence of disease, injury, or drugs   Patients may experience social/ emotional problems secondary to disease, injury, or drugs; for example, they may be found to have some form of cerebral disease (such as brain tumor), stroke, damage secondary to advanced syphilis or chronic alcohol ingestion, or acute or chronic dysfunction after ingestion of hallucinatory drugs.[19,20]

Health-care advocates working with these patients must have all the interpersonal skills to be able to assist the patient in reestablishing anchors with reality. In addition, however, advocates also have the tools of science and technology on their side. Although some patients may have permanent dysfunction subsequent to the cerebral insult, there are therapeutic measures that can be brought immediately to bear that may reduce progression of the process and relieve some of the source of the behavioral difficulty.

Psychologically, such situations as these are somewhat easier for health-care advocates and the family to "make sense out of." Unlike some of the primary life-enhancing situations discussed previously, the advocate, patient, and family have the benefit of being able to say, "This behavior is a result of *that* having happened." The influence of a tumor or a toxin can be more easily visualized than the influence of social dynamics and anxiety on behavioral function. Feelings of guilt in response to the role that familial dynamics play in certain anxiety reactions are not so prevalent in these situations. This fact contributes to a less emotionally loaded process in working with patients and their relatives. Fear of pitching in and helping is seen less frequently in family members when they neither perceive nor are led to believe that they, in some subtle or straightforward way, have contributed to the problem. On the other hand, health-care advocates need to be sensitive to circumstances in which organic conditions might be associated with a high degree of guilt—for example, when brain injury has resulted from an accident or assault in which a family member has been involved, inappropriate responsibility taking for the drinking problem of the patient by the spouse, and drug overdosage in a suicidal attempt.

Even though more concrete causes are operating in these kinds of life-enhancing situations, health-care advocates must nonetheless explore with the patient or family the personal characteristics of the patient in the present or prior to the damaging circumstances. A person's previous personal style substantially influences the specific form or intensity of behavioral expression, even though there is a precipitating physical cause. Knowing something of the patient's previous frame of reference gives the advocate some beginning structure within which the patient's seemingly bizarre reactions can be understood.

CASE IN POINT

Ralph was admitted to the hospital after slipping in the shower and suffering a moderate concussion. Physically, he seemed to be progressing well, but his overt behavior was causing concern. He could not remember where he laid things down. He would verge on panic and insist that the staff tell him where his things were. At times he waxed into a paranoid style, suggesting that someone had taken things from him.

When these observations were discussed with Ralph, he replied that he had "simply never been like this before." A conference with his wife revealed a different perception, however. She explained that, for all their married life, Ralph had relied on her to have everything in place. She described him as "not even able to find his clean socks if they weren't on the same side of the drawer." She was less concerned about his behavior than was the staff. She found it "a little extreme" at that time but assured the staff that he would probably do better when he got home.

Temporary cerebral disruption together with unfamiliar surroundings had exaggerated his dependent style of relying on others to keep his life in order. Ralph did do better at home.

As this case suggests, all patients with various acute and chronic brain dysfunctions are able to organize themselves better and to make sense out of their disturbed perceptions when their immediate life space is highly structured. The structuring of external reality seems to be a necessary precursor to the gradual regaining of more organized internal perceptual structure. This pattern is similarly observed in normal early childhood development.[21] The health-care advocate who is sensitive to the patient's difficulty with memory, orientation to time and space, and making appropriate judgments will work with the staff or family to develop a helpful, structured social milieu. The advocate recognizes that such structuring is not intended to increase dependency in the patient. On the contrary, in such a structured environment tailored to the individual patient's needs, independent functions can be more easily grappled with by the patient. With increasing gains in responsibility taking and autonomous function, less structure is required. The family's or patient's perception of this structure being "childlike" can be prevented by sharing along the way the reasons and the goals for the process. Even though a patient may appear unable to understand such logic because of verbal and motoric difficulties, the experienced health-care advocate is sensitive to the fact that a patient may be more able to process verbal input than to express verbal output.

In working with patients who have used consciousness-altering drugs heavily, health-care advocates need to be particularly aware of the unique "gapping" in memory function or "flashbacks," which may persist for a lengthy period of time. Anxiety can be high for these patients as they attempt to reengage with academic functions or an occupation requiring symbol sequencing, as demanded in reading and mathematical computations. Anyone attempting to provide a therapeutic social milieu for young adults who have spent the majority of their adolescent years "into drugs" also should keep in mind that many of the usual developmental tasks of these years may have been sketchily experienced. Both in an individual interpersonal helping relationship or social-group process, such patients may have to be assisted in grappling with adolescent problems for the first time.

Our clinical experience with youthful chronic marijuana smokers coincides with what is now being described in the popular magazines as the pot-induced personality profile—a complex of behaviors that is similar to the organic brain syndrome seen in a geriatric popoulation. Even when the health-care advocate enlists the cooperation of the young patient to discontinue marijuana use, both must be prepared to "wait out" the lengthy period of time for the cannabinoids to metabolize. In the meantime, the knowledgable advocate must patiently support the person through hopefully diminishing impaired judgment, short attention span, low frustration tolerance, resistance to authority, and periodic stubborn denial that anything is at all "out of kilter" or that they need ongoing help. On the outpatient basis, we have found that very frequent, scheduled brief contacts focused on structured and attainable short-term goals are more effective than open-ended "talk sessions" that last more than a half hour.

Because health-care workers are so used to looking for causes of patients' difficulties in the area of "what they have brought with them," it is easy to become insensitive to what the "cure" might be contributing to the behavior problem. As has been reviewed throughout the text, interpersonal and setting variables can affect a patient's behavior, but so also can such things as medications that the patient is receiving as treatment within the setting. Because of the enormous variety of drugs that are known to have behavioral side effects and the infinite number of patients who respond differentially, the subject is impossible to cover here. However, the perceptive health-care advocate will always act to rule out prescribed-drug reactions immediately when confronted with precipitous *or* gradual changes in the patient's mood or perceptual organization abilities.

Indirect influence of disease and injury   Another group of patients commonly requiring a secondary life-enhancing focus are those who have sought care for disease or injury that in itself has no direct relationship to cerebral dysfunction. However, the stress impact of the event or the treatment measures taken can precipitate behaviors that frighten, mystify, and frustrate those around them.[22]

As discussed previously concerning life-saving and life-sustaining situations, the meaning that a life-threatening event or physically disfiguring condition has for a patient is critical to understand. Many of the precipitous episodes of high anxiety, often bordering on psychosis, can be avoided by sensitively listening to the patient and providing the interpersonal opportunity for working the anxiety through.

In addition, health-care advocates need to be aware that concern for a patient's full or adaptive recovery often requires actions that extend beyond the walls of the inpatient setting. This is particularly evident with patients who, on discharge, have to face extraordinarily long periods of recuperation at home or social readjustments in the face of physical incapacities.

CASE IN POINT

One afternoon two years ago, Trina and Desiree decided to ride on Trina's bike. Trina, age 8, knew she was breaking a family ground rule to not ride double on the bike, but asked her 4-year-old sister nonetheless and Desiree complied.

While riding in front of their home, they were struck by a car. Trina, who sustained a broken pelvis and a minor head injury, became conscious before the rescue helicopter came, thus remembering the life-saving events. Desiree was initially not to be found when the helpers first came to the scene—her small body was wrapped up under the chassis of the car. She did not recall anything of the accident or postaccident events until she awoke in a hospital bed several doors down from her sister.

Trina's physical recuperation was uneventful. Upon discharge from the hospital, her only remaining scar was on her heel, where a piece of embedded tennis shoe had had to be removed. Psychologically, however, Trina suffered both immediate and chronic guilt—for breaking a parental ground rule and from feeling responsible for her sister's very serious leg injuries, which would impair and scar her for life. While in the emergency room and in the hospital ward, Trina was obsessed with concerns for her sister's safety. Not until she and her sister were placed in the same room would she accept her ever-present parents' verbal assurances. Desiree, on the other hand, experienced loneliness whenever a parent was not present; often she was irritable, quite the contrary to her usual cheerful, vivacious self. Both experienced bad dreams.

At the time of discharge, it appeared that the following would be the medical concerns of the future: Desiree would require periodic surgery on her legs for grafting and stabilization of the right knee joint; Trina would have no ongoing difficulty, even though one of the doctors intimated that she might have trouble in her childbearing years as a result of her broken pelvis.

Upon return home, the bad dreams stopped. Trina's anxiety in relation to the accident expressed itself for a brief period during times she walked to and from school, when she would fall to the ground if a car came too close or she heard squealing brakes. Her brother's walking her to and from school for a while seemed to help her cope. As the months ensued, leaving the life-saving and life-sustaining functions of helpers behind, medical bills and legal expenses accumulated; settlement about the accident was difficult and into litigation. A troubled marriage between the parents was precipitated into divorce.

Trina, now 10 years old, and Desiree, now 6 years old, are strikingly different in their responses to the accident and resultant injuries. Trina is quiet, almost sullen, still taking over-responsibility for what happened, the resolution of her guilt hampered by ongoing legal depositions and court continuances keeping the memories ever alive. As well, Desiree's ever-present scars and difficulty in running keep the fact of the accident in constant reminder. Desiree, on the other hand, has returned to being her cheerful self, having the utmost faith that the doctors are going to make her legs better and beautiful someday. The fact that this will not happen is known to all of the family except her. They do not wish to confront her with that brutal fact and all dread the day when the permanence of her disfigurement intrudes on her self-concept and self-esteem. This year in school, however, Desiree refuses to wear skirts and insists on slacks so the other children will not call her "chicken legs," as they did the year before. This year, the parents did not tell the teacher about the accident so that "it would not become an issue." Whereas Desiree yet does not experience the depressive postaccident reaction as does her older sister, they both share similar anger and depression over their parents' divorce. Depression and anger about what has happened, and is yet to be faced by their daughters as they grow into young women, plague both parents—presently their common bond of emotion. Both parents are over the phase of irrationally blaming each other. They are focused, as are the children, in getting the court business over and settled so they can satisfy their need for retribution of their many losses and get on with the task of both forgetting and preparing for the psychological crises that yet lie ahead. Close follow-up of this family after hospital discharge was obviously imperative, although such follow-up frequently does not happen.

In this case, a considerable life-enhancing helping function is still necessary now and over time; had it begun earlier and been coordinated from the central base of the original caregivers, the overall losses may not have been as great or at least not so deeply felt. At best, an already troubled marriage may perhaps have found the necessary assistance to utilize the crisis as a way to develop a more healthy organization rather than having the crisis lead to permanent disorganization.

Public-health nurse follow-up is a resource of traditional value when ongoing medications, treatments, and psychological support are at issue. Ideally, more effective life-enhancing care is possible if a continuity-of-health-care advocate begins an interpersonally focused discharge process with the patient in the inpatient setting and maintains the interpersonal relationship within the home. Allowing an inpatient open awareness to the adjustments still ahead but simultaneously providing continuity of support prevents two phenomena frequently seen: (1) anxiety reactions of the patient prior to discharge that often are expressed as suddenly "getting worse," and (2) depressive reactions of the patient after discharge—reactions in response not only to loss of function but also to the loss of 24-hour support.

The influence of developmental deviation   Developmental deviation is a broad concept. It is used to describe a variety of conditions stemming from genetic, prenatal, postnatal, and early childhood circumstances that lead to a level of ability at deviance with normal growth and function. The deviation may manifest itself in fine and gross motor function, cerebral neural deficits, or congenital organ defects. Any one or more of these effects may be manifest in the child or adult, depending on the causative factors—for example, genetic patterning, metabolic imbalances, nutritional deficiencies in the prenatal and postnatal periods, or birth anoxia or trauma. Intellectual retardation may be an interacting difficulty, depending on the site and extent of cerebral damage.

Health-care advocates have a long tradition in the evaluation and diagnosis of infants and children with these difficulties. However, only within the recent past have health-care advocates been expected to become more actively involved in (1) developing remedial programs for these children and (2) assisting parents to develop more life-enhancing family interaction that provides for the inclusion of the child.

This is a complex field and worthy of the many fine texts that have been written concerning the humanistic approaches required.[23,24] It is a field of endeavor that requires a strong base in child development and early detection know-how, as well as solid interpersonal skills; that is, the helping process requires the ability to be openly factual and the skill to convey the available facts to parents in a way that allows them understanding and avenues by which they can act helpfully in their child's behalf.

Health-care settings in which advocates commonly interact with the parents of a child with a developmental deviation or with the child, or with both are obstetrical units, pediatric outpatient offices, evaluation clinics for children, pediatric inpatient units, and institutions for the retarded. Since the recent advent of home-care "normalization" programs, in contrast to institutionalization, increasing numbers of older children and young adults with developmental deviations will be experienced within general health-care settings.

Social/emotional difficulties that the health-care advocate might expect to encounter most often in working with parents and their children with developmental difficulties are feelings of guilt and responsibility for causation, marital discord, child abuse and neglect, and adjustment reactions of the child as influenced by overprotection, rejection, inability of parents to provide an appropriate social milieu, or overestimations or underestimations of the child's developmental ability.

Using the "Behavioral Expert"

Evaluation assistance   One of the purposes of this text has been to provide health-care workers some ways of evaluating their work situations so that they can better understand their patients and themselves. Through a framework for analysis and case-in-point examples, it is hoped that advocates increasingly appreciate that there are things that they can do in evaluation before engaging the behavioral expert to come in and solve the mystery. At the same time, however, we have emphasized that when health-care advocates sense that a situation is taking them over their head, so to speak, they call for help.

When advocates do call for assistance, the behavioral specialist may use a consultation approach with the health-care advocate or total staff concerned with the patient's care. Sometimes the specialist may find it necessary to relate directly to the patient or family for the increased data that the situation may require. Depending on the individual circumstance, the specialist, if a clinical psychologist, may wish to utilize formal testing procedures.

From time to time, an advocate may wish to refer the patient directly for testing services. In making an appropriate and maximally useful referral, the advocate might keep a number of things in mind. First, psychological tests are not magic. Essentially, they are instruments that require that responses be elicited from the patient in systematic and more or less structured ways.[25] Subsequently, these responses are compared to standardized norms, that is, the responses of a group of other persons who have taken the tests previously. The degree or kind of deviation from the responses of this group of "normal" other people provides a measure from which to infer the degree of pathology or the abilities of the patient in the face of certain tasks.

However, the patient's responses to the test stimuli—whether they be questions, problems to solve, pictures, or designs—are interpreted by the clinician within the total context of the testing situation; that is, the clinician attends not only to the number and quality of the test responses but also to the patient's "style" in approaching tasks. Conversational, interpersonal behavior during the testing session is also utilized by the clinician as valuable data. Thus, interpretation of a testing situation provides a more composite, meaningful picture of the patient than would be obtained simply from a set of numerical scores. If there is any magic in psychological testing, it lies in the combined integrating and interpersonal abilities that reside within the clinician, not in the tests per se.

Second, psychological testing is an expensive enterprise with regard to time and should be selectively requested. Generally, it is indicated when there is no other way to elicit the information that the advocate wishes to obtain. For example, the advocate may sense that the patient is experiencing a thought disorder but be unsure of the exact nature of the perceptual distortion. Some patients consciously and unconsciously guard their thought processes, and conversationally it may be difficult to understand fully the gaps or distortions; or the advocate may suspect that the patient's behavior reflects fairly deep-seated social/emotional conflict but finds the patient unable to talk openly about the anxiety. Sometimes, there is a question about the full range of the patient's intellectual ability and how this ability might be affected by a disease process or trauma. In the rehabilitative phases of care, requests for a profile of a patient's occupational interests and abilities may be made.

Third, to the extent that advocates can specifically and comprehensively state what they want to know, the psychologist can provide more realistic and useful feedback. Psychologists are generally disconcerted when a simple diagnostic category is asked for in the test request. Similarly it is not enough to request that the testing provide only etiological statements; for example, "Tell me whether the patient is organic." Psychologists view tests as but one set of tools in developing a comprehensive picture of the patient as an integrated being. As Korchin and Schuldberg states: "Clinical diagnosis, in the restricted sense, may be included, but more usually the intent is description and prediction toward the ends of planning, executing, and evaluating therapeutic interventions, and predicting future behavior."[26]

Notes about psychotherapy   Advocates not only reach out for the behavioral expert to assist in evaluation, they also often refer the patient for psychotherapy. Most often, referral occurs when the advocate's time or skill level is not adequate to the patient's need.

Volumes have been written about the theory and practice of psychotherapy that can be reviewed for an in-depth understanding. However, health-care advocates should be aware of several essential aspects of this sometimes mysterious process.[27] Essentially, psychotherapy is a defined relationship between the helper and the patient or a group of patients. It involves an interpersonal process, a fact that holds true regardless of the different theoretical orientations and terminology utilized in understanding what is going on with the patient or the therapist or the interaction between the two of them. It is a process that concerns itself with the patient's struggle to derive fulfilling meaning and more effective ways to become a part of the mainstream of life. The process may have a series of goals as patients struggle with what they want to experience for themselves in the outside world; yet, the ultimate goal of psychotherapy involves the following, in Taft's words:

> To conquer the problem of living then, insofar as this is possible, is to learn to accept it as a process, to achieve a freedom and a balance which permits the shattering of any particular wholeness, without mistaking it for total disruption and finds in the break-up of the old, not merely loss but the material for new creation.[28]

The many ways that we have suggested that health-care advocates may effect a humanistic environment and relate more therapeutically to patients within the health-care milieu are derived from the principles that make psychotherapy a helpful process. Therefore, at this point, you should have a fairly good grasp of the notion that what goes on between patient and helper in a variety of settings and encounters also goes on within formal psychotherapy.

What makes formal psychotherapy different from what we have suggested that advocates might do in their everyday work? Structurally, it is different. It involves the therapist's commitment to a special time and place to which the patient can come, having the reassurance that the therapist will be there for a dependable period of time. This structure allows a microcosm of experience in which the patient can try out the expression of old fears simultaneously with exploring new awareness of thought, feeling, and actions. Trying to extract interpersonal understanding "on the run" or in bits and pieces within the busy health-care setting or within a harried home-based environment is energy depleting for some persons. The structure of the psychotherapeutic hour, together with its commitment to dependability, allows an in-depth focus on the patient's central concerns in life.

The patient is the one who ultimately decides what the definition of help is to be. Therefore, psychotherapy as just described may not be what the patient wants, even though that might seem to be indicated. Psychotherapy does not insist or demand that a patient come for the help. It is not something done "to" people. If it is ethically and effectively practiced, it is done *with* people, with a critical starting point being the patient's desire to have the experience.

Tertiary Life-Enhancing Functions

Today, there is a pendulum swing to tear down or empty our institutions that have provided residential care for those with social/emotional problems, chronic brain disease, and developmental disabilities.[29] *Normalization* is now a vogue term. For example, parents who but a few years ago were being counseled long and hard concerning institutionalizing their child are now being counseled concerning the benefits that can ensue if the child is returned home and attends a community-based day-center program. Normalization is not a new approach. The mental-health field has been attempting this home-based noninstitutional shift for some years. However, many patients, long alienated from family ties, have only moved as far as a nursing home or inner-city boarding homes. Finding appropriate and high-quality residential settings for some children and adults is now a difficult task. We are not so sure that it should be a difficult process and are suspicious of the motives for the decline in institutional emphasis.

Our major concern lies with past experience with institutional settings and the struggles that have occurred in bringing them in line with even the most basic definition of humane care. We wonder if the present swing to normalization and home-based programs has come about because it is indeed good for all patients, or because legislators and professionals have failed to do something about the chronic inability of our culture to develop group living experiences that are humane and life enhancing.

We also ponder, in view of the swing toward community normalization, what the plight will be for those institutions that are left. It is always hard to be on the short end of the financial stick when the "in" programs are receiving the lion's share. The public may also come to believe that such institutions no longer exist, thus eroding the public concern and support so hard fought for in the past 30 years; but it is not just the public who lose sight and touch with institutions. We have educated a generation of young professionals who have never been inside an institution that cares for human beings—young or old—beyond inner-city hospital or clinic walls.

Our philosophy has always supported the belief that a community and family base is the best on which to nurture and experience the most humane and enhancing life throughout the life cycle of health, illness, existential struggles, aging, and death; but that is an ideal. The real world requires at present and will in the future some persons of all ages to be cared for in sites other than home and the normal mainstream of the community. What can health-care advocates do about that?

Tertiary functions in the life-enhancing dimension of care involve what health-care advocates can do to prevent dehumanizing practices in residential care giving.[30] Following is a list of specific activities that are believed to be needed in taking the first step—increasing one's awareness of the problem:

1. *Familiarize yourself with your local and state residential centers, hospitals, and nursing homes.* Private settings are more difficult to get into for observation than public institutions. Persons working in any of these settings will be less rejecting and threatened by your wanting to visit if you do it in the context of an educational field trip with instructors going along. Many of them have never been inside some of these settings either. However, the clearest picture of what actually goes on and how patients are treated can best be experienced by doing volunteer work within the walls. Institutions have a way of putting their best foot forward for visitors.
2. *Find out how much money is being given to public-supported institutions for the number of patients for whom they provide care, as contrasted with community programs. Attempt to determine how within the institutions the money is actually being spent.* To request examination of how public tax monies are spent by our agencies and institutions is supposedly a taxpayer's privilege; yet, resistance will probably be met. Observe carefully the kind of resistance that you are confronted with and from whom it comes. Appraisal of fund utilization is often difficult to obtain, even when one believes oneself to be in an administrative position that would give free access to such data. Following is a case in point from our own experience in which resistance was met in finding out how money was actually being spent in a large mental hospital.

CASE IN POINT

A request came through the central office for approval of the development of a practical nursing program at a large state mental hospital. To develop this program, considerable nursing staff monies would have to be moved from direct patient care to the educational division. The request was responded to with a plan first to appraise the total hospital budget to learn how funds were being utilized.

From a review of the formal line-item budget, it initially appeared that actualizing the hypothesized benefits from the presence of students and educational training might be feasible; yet, observations of the hospital milieu and comments from discussions with attendant and staff-level nurses suggested that something was askew. Closer examination of vouchers and actual use of line-item funds was requested. This request stimulated intense resistance at the hospital level.

With regard to the nursing budget, formal administrative pressure was required to obtain the necessary data. Several administrative nursing personnel were found to be utilizing the bulk of the presently allotted nursing education money to attend national conferences. Staff at the front lines of patient care derived no in-service education benefit from these expenditures. Other funds line-itemed for direct patient comfort (e.g., clothing and bed linen) were found to be frequently "in excess" and to have been transferred into administrative function; yet, a survey of the wards indicated that, at that moment, the hospital was 3,000 sheets short of what was necessary to provide patients with clean linen once each week.

Simultaneously, other divisions of the hospital were asked to begin a formal permission procedure for expenditures over $100. This request was to allow a time-limited survey on priorities being used. The irony of the hospital's priorities showed itself. In the face of shortages of clothing and sheets, the farm division requested several thousand dollars for hospital staff to accompany their prize-winning Hereford cattle to the state fair.

Both the nursing-education program request and the cattle-entourage request were denied. Both divisions were asked to reevaluate their program priorities in light of an overriding goal of humanistic care for patients. The director of nurses resigned in a huff.

---

3. *Request instructors to assist you in developing a group seminar concerning the design and maintenance of life space for patients.* In part, students experience their clinical work in a peripheral way; that is, the setting that houses patients is there when students come for their practicum experience and is there when they leave. Rarely is the opportunity available both to participate in and feel responsible for maintaining the underlying framework of the patients' life space. Following is a problem situation and a suggested task that can be the central focus of a seminar.[31]

"20 ROW" PROBLEM

The "20 Row" of buildings lay at the east end of a large state mental hospital. Each building was identical, housing 95 patients each. Patients were segregated into a men's and women's building. Ages of the patients ranged from 49 to 74 years. Patient records as to original diagnosis and entry problem were unavailable within the buildings but could be obtained from central administration microfilm. All patients had been hospitalized in these buildings or other divisions of the hospital for at least five years. All were ambulatory and wearing state-hospital clothes.

The buildings provided the space of a typical high school gymnasium. Each was divided in half by a full wall. On one side of each building were 95 beds, so close together that patients had to get in over the ends; beds were unmarked with names. No storage for individual goods was provided. At the end of the bedroom was a large linen closet from which clothing and linen were dispensed. On the other side of the wall were 95 rocking chairs and an eating area at one end. Enough tables and chairs were provided for approximately 25 patients at a time to eat in shifts. At the opposite end were an enclosed nursing station and several offices for professional personnel.

The attendant staff was comprised of four persons on day, two on evening, and one on night shift. A registered nurse made rounds once each shift and was available by phone in an emergency. A psychiatrist was assigned to an entire hospital division of which 20 Row was a part. Her offices were elsewhere. A psychologist and social worker were similarly assigned to the buildings. These personnel were rarely, if ever, seen by the attendant staff. Once each week, maintenance personnel came by to assist attendants to "scrub the place down," a procedure that consisted of stripping beds and hosing down each side. On the east side of the hospital grounds, the smell of urine always heralded one's approach to 20 Row.

Hypothesize that the attendants from 20 Row have approached you for a definite plan in bringing more humane care to these patients. Available to you are the following options that place limits on the possible solutions to the problem. Take each option, beginning with the level 0, and work each one through in "think tank" fashion:

Level 0 option. You have only the request of the attendants and the blessings of the supervising nurse to "do anything." No money is available. Specific feedback from the division psychiatrist, social worker, and psychologist indicates that they do not wish to be involved.

Level I option. You have the request of the attendants plus the willingness of the professional peripheral staff to "sit down and talk about what we might be able to do." You still do not have any money to spend.

Level II option. You have the request of the attendants, the support of the assigned peripheral staff, and the blessings of the central administration to cooperate in anything that you believe would be the most effective plan. Funds will be forthcoming if the budget proposal is "reasonable" in meeting a basic level of humane care more life-enhancing and self-satisfying than the patients have been experiencing.

At the conclusion of this think-tank experiment, evaluate just how much "training" is actually required to develop humane, life-enhancing spaces for human beings, whatever their problems.

At this juncture it should be apparent that the key to carrying out tertiary life-enhancing functions lies within health-care workers themselves. If this text has had any meaning at all, the health-care worker is aware that, between common sense, a fine evaluative ability carried around in one's head, and a humanistic sensitivity carried in one's total being, no one should have to be told how to respect human dignity and what to do about it.

Summary

Life-enhancing functions are in some measure a part of every helping contact. However, in certain situations, a more specific function can be clearly delineated and consciously applied. These situations are those in which the patients' problems are (1) primarly related to social/emotional difficulties in living and are not disease related and (2) secondary to bodily insults and deviation in normal physiological development.

In primary life-enhancing functions, almost total reliance is placed on the interpersonal relationship and the person of the helper as the critical therapeutic force. Within secondary life-enhancing situations, no less importance is given to the interpersonal process in helping. However, integrated within secondary situations must be a high degree of knowledge as to organic cerebral dysfunction and the psychological effects of threats to physical survival, physical disfigurement, and incapacitation.

The broadest level of the life-enhancing dimension is that of tertiary functions— that is, those commonsense behaviors that go into the development of humane group living experiences for patients needing, or being left to, residential care. Significant to this process are those behaviors in which health-care advocates must engage with administrators and "fundholders" to ensure living environments that are conducive to patients' maintaining and regaining socially productive and self-satisfying interpersonal skills.

Health-care workers inclined to work in life-enhancing settings will have no easy task, albeit a rewarding one. With the exception of those settings with a secondary focus, there is little well-defined structural evidence for cause and little technology available for cure. Most often, the relationship is all. Thus, it behooves the health-care advocate to become a serious student of self as well as others.

Working in life-enhancing situations requires a high degree of trust in oneself and the essential integrity and potential of the patient. At times this faith is difficult, particularly when patients seem to resist knowing themselves or being known by others. At other times, this faith seems difficult as one ponders whether one is "old enough" to struggle with the patient through the existential crises that neither have been experienced for oneself nor are desirable destinies to consider as one's own.

However, struggling with another to figure out life-enhancing goals and experiences to reach those goals can be a maturing, broadening adventure. Perhaps in no other health-care situations can one continue to learn that pain does not come just from disease or injury and joy does not emerge simply from quantities of experience and material things. As a dynamic helping process ensues between two persons, one increasingly appreciates the value of quality humanistic relationships and how barren everyone is without them.

Life-enhancing experiences have high utilization as situations in which beginning helpers can struggle to grow and try out their personhood. Within an advocacy model of humanistic helping, no student or instructor should fear that patients are at the mercy of another—novice though one may be. As we will review in Chapter 12, students are found to fear interpersonal involvement less than the feeling of distance from where they sensitively perceive involvement is needed.

REFERENCE NOTES

1. Francine Sobey, *The Non-Professional Revolution in Mental Health* (New York: Columbia University Press, 1970).
2. See Rosenhan's study in which "pseudopatients" (he and seven other "sane" professionals) get themselves admitted to 12 different mental hospitals in the United States by alleging "schizo-

phrenic" symptoms. None was detected as sane postadmission after they dropped their facade—except by patients. On discharge, all the pseudopatients except one were labeled as having "schizophrenia in remission." D. L. Rosenhan, "On Being Sane in Insane Places," *Science* 79 (19 January 1973): 250–58.

3. Thomas Szasz, *The Myth of Mental Illness: Foundations of a Theory of Mental Illness* (New York: Harper & Row, 1963).

4. The "DSM III" is common jargon in the medical profession and refers to *The Diagnostic and Statistical Manual of Disorders*, 3rd ed. (Washington, D.C.: American Psychiatric Association, 1980). It would be well to familiarize oneself thoroughly with this manual to appreciate the frame of reference about behavior that psychiatrists are using when they discuss "abnormal behavior" of adults and children. All of the health-insurance companies providing mental-health coverage require the service provider to diagnostically categorize patients according to the criteria in this manual.

5. Thomas H. Holmes and Richard H. Rahe, "The Social Readjustment Rating Scale," *Journal of Psychosomatic Research* 11 (1967): 213–18. Within this easily read and highly significant article is the social-readjustment-rating questionnaire, which can be a valuable sensitization guide to doing interviews with patients in both life-sustaining and life-enhancing settings. Holmes and Rahe's work says essentially what Selye's stress theory says: stressors come in many forms, many of them seemingly positive; for example, change, whether positive or negative, creates a higher stress profile. This theory correlates with the old developmental hypothesis that any change, even in the direction of positive growth, creates a certain amount of anxiety.

6. Unless health-care advocates have obtained formal, in-depth education beyond their regular curriculum, it is not recommended that they attempt to counsel people concerning sexual dysfunction. Traditional professional health-care education adequately teaches anatomy, the physiology of conception and fetal development, and disease processes of the reproductive system. However, most health-care workers know only as much about the dynamic interrelationship of physiological and social/emotional behavior in sexual experience as they have learned in their own personal growth and development. An outstanding text as a starting point in enhancing both personal and professional learning is Helen Singer Kaplan, *The Illustrated Manual of Sex Therapy* (New York: Quadrangle/New York Times, 1975).

7. Readers might enjoy Carl R. Rogers, *Becoming Partners: Marriage and Its Alternatives* (New York: Delacorte Press, 1972). For marrieds or unmarrieds, see William H. Masters and Virginia E. Johnson, *The Pleasure Bond: A New Look at Sexuality and Commitment* (Boston: Little, Brown, 1974). This little-known book for the general public is required reading for many of our patients. The final chapter—"Commitment"—is one of the finest definitions of the concept you will find.

8. For a complete review of Seeman's alienation theory, see the work of Melvin Seeman as reported in *Mental Health Program Reports, 4* (Washington, D.C.: U.S. Department of Health, Education and Welfare, National Institute of Mental Health, January 1970), pp. 127–41.

9. Available throughout the country since the mid-1960s are a number of groups that focus on wellness and enhancement of function through increased awareness of self. They are not all the same in the processes that they use. The following references will provide an overview of the various approaches: Arthur Burton, *Encounter* (San Francisco: Jossey-Bass, 1970); Robert T. Golembiewski and Arthur Blumberg, eds., *Sensitivity Training and the Laboratory Approach* (Itasca, Ill.: F. E. Peacock, 1970); Muriel James and Dorothy Jongeward, *Born to Win: Transactional Analysis with Gestalt Experiments* (Reading, Mass.: Addison-Wesley, 1973) (a kind of do-it-yourself manual and fun to read); and John B. Enright, "Awareness Training in the Mental Health Professions," in *Gestalt Therapy Now*, eds. Joen Fagen and Irma Lee Shepherd (Palo Alto, Calif.: Science & Behavior Books, 1970), pp. 263–73.

10. Child abuse is a significant national problem on which attention is now highly focused. Every health-care worker should be aware particularly of its early detection and how to go about dealing with it in advocacy fashion. Check your local and state laws. Also, the following will give a comprehensive review of the field as it early evolved: Vincent J. Fontana, *Somewhere a Child Is Crying*

(New York: Macmillan, 1973); J. C. Holter and S. B. Friedman, "Child Abuse: Early Casefinding in the Emergency Department," *Pediatrics* 42 (1968): 128–38; C. Henry Kempe and R. E. Helfer, eds., *Helping the Battered Child and His Family* (Philadelphia: Lippincott, 1971); Aaron R. Rausen, ed., "Symposium on Child Abuse, Part II," *Pediatrics* 51 (suppl.) (April 1973). Copies of this supplement may be ordered from the American Academy for Pediatrics, 1801 Hinman Avenue, Evanston, Ill. 60204.

11. "The Battle over Abortion," *Time*, 6 April 1981, pp. 20–28. This article will provide a comprehensive summary of America's most volatile political and emotional issue. Abortion counseling is one of the most difficult and sensitive helping processes and is not for the uninformed novice in any of the helping professions.

12. A. B. Downing, ed., *Euthanasia and the Right to Death* (New York: Humanities Press, 1970).

13. One of the best overviews concerning depressive disorders and their effect on self-concept is to be found in Hagop S. Akiskal and William T. McKinney, Jr., "Depressive Disorders: Toward a Unified Hypothesis," *Science* 182 (5 October 1973): 20–29. This article is particularly relevant in that it demonstrates what we have been stressing throughout the text: that many factors, such as clinical, experimental, genetic, biochemical, and neurophysiological data, must be integrated for one to appreciate certain behavioral reactions. It has an impressive bibliography. Also see Carl P. Malmquist, "Depressions in Childhood and Adolescence; Part I," *New England Journal of Medicine* 284 (22 April 1971): 887–893; ibid., "Part II," *New England Journal of Medicine* 285 (29 April 1971): 955–61.

14. With the increased incidence of drug usage on high school and college campuses, many preclinical students have had experience with their peers' perceptual distortions and episodes of "freaking out." Such behavior is characterized by the panic that ensues from loss of perceptual anchors in the external world and an awareness of inner phenomena that is unfamiliar and frightening.

15. In addition to review of the DSM III descriptions of psychotic conditions (see note 4), see E. Robert Sinnett, Nancy Barnett, and Leon Rappoport, "Coping with Abnormal Behavior: A Social Psychological Approach," *Professional Psychology* 3 (Summer 1972): 222–30.

16. This study was conducted at the University of Missouri, School of Nursing, Department of Continuing Education, Columbia, Missouri.

17. Not all patients who are experiencing perceptually disordered behavior require inpatient care, but, whether inpatient or outpatient care is the focus, a fully effective helping process concerns itself with the majority of hours that the patient spends not involved in a one-to-one relationship with the primary caregiver.

18. Jay Haley, *Leaving Home: The Therapy of Disturbed Young People* (New York: McGraw-Hill, 1980), p. 20. This text is a must for anyone working with families, even when the identified patient is not as bizarre as the patients about whom Haley writes. His view is that the most therapeutic intervention with families is directed at the basic organizational structure. He states, "To overlook the organizational situation can lead to naive interventions which prevent change or even make matters worse. In fact, families will make use of a naive clinician to stabilize and avoid change" (p. 29). Also see Cloé Madanes, *Strategic Family Therapy* (San Francisco: Jossey-Bass, 1981). This book is an excellent reference when working with marital pairs and parent/child problems.

19. Although the following is an older reference, students cannot go wrong in reviewing the comprehensive collection of articles on organically induced behavioral disorders in Silvano Arieti, ed., *American Handbook of Psychiatry* (New York: Basic Books, 1959), vol. 2, pp. 1003–1316.

20. For a comprehensive reference on the full-spectrum of drug use, review James C. Coleman, *Abnormal Psychology and Modern Life*, 5th ed. (Glenview, Ill.: Scott, Foresman, 1976), chap. 12.

21. Those advocates working with persons experiencing highly disorganized thinking and motoric behavior would do well to review their child-development material. Much of this behavior is regressive to earlier levels of development that were appropriate to another chronological age and perhaps appropriate to nuclear-family organizational functioning in that patient's family. Clues to understanding can be obtained in using a developmental view. Likewise, therapeutic interventions based on a developmental framework assist in keeping interventions appropriate to the patient's current status.

22. Events that imply a close brush with death are highly stressful both during and after the fact. Be highly watchful in the immediate and long-term postoperative period of those patients who have experienced open-heart surgery. The high incidence of disruptive behavior in these situations is just now receiving documentation. Reactions may vary but tend to involve an agitated/depressive expression of existential conflict. Also keep in mind that many patients are not in the best of mental health when a sudden injury, assault, or physical disease occurs.

23. A particularly fine book that speaks simply and directly to the heart of the matter of needing to work humanistically with parents is Eugene T. McDonald, *Understand Those Feeling* (Pittsburgh: Stanwix House, 1962). See also the classic book of Alan O. Ross, *The Exceptional Child in the Family* (New York: Grune & Stratton, 1964).

24. See the following works edited by Jerome Hellmuth: *Exceptional Infant: Studies in Abnormalities*, vol. 2 (New York: Brunner/Mazel, 1970); *Cognitive Studies: Deficits in Cognition*, vol. 2 (Brunner/Mazel, 1971); and *Disadvantaged Child: Compensatory Education, A National Debate*, vol. 3 (Brunner/Mazel, 1970).

25. The following collection of classic references should provide a more than adequate overview of psychological testing: David Rappaport, Merton M. Gill, and Roy Shafer, *Diagnostic Psychological Testing* (New York: International Universities Press, 1968); Roy Shafer, *The Clinical Application of Psychological Tests* (New York: International Universities Press, 1951); Molly Harrower, "Differential Diagnosis," in *Handbook of Clinical Psychology*, ed. Benjamin Wolman (New York: McGraw-Hill, 1965), pp. 381–402; Gerald Solomons and Hope C. Solomons, "The Physician and Psychological Appraisal," *Developmental Medicine and Child Neurology* 15 (1973): 95–103; Irving B. Weiner and Robert W. Goldberg, "Psychological Testing of Children," *Pediatric Clinics of North America* 21 (February 1974): 175–94. All you ever wanted to know about the status of psychological testing—and much more—is found in a special issue of *The American Psychologist* 36, no. 10 (October 1981): "Testing: Concepts, Policy, Practice and Research."

26. Sheldon J. Korchin and David Schuldberg, "The Future of Clinical Assessment," *The American Psychologist* 36, no. 10 (October 1981): 1147. See also Michael D. Cox, Francisco X. Barrios, and Lance E. Trexler, "Psychological Evaluation," in *A Clinician's Manual of Mental Health Care: A Multidisciplinary Approach*, eds. H. Steven Moffic and George L. Adams (Menlo Park, Calif.: Addison-Wesley, 1982), chap. 8, pp. 76–90.

27. See Sheldon J. Korchin, *Modern Clinical Psychology* (New York: Basic Books, 1976). An excellent, easily read text that covers the various psychotherapeutic orientations, as well as the overall philosophies and functions of the clinical psychologist. As required reading in fully understanding the patient/therapist relationship, see Rachel T. Hare-Mustin et al., "Rights of Clients, Responsibilities of Therapists," *American Psychologist* 34, no. 1 (January 1979): 3–16. This article deals with four critical issues in the therapy relationship: providing patients with information in order to make informed decisions about therapy; therapy contracts; responding to challenges about therapist competence; and responding to patient complaints.

28. Jesse Taft, *The Dynamics of Therapy in a Controlled Relationship* (Gloucester, Mass.: Peter Smith, 1973), pp. 286–87. This is one of our favorite books. It speaks to "process" like no other book we know. We suggest that you first read the last chapter, "The Forces That Make for Therapy." Taft originally wrote this book in 1933. See also Anita J. Faatz, "Reflections on the Meaning of Process," *Social Casework* (October 1963): 458–63.

29. With the beginning of the community mental-health center movement in the early 1960s, many mental hospitals were renovated and cleared of chronic patients, who were returned to the community.

30. The following books are classic and highly relevant at this time: John Cumming and Elaine Cumming, *Ego and Milieu* (New York: Atherton Press, 1962); Milton Greenblatt, Daniel J. Levinson, and Richard H. Williams, eds.: *The Patient and the Mental Hospital* (New York: Free Press, 1957); Milton Greenblatt, Richard H. York, and Esther Lucille Brown, *From Custodial to Therapeutic Patient Care in Mental Hospitals* (New York: Russell Sage Foundation, 1955); National Institute of Mental Health, *Mental Health: Principles and Training Techniques in Nursing*

Home Care. DHEW Publication no. HSM 73-9046 (Washington, D.C.: Department of Health, Education and Welfare, 1972). For a text concerning the residential care of children, see Albert E. Trieschman, James K. Whittaker, and Larry K. Brendtro, *The Other 23 Hours* (Chicago: Aldine, 1969).

31. The "20 Row" problem is a real situation from our experience. It did have a solution at level 0.

Humanistic Advocacy as Burnout Prevention

Chapter 10

Existential Burnout:
A Social/Cultural Phenomenon

A recent editorial entitled "The Burnout of Almost Everyone"[1] pointed up the fact that the term *burnout* has become a very "in" concept in the 1980s. It is no longer a concept belonging to the professions, which originally used it to describe a complex job-related stress syndrome. The term *burnout* is now heard frequently in social conversation as simple jargon referring to low motivation, sour attitude, and a grim sense of the future. A weary-looking 8-year-old patient recently defined the idiom during his after-school psychotherapy appointment:

> Andrew: I'm burned out on trying to do good in school. And I'm real burned out on trying to keep my sister out of my room. I'd still rather be a dinosaur than a kid.
>
> Therapist: What's this "burned out" stuff? I don't see any burns on your outsides.
>
> Andrew: (Angrily) God, you dummy. Didn't you hear me? I'm tired, tired, tired of trying anything. Nothing ever turns out.
>
> Therapist: You sound real discouraged today.
>
> Andrew: What does "discouraged" mean?

To clarify some of the psychobabble surrounding burnout, in this unit we will discuss the concept from two viewpoints: (1) as a *social/cultural stress phenomenon* related to developmental and existential issues and (2) as a specific *job-related stress reaction* affecting helpers in health-care situations.

Many patients, seemingly well functioning socially and in the job market, sound a lot like Andrew when they initially seek help in life-enhancing situations. It is difficult to put your finger on what they are saying specifically. Something seems amiss for them in terms of hitting the mark between what they think they want in life, how to get it, and feeling good about the whole process, whether things pan out or not.

For many people, "burned out" describes a depressed state in response to finding out that, no matter how prolonged their adolescence, one day they must face the full demands of mature functioning. For others, "burned out" describes a feeling of despair in reaction to the realization that, for all their trying to carry out a responsible adult role, they never seem to get ahead or to where they believe they should be after all the effort.

As reviewed in Chapter 3, these situations reflect generalized existential anxiety about the meaning of life and must be understood within the context of our culture in the here and now. The following are a few contemporary cultural paradoxes that can be forerunners to social/cultural burnout symptoms:

One is supposed to "do good" in school so one can get into college and "do good" in college so one can get an exceptional job. Yet, college graduates today may obtain no better jobs than their lesser-educated peers unless they majored in one of the high technologies, such as computers, business accounting, or geology. What if these areas are genuinely not one's interest?

One is supposed to find a "good" mate, buy a nice home, establish a "good" family, and provide for them better than one's parents did for one. Yet, in many parts of the country, the divorce rate soars into the 50 percent bracket, and, in some schools, 70 percent of the children are from single-parent families.[2]

One is supposed to be patriotic and go off to war to serve one's country in the tradition of one's forefathers in the wars to keep America safe. Yet, the response to Vietnam veterans was nonsupportive of their effort or of their massive problems in readjustment. Meanwhile, America becomes increasingly unsafe from an outrageous civilian crime rate.

For many, the existential burnout syndrome occurs after trying and feeling that they have thoroughly failed. This reaction is commonly seen in situations of business failure, death of a loved one, divorce, or when a patient becomes informed of a serious illness and believes there is no hope. Also of great concern are those, particularly in the younger population, who experience "burnout-before-the-fact": the group that keeps so many options open to avoid failure at all costs that there is never a commitment to anything or anyone.

At the risk of overgeneralization, the majority of persons caught in these existential webs may be described as victims of culturally induced expectations about life's payoffs that did not evolve as they had fantasized. The emotional pain and turmoil in facing this reality is nonetheless very wrenching, for a less than desirable outcome of one's labors strikes at one's beliefs about what the world should be.

While the surface symptoms of existential burnout are similar to the job-related burnout syndrome, we see a significant underlying difference. In working with existentially burned-out people, it has been our experience that very close beneath the surface demeanor of despair and discouragement are exceptionally strong feelings of rage and resentment. With people suffering the job-related burnout response, anger and resentment are often the most difficult emotions to mobilize. Further, with those who are in existential burnout, their anger seems much more to derive from a view that life should really be like a sit-com TV drama and from the fact that no one person or "system" can be found to blame for their having been led down the primrose path. In contrast, burned out health-care workers tend to be overaware of the existential realities of life and often have lost even the most minimal capacity for anger at the pain of life and ultimate death.

In bringing a helping process to bear with people experiencing the despair and/or resentment of existential burnout, one must of course keep in mind each person's unique frame of reference. However, the helper is on fairly safe ground in assisting them to focus on and begin restructuring their attitudes and behavior in several general areas. These areas constitute key *psychological maintenance needs* that are necessary for the healthy survival of all human beings. Coleman summarizes these maintenance needs as (1) curiosity, understanding, order, and predictability; (2) adequacy, competence, and security; (3) love, belonging, and approval; (4) self-esteem, worth, and identity; (5) values, meaning, and hope.[3]

As we shall see in the final chapter, some students in the health-care field, as well as some seasoned professionals, have inadequately met these needs in everyday life, and their unmet needs are a part of their job-related burnout syndrome. Therefore, readers are encouraged to evaluate their own present attitudes and beliefs, keeping in mind that, to the extent that their own "existential house" is in order, they are less vulnerable to the subtle sabotaging effects of a burnout phenomenon arising within their professional setting.

The Need To Feel in Control

It is a fact that people cannot thoroughly control their life's experience or their ultimate destiny. Kopp describes this core reality succinctly:

> No matter what the species, no creature is in a position to control its own life. Of all life forms, only human beings additionally are able to be aware of their predicament. We are free to know that too soon we will die, and that after a short while no one will even remember our having lived.[4]

Yet, it is also a fact that human beings from early on try to be in control in face of the ultimate impossibility of achieving total control and, as adults, encourage their children to keep trying to do so. For example, long before a child's loss of innocence about the length of life and the meaning of death, one observes them working methodically to develop physical, emotional, and social functions that give them a sense of order, predictability, and control of their ever-increasing life space. As verbal functions become more expressive, we experience children asking questions at every turn to further understanding, to reduce the confusion of ambiguity, and thereby to reduce the stress of not knowing. In these early years, it is literally a matter of survival, for no one could endure the chaotic experience of a vast world of stimuli that could not be organized, understood, and manipulated in any way. Nor would the young achieve the essential ability to take care of themselves and others in future generations if they had not learned to control key functions and situations effectively. As Coleman says: "Unless we can see order and predictability in our environment, we cannot work out intelligent responses to it."[5]

Along the course of life, through the varying stages of childhood and adolescence in particular, there are minicrises in coming to terms with the awareness that things in life do not stay the same (including one's physical body) and that new modes of thinking and adapting must occur. Kopp states:

> The child needs to let go of a fairy-tale belief in how things work. The adolescent must abandon a romantically idealized vision of how things *should* work. Though at different levels, each must learn to make room for the role of chance.[6]

Hanging onto an adolescent percept of the world well into adulthood may seem like a lesser price to pay than the turmoil of growth in facing the world as it is with all its imperfections. However, as the growing body of literature concerning adult developmental crises proposes, somewhere along the line before death, the illusions of ultimate control are faced. At such points of existential crises, humans have two options: *regression* in despair to a state of no longer trying or *progression*, which consists of making the best of it by means of a realistic sense of mastery and responsibility within the limits present at the time. Obviously, the latter is the preferred option; in addition to the survival need that progression fulfills at the time, this approach to life also contributes to longevity.[7]

Against the backdrop of shared knowledge that the plans of humans are likely to be marred by chance events, the health-care advocate still can do much to assist people (patients and other health-care workers) who are immobilized in existential burnout. In general, one can begin to explore with people those areas in which they can either assume more control of their own lives or begin to take more charge of their experience.

For some people, new or increased information helps them gain an increased sense of mastery over their lives. This premise has been the basis of health education and preventive-medicine programs for years; that is, give people the necessary tools and knowledge so they can be more in charge of themselves in intelligent, health-preserving ways. As expressed in Chapter 3, knowledge is power, and sharing such power assists people in feeling a critical sense of being in control.

For others, new learning must include strategies for being more effective in life management, and these strategies must be practiced within a sustaining, supportive environment until the new approaches are integrated into the life style, and patients can carry them out on their own. Whether one attempts to help a patient or family dealing with a chronic physical illness or responds to the existentially stressed patient in a psychotherapeutic setting, the need for continuity until some sense of personal mastery is achieved is vital to the overall helping process.

The Need To Feel Adequate

A necessary extension of the feeling of being in control is the feeling that one is adequate, capable, and competent to handle everyday life situations. It is not enough simply to be "in control" unless one also feels that one is successful at it. Doggedly staying in control with gritted teeth, or "just hanging in there" is not equivalent to success in getting through life. Feeling adequate involves not having to question whether one is succeeding or failing on a minute-to-minute or day-to-day basis. People who present themselves as anxiously aware of their need to hang on and expend excessive energy on control issues become vulnerable to narrowed perceptions of the world and are precarious in their ability to ward off massive existential despair.

To a large degree, the roots of feelings of adequacy and success lie in the early phases of intellectual and social development, when feedback from significant others and the impact of social experiences forged our initial self-concepts. The sense of adequacy or inadequacy is often a perceptual phenomenon carried far beyond this initial experience. Some adults carry a childhood perceptual script of inadequacy throughout their lifetimes; other adults have corrective experiences as they integrate new feedback in their later development—for example, an interested employer or teacher; a supportive, loving mate; or a warm, humanistic health-care advocate.

Early feelings of inadequacy can also be overcome by developing competencies in areas in which one wants to achieve, whether these be social, emotional, or economic. This fact again highlights the importance of learning and "being in the know" so that one feels more secure (less negatively stressed) in relating. Clearly, the stress-reducing effect of feeling competent is seen in the psychotherapeutic encounter when one experiences the improved affect and self-concept of adolescents as they begin their first remunerative employment; when one teaches prenatal classes and later observes the aura of adequacy emanating from the more competent new mother and father; or when one teaches beginning health-care advocates and notes their increasing ease during patient interactions as their skill grows.

Selye[8] proposed that one of the critical experiences in life that seems to ward off deleterious effects of stress is the attitudinally based feeling that one is a success. Just as having a sense of mastery in life contributes to longevity, so do successful people tend to live longer. In addition to the characteristic of mastery that successful people possess, there are many accrued benefits of success through achievement that can be perceived as stress reducers. For example, persons who experience success with accompanying monetary resources and power positions are more likely to be able to take time off and to purchase convenience/relaxation items or services to reduce tension. Exceptions to this principle are the hard-driving, Type A executive personalities described by Friedman[9,10] who, in spite of outward success (prestige, power, money), unrelentlessly live each day as if every imperfection in oneself, others, and the world must be righted.

The discrepancy between the successful person who lives longer and is less negatively stressed and those who continue to push themselves and others in spite of "success" points to the perceptual/attitudinal nature of the concepts of adequacy, competence, and success. Our own beginning research concerning people's self-definitions of success also demonstrates this connection. At present such research is concerned only with those persons—regardless of age, sex, ethnicity, or social/economic achievement—who consider themselves "successful." For example, in selecting subjects to explore what determinants are being used in self-definition, we use only those persons who respond yes to the simple question "Do you consider yourself a success?"

Although the data are too rudimentary at this time for amplified results, it is interesting to note that "outside appearances" (for example, economic status, employment position, or social circle) have no predictive power as to how a person will answer the initial question. Further, we are noting a tendency with most of our self-defined "successes" to express a feeling of satisfaction with themselves, their jobs, and significant others in their life. This tendency is in contrast to persons whom we call the "yes-butters"—those who equivocate later in the interview and break down their perception of success into discrete segments of their life rather than perceiving themselves as a gestalt of success. Our preliminary research premise is that genuinely successful people achieve a personal sense of fulfillment for themselves in work *and* love *and* play. How they have achieved this sense of fulfillment and are able to sustain the perception is yet to be discovered.

The Need To Feel One Belongs

People who are alienated from a sense of belonging to family, job, or social-play group are excluded from opportunities for love, approval, and making productive contributions to others. The anxiety and/or boredom of loneliness, absence of job satisfaction, and self-doubts about personal meaning or worth are all negative stressors leading to the apathy and despair of interpersonal burnout. For some time it has been known that, in the early developmental years, the unfulfilled need to belong is a vital factor in anaclitic depression and in the capacity for an infant to survive. More recent statistics concerning the health and life span of single males at any age points to the positive effects on mental and physical health of feeling attached and having meaning to another or to a group.[11]

So far in our success research, we have found our subjects to be fairly autonomous individuals—that is, having a well-defined sense of self, having an appropriate sense of coming and going as they please, and not excessively needing others in order to feel comfortable. Yet, so far, none of the "successful" subjects has been found to be an alienated loner. In fact, a common expression among them is "we could not have done it alone," as they give examples of key people in their present environs or along the way whom they perceive as critical to their success. Many of their comments sound akin to Selye's third ingredient in his recipe for the best antidote to life's stresses: altruistic egoism—that is, "looking out for oneself by being necessary to others, and thus earning their goodwill."[12]

The fulfillment of the need to belong is always important to evaluate in understanding a person's job dissatisfaction and/or burnout syndrome. When a person looks to the job setting as a substitute for love, approval, and belonging that are absent in family and social life, they find that little resolution can occur strictly within that setting. The fact that employers realize how employees look to their work setting to meet such needs has resulted in extracurricular social programs, such as retreats, athletic programs, and other social opportunities. However, it has been our experience that such in-house programming can have a backlash effect, particularly when employees approach retirement and must begin to face the responsibility for filling their own social/emotional needs. In our employee-assistance counseling experience, what superficially may appear to be work-related burnout is often not the case, as is shown when social/emotional issues at home base become less stressed and more satisfying. Further, to avoid overdependency on the work situation, we encourage the development of social/emotional resources within the family and the community at large concurrently with the use of company programs.

The Need To Feel Worthy

Unless people become chronically wounded with respect to negative perceptions of themselves and others, one generally observes human beings of any age striving to keep intact their sense of self-esteem. All of the previously mentioned maintenance needs are absolutely critical if one is to feel good about oneself and perceive oneself as worthy of the love and respect of others.

Even though the antecedents of self-esteem lie in early childhood development, there comes a time in adult life when people become "their own good parent," so to speak. That means that people come to disregard unrealistic scripts about themselves and endeavor to structure and participate in esteem-raising enterprises. For most of us, this "self-parenting" requires a point in time when we give up the futile search for exclusively external sources of self-esteem.

Self-esteem is present as a very real sensation when one can say in one form or another:

Because I more realistically understand and can make more sense out of the chaos of my life space, I can rely upon myself to make less childlike, naive responses to situations. As I increasingly can trust my intellect and judgment, I feel more adequate, less helpless, and less at the direction (or mercy) of others. My awareness will assist me to evaluate what further competencies are needed by me, and I'll seek those so I feel more secure and less pressured by self-doubts. To accomplish this, I know I need other people to experience and to learn from. If my family or work situation does not provide me the sense of approval, belonging, or the potential for learning new competencies, I will appropriately seek out new experiences in which my needs might be more effectively met. In this seeking, I feel comfortable about myself, my risk taking, and my growth process, and I thereby positively respect the worth I can be to others as well as myself.

The Need To Feel Life Has Meaning

Menninger[13] describes values as guideposts against which one evaluates direction and risk taking. Values are imperative to the psychological-maintenance-need system, as they serve to clarify the purpose and meaning of life, in addition to their traditional function of setting standards of culturally acceptable behavior. Values may be seen in the acts or choices present in the repertoire of here-and-now behavior. A positive value system has features of optimism about the future, giving rise to a sense of hope.

People who are experiencing chronic existential burnout and no longer are flailing against the perceived injustice of life's imperfections often present themselves as flat, affectless, and planless. In the absence of evidence that they may be experiencing undetected physical illness, acute depression,[14] or chronic drug abuse, one must be prepared to take on the task of exploring their total outlook on life and encouraging them to find some hope and meaning from which to mobilize motivational energy. Coleman emphasizes the vital link between motivation and values, hope, and the meaning of life:

> Values, meaning and hope appear to act as catalysts; in their presence energy is mobilized, competencies are developed and used, and satisfactions are achieved. Without them life seems futile and the individual is bored and enervated.[15]

Conclusion

Helping those experiencing existential burnout is one of the most difficult helping situations the health-care advocate will encounter, as it requires the victim of burnout to discover or rediscover the self within. Such discovery needs support from others. Here is where the advocacy model can be useful, for it essentially stipulates that, instead of doing battle alone to gain one's ends in the world, one must enlist cooperation with yet full recognition that one may fail. In the patient/helper partnership that the advocacy model espouses, a model for cooperation is constructed as well as a support system in case goals are failed and help is needed by both to begin again.

REFERENCE NOTES

1. Lance Morrow, "The Burnout of Almost Everyone," *Time*, 21 September 1981, p. 84.
2. Judith S. Wallerstein and Joan Berlin Kelly, *Surviving the Breakup: How Children and Parents Cope with Divorce* (New York: Basic Books, 1980).
3. James C. Coleman, *Abnormal Psychology and Modern Life*, 5th ed. (Glenview, Ill.: Scott, Foresman, 1976), p. 101–104.
4. Sheldon Kopp, *An End to Innocence: Facing Life Without Illusions* (New York: Bantam Books, 1981), p. 167. Kopp's book can be read through the eyes of the patient or the helper with respect to recognizing and working through existential burnout. Of particular importance are Kopp's candid comments on his own experience with serious neurosurgery and a subsequent heart attack after he believed the former crisis to be resolved.
5. Coleman, *Abnormal Psychology*, p. 101.
6. Kopp, *End to Innocence*, p. 49.
7. Robert N. Butler and Myrna I. Lewis, *Aging and Mental Health: Positive Psychosocial Approaches* (St. Louis: C. V. Mosby, 1973).
8. For an outstanding interview with Han Selye, see Laurence Cherry, "On the Real Benefits of Eustress," *Psychology Today* 11, no. 10 (March 1978): 60–69. *Eustress* is Selye's word for the "good" kind of stress that can come about by the conversion of negative stress into positive experience through attitude change.
9. See Meyer Friedman and Ray H. Rosenman, *Type A Behavior and Your Heart* (New York: Fawcett Crest Books, 1974).
10. Contrast Friedman with the recent comprehensive review of treatment of heart conditions, "Taming the No. 1 Killer," *Time*, 1 June 1981, pp. 52–59. Friedman's research emphasizes prevention, treatment, and recovery of coronary conditions with high consideration for attitudinal and life-style changes that are similar to Selye's formulations (see Cherry, "On the Real Benefits of Eustress"). The *Time* article exclusively emphasizes modern medicine's technological progress in drug and surgical treatment.
11. Letitia Anne Peplau and Daniel Perlman, *Loneliness: A Source Book of Current Theory, Research, and Therapy* (New York: Wiley, 1982).
12. Selye's complete recipe for the best antidote to the stresses of life is (a) "seek your own stress level, to decide whether you're a racehorse or a turtle and to live your life accordingly"; (b) "choose your goals and make sure they're really your own, and not imposed on you by an overhelpful mother or teacher"; and (c) "altruistic egoism—looking out for oneself by being necessary to others, and thus earning their goodwill." See Cherry, "On the Real Benefits of Eustress," p. 70.
13. Karl A. Menninger with Paul W. Pruyser, "Morals, Values, and Mental Health" in Albert Deutsch and Helen Fishman, eds., *The Encyclopedia of Mental Health* (New York: Watts, 1963), vol. 4, pp. 1244–45.
14. John Bowlby, *Attachment and Loss*, vol. 3, *Loss: Sadness and Depression* (New York: Basic Books, 1980).
15. Coleman, *Abnormal Psychology*, p. 104.

Chapter 11

Professional Burnout:
A Job-Related Stress Reaction

Health-care workers, like other humans, can be vulnerable to existential burnout, as previously described. Helpers share the same planet and contemporary culture as their patients, and must resolve the same paradoxical dilemmas that life affords everyone else. The assumption is, however, that helpers are somewhat "healthier" and "stronger" because of their rich knowledge about how to be healthy and how to treat illness in the prevention of death. In some respects, this assumption is true, and many helpers do utilize what they know and share with patients in maintaining and enhancing their own health. Many helpers, however, cling to an illusion of immunity, believing that what happens to their patients will never happen to them, and, if it does, show reluctance to seek out appropriate aid at the first signs of serious difficulty.

CASE IN POINT

Jennifer sought psychotherapy at the insistence of her mother. Jennifer was in her final year of a baccalaureate nursing program and already seemed burned out. She had difficulty expressing why she had come for the first interview, except that her mother had wanted her to. She was from a prominent medical family: Her father was a well-respected, hardworking

M.D. in private practice; her mother had formerly worked as an R.N. and now was taking continuing-education courses; her brother was a graduate student in biochemistry.

Behind the initial affectless demeanor of a young woman with an outstanding academic and clinical record lay a tragic story of family burnout. First, Jennifer revealed her history of drug usage with her peers. She had already dropped this social group and had discontinued drugs a few months before on her own as she began to realize negative consequences in her study habits and clinical functioning. Then, Jennifer explored her serious concern about her parents' severe depressions, reported to be related to chronic marital discord. Jennifer felt simultaneously impotent and responsible for helping them. Finally, several sessions later, she tearfully talked of her brother's terminal carcinoma, now in remission but, ultimately and in the near future, fatal. Helping the entire family to face Don's death and dying with him involved breaking through illusions into highly defended pain. But this approach diffused the lonely individual paths of destruction that each family member had been walking on for three years.

Jennifer has long since graduated, and we hear from her at times as she enthusiastically describes her work as a beginning professional. She no longer is carrying the excess burden of existential dilemma stemming from her family situation. The tragedy of her young brother's dying is still real, but she is no longer caught in trying to keep herself or her parents from facing reality. Energy previously trapped in denial is now freed up to relate with them openly and recreationally. She understands that she can no longer carry her wish to "right a wrong" into helping situations with others. She is better equipped and more competent to help others face and work through tragedy, assisting them to avoid ineffective defensive postures that become destructive and immobilizing. She also is aware that, while she has more effectively worked out her personal and family situation, she is still vulnerable to professional burnout because she has chosen a stressful occupation. In other words, in helping Jennifer to develop a reparative course of self-advocacy, we believe her to be better prepared to identify, evaluate, and help others trapped in existential burnout. She can stay close to people without experiencing negative stress and getting caught in avoidance traps so common in job-related burnout.

Stages of Professional Burnout

Before reviewing the stages of job-related burnout, it is important to reiterate some comments about anxiety and stress. First, stress in life is ever present; in its simplest definition, stress is any adjustive demand placed on the individual, whether unpleasant or pleasant. In discussing burnout, we are not concerned with "normal" stressors or even occasional spurts of anxiety or self-doubt. These occasions are unavoidable and even necessary to motivation, self-reflection, risk taking, and growth. What we are concerned about are instances when stress exceeds the optimal level for individuals and when decompensation of effective behavior begins in response to perceived excessive demands.

These severe stress reactions are likened by many authors[1] to the biological model of Selye, which involves three basic stages: (1) an alarm/mobilization state, (2) a resistance state, and (3) an exhaustion state. Although initially a biological model, behavioral correlates reflected in personality variables are apparent in this model as one observes the highly stressed person attempting to cope. For example, in the beginning of the *alarm state*, one observes persons heightened in their awareness and behaving in such a way as to suggest they are dealing with an emergency—that is, the "flight-or-fight" response. In the beginning phases of this state, the person may appear to be a highly energized, "good" worker. Beginners in the health-care professions or very new employees may respond initially in this manner to the stress of a new job, but, over time, as they feel more oriented and secure in their role, this behavior drops off. What happens is that, in response to the initial alarm state, effective coping mechanisms come into play and the person's stress level drops to the optimal level. But what if the negative stressors that led to the initial reaction remained, and new ones came into the situation that caused feelings of being overpowered to ensue?

CASE IN POINT

Leslie's first job interviews after graduation were grueling for her. She wanted the staff-nurse position on one particular unit very much because she liked psychiatric nursing and she trusted the head nurse to be supportive of her since the head nurse had previously helped Leslie when she was a student on the service. Leslie knew, however, that many more experienced nurses were vying for the position. Leslie eventually obtained the position she wanted. Although she was enthusiastic for a short time, her anxiety mounted because of her uncertainty that she could perform as capably as she had envisioned.

This anxiety state was not overwhelming, and, as the weeks of orientation went by, Leslie's initial alarm state diminished. Events of the fifth week, however, propelled Leslie into another alarm state. The head nurse resigned unexpectedly, and a new, unknown replacement was perceived by Leslie as placing a highly stressful demand upon her still-fragile beginning experience. In the transition, the unit organization and structure floundered, as did Leslie, who had few background experiences to help her weather uncertainty. More experienced staff tended to disregard Leslie's concerns about her performance and her apprehensions about a replacement. After work, she began to experience a pattern of gastrointestinal upsets and vague headaches that were not her usual style.

When the new head nurse arrived, many changes in philosophy and routine began to occur. Leslie had difficulty with these changes because her duties did not seem like the same job she had initially wanted so much. In addition, she did not like the new head nurse, believing her to be not as supportive as she wished. Yet, Leslie felt she had no options since she believed she should not change jobs so soon in her budding career.

In the above example, the second alarm state, common to beginners, did not diminish and, in its chronicity, the signs and symptoms of decompensation—the *resistance state*—began to occur. In this state, we observe persons to be coping, but finding it necessary to use considerable energy to keep themselves or the situation on keel and to avoid psychological disintegration. In Leslie's case, she lost her enthusiasm for the position she had earlier referred to as her "plum of a job"; she began to use the psychological defense mechanism of rationalization: "What did I expect anyhow, to go right out of school and get what I want? Everybody tells me I'm lucky just to have a job at that hospital." Though superficially protecting herself from the pain of disappointment, her enthusiasm dwindled and became expressed in her gradual withdrawal from patient interactions and failure to make contributions in staff conferences. She began taking sick days as her headaches intensified. She felt that her repeated attempts to talk about her chronic dissatisfaction with her co-workers and the new head nurse were ineffective. She stopped trying.

When Leslie stopped trying to communicate her needs and "make something happen," withdrawing not just from patients but from the work situation per se, she had psychologically and physically moved into the *exhaustion state*. This is the phase of chronic stress reactions in which coping mechanisms have failed and the human being feels lost, helpless, and depleted. Daley states that "the worker is now faced with two choices: either get out of the job or break down."[2] For some professionals, enough adaptive energy remains to take the risk of "getting out": for others, the psychological damage has become so severe in the chronic phases of the exhaustion state that perceptual and thinking disorders ensue. In such a state, people have often lost sight of their own decreased efficiency and effectiveness or their extreme use of defense mechanisms to help restructure their overpowering reality (for example, projection, displacement, reaction formation, denial).

The above stages and the case in point suffice for theoretical purposes. However, it is important to keep in mind that the stages of burnout may not follow exactly as outlined in theory; neither can one expect a single set of behavioral correlates at each stage to apply to everyone. For example, some professionals may leave a job situation when they begin to experience the chronic effects of the alarm state and immediately take a new position in which they are confronted with the same stress variables. In the new situation, one might observe this health-care worker to experience quickly the signs and symptoms of the stagnated secondary resistance state without demonstrating a preliminary alarm state. The professional's own personality and the coping mechanisms that have been utilized over a lifetime will be highlighted in the attempt to deal with highly stressful health-care situations.

A further characteristic of the job-related burnout syndrome as it occurs in "real life" is that it is an insidious, subtle process not always accompanied by the succinctness, drama, or forewarning described theoretically. From our contacts with hundreds of health-care employees and supervisors attending workshops on stress and burnout, we have found that the recognition of burnout in others is often an easier process than recognition of it in oneself. Mannon's study of emergency medical technicians revealed similar findings:

> My own personal observations and interviews at County Hospital revealed that the feelings associated with burnout are vague and not clearly explainable to outsiders. An EMT or paramedic would admit to me that he or she felt burned out but would be unable to pinpoint the reason or identify the exact emotions, attitudes, and states of mind that accompanied this feeling.[3]

Signs of Job-Related Burnout

Following is a list of behavioral signs and symptoms of job-related stress compiled from workshop participants in different states throughout the country. Some of the material was derived from what health-care workers "on the front lines" described as happening to themselves or co-workers; some of the material was derived from what nursing supervisors observed to happen with their employees.

1. Lack of enthusiasm about going to work, experienced as vague, diffuse feelings of dread
2. Feeling that what used to be a challenge no longer "turns one on"
3. Feelings that tasks that used to come "naturally" are now forced or are preceded by unexpected feelings of free-floating anxiety
4. Procrastination about doing things that used to be tackled without hesitation
5. Irritability with patients and/or co-workers concerning petty deviations from expected behavior or procedural policy
6. Sharing frustrations about work, family, or social life with patients
7. Increasing physical distance from patients
8. Increasing physical distance from co-workers—for example, too busy to go on a break, excuses in response to invitations to go to lunch with others
9. Change in the way one talks about patients, increasingly referring to them as "cases" or as a collection of symptoms
10. Feeling put down or self-righteous when receiving feedback from supervisors or co-workers that one's performance is declining
11. Increasing desire to take a sick day to "get away from it all"
12. Increasing preoccupation while at work with being someplace else or with someone else
13. Increasing and/or extremes of emotional reaction to dying and death of patients—for example, uncontrolled weeping, anger, or development of stoney-cold responses
14. Beginning to feel that the helping process is simply futile and that one no longer can have a positive impact on situations
15. Feelings of immobilizing fatigue when one comes home from work in face of no physical illness or increase in work load
16. Development of minor physical complaints that one's physician says are stress related
17. Inability to leave work issues at work—for example, bringing paper work home more often, more frequently going into work on days off to get "caught up"
18. Feedback from friends and family that one is talking more about job frustrations at home or during social events
19. Change in one's "need to relax" habits—for example, increase in the need to drink, take drugs, or smoke to unwind; increased need to nap before bridging into home or social activities; increase in preferring to stay home; refusing to participate in usual outside activities

20. Alteration in sleep habits—for example, difficulty getting to sleep; dreams preoc-
    cupied with work issues; early morning awakening; feeling tired upon arising
21. Change in eating habits—for example, diminished appetite or eating more, with
    accompanying weight gain
22. Diminished sexual drive

Evaluating Your Own Burnout

As previously mentioned, it may be easier to pick up signs of burnout in others before
recognizing burnout in yourself. Whether a comment from a friend, mate, or supervisor signals you to self-evaluation, or whether you yourself have a hunch you are
"burning out," do nothing until you sit down and take a long objective look at where
your unique stress points might be. It is all too easy to seek out crash cures in a
piecemeal, impulsive fashion, failing to identify target sources of stress that require a
more comprehensive approach, leading to a serious commitment to life-style change.

Before assuming that the work situation is the culprit, we suggest taking an in-
depth look at two areas: your personal life and your physical health. Consider the
following questions:

How is my physical health?
Might I possibly have the beginning symptoms of a disease process that I have failed to
    have medically checked?
Have I been pushing myself to go to work with minor illnesses when I should have
    taken a sick day to fully recover?
Have I gone back to work "too soon" in the past three to six months after a major
    illness or surgery?
Are my eating habits erratic? Do I frequently skip breakfast or lunch or tend to eat on
    the run?
Am I frequently on a crash-diet regimen to lose weight? In general, am I taking in
    adequate nutrients regardless of the number of calories?
Am I using or abusing any medications that contribute to "drug hangover"?
Am I allowing myself adequate sleep?

How is my personal life?
Have I had a recent personal crisis (marital crisis; loss of a significant person; illness of
    a child, mate, sibling or parent; financial loss, and so on)?
Have I been experiencing chronic, unresolvable discord or lack of communication with
    a significant other?
Have I recently changed my living arrangements radically (moved to a new residence,
    acquired a live-in mate, recently been married)?
Is my sexual life comfortable and fulfilling?
Am I attempting to do "too much" after work hours (too much partying, carrying a
    college load, single parenting without adequate supports)?

If one or more of the above situations are unrecognized as a source of stress, one can well imagine the compounded stress load if one willy-nilly changed jobs in the belief that one's work was the culprit. Yet, we do know that the work situation indeed might be just that. In evaluating one's work situation, it is important to sort out the stressors as to recent temporary adjustive demands versus global adaptations that relate more to one's personal style, attitude, and basic competency. First, evaluate what are considered temporary adjustive demands, from which one might expect a return to optimal stress levels within a relatively short period of time:

What recent changes have occurred within the work setting?
Have I been promoted recently or received a requested transfer?
Have I recently changed my shift (even if I requested it) or changed my rotation of days off?
Have there been recent changes in administration, program philosophy, or budget?
Has there been a recent turnover of significant staff on whom I had come to rely?
Have patient loads recently increased?
Has there been an increase in the number of patients dying whom I had come to know?
Has there been a change in overtime requirements due to temporary staff shortages?

Next, consider the following questions to ferret out some of the more elusive stress points that may be operating and compounding over time:

Am I in the best job situation for myself?
Some people do not "know" themselves adequately to determine the kind of job they fit with best. Subtle conflict between job characteristics and personality styles can lead to vague, chronic dissatisfaction. There may be nothing inherently wrong with either the job or oneself but simply an inappropriate fit. The conflict may be with respect to the kinds of tasks expected; it may also involve a sharp difference in values. In a review of four major texts concerning job-related professional burnout, Chance attempted to answer the question of what causes burnout. He stated:

The authors of these books agree that the immediate cause is a mismatch between effort and results. Burnout victims start out full of fire and good intentions, but their efforts are not repaid in kind. The reality is that it is very difficult to help people. Add to that low pay, impossible workloads, miles of red tape, inadequate training, low prestige, and ungrateful clients. There is, moreover, the fact that society at large does not really understand what the helping professions are all about.[4]

Is the job stimulating enough and/or meeting my achievement needs?
Occasionally one does not recognize that the job is not challenging enough, and what seems like burnout is actually boredom. Many people begin to get dissatisfied

because a job is too easy. Such a situation, compounded with being in a "dead-end" position without chance for advancement, creates chronic frustration.

Do I have the essential competencies for the job?

Just as many people take positions for which they are overqualified and thereby experience negative boredom stressors, many take positions for which they are underqualified and experience chronic insecurity stressors. Inadequacy is a difficult aspect of the self to face openly, but a vital one to investigate. If you feel inadequate, clarify your perceptions with your supervisor. If you lack expertise, do something to improve your skill level. Even if your supervisor believes you to be functioning adequately, seek out educational experiences that provide you with a greater sense of security.

Am I expecting too much nurturance from my job?

We have already discussed that one can run into emotional trouble if one expects life at work to make up for gaps in one's social/emotional life with friends, lovers, and family. A helping profession demands much giving to others. Expectations that one's work life can give back the measure one needs from others is a quick path to job burnout and existential despair.

Am I attempting to give more than the job requires?

Be certain of your job description and the realistic expectations of your employer. Avoid underpaying situations unless you are desperate. Avoid the unhealthy habit of self-sacrifice in order to be the "nice guy." Carefully evaluate how much you are trying to "save everyone." Unrealistic rescuers often end up being the victim of their perceptions of being underappreciated and overused. Such interpersonal martyrs eventually are resented by co-workers, which further decreases the chance to obtain the approval so desperately sought through giving too much.

Am I utilizing others enough in assisting me to carry out my work?

Health care is a cooperative enterprise if it is to be maximally effective and minimally stressful. If one is a go-it-aloner, the job can be much more stressful than if one has learned interpersonal trust and the value of mutual interdependency with co-workers and patients. The advocacy model for working with patients as emphasized throughout the text can reduce the stress of feeling overresponsible in one's day-to-day work.

Am I facing realistically that being a helper in the health-care field will always be a stressful occupation?

Burnout is a hazard for everyone, no matter how good the job fit, for we are in the high-risk business of helping others with serious problems in the physical/social/emotional spheres of life. The risk has to be faced if we want to stay in the field; however, the risks can be minimized if we are serious in becoming, as Heidegger expresses, "active guardians of our existence."[5]

Am I in a work situation that is aware of the burnout phenomenon and takes active steps along with myself to prevent its occurrence?

As discussed throughout the text, there are innumerable characteristic patterns within traditional health-care settings that directly and indirectly contribute to staff or patient burnout. Again, we strongly encourage health-care workers to advocate assertively for conditions that enhance rather than detract from patient and helper strivings to be healthy. However, there comes a time in some situations when the system is simply unresponsive, and it is the wise, self-advocating helper who resigns out of humanistic conviction and before a state of irreparable exhaustion develops.

The above evaluative questions have considerable usefulness in generally exploring where to start tackling a burnout syndrome. In our psychotherapy experience, however, we have found that many "successful" professional clients (for example, nurses, doctors, social workers) have lost touch with just how brutally they push their bodies and minds day after day. In addition to exploring the above issues with them, we ask them to keep a diary of their activities and bring it into the next session for mutual review. Following is an excerpt from a typical week's diary of a 35-year-old female psychiatrist who initially sought psychotherapy because of depressed feelings in response to a marital problem.

CASE IN POINT

Wednesday

8 P.M. Finished with hospital visits. Home by 8:30. Husband at med library. Grab a sandwich. Contact answering service. No calls. Open mail and pay a few bills. Bed by 10:30. Husband comes home at 10:45. Bad mood.

11:30 P.M. Emergency call from patient—upset because her best girlfriend's husband just killed himself after girlfriend filed assault charges against him for beating her. Concerned about patient as her father killed himself two years ago and it's still rough going for her. Bed midnite.

Thursday

6:30 A.M. Work on papers and dictate reports. Fix breakfast and straighten up house. Talk to husband about my schedule the next two days. Short day today so can fly out to Durango tonight for consultation Friday.

9:00 A.M. Appointment at my gyn doctor—overdue Pap test.

9:30 A.M. Call Anna (secretary)—have four calls to make. No time. See patients in office 10–2.

10 A.M. Patient—very upset about need to put her husband into nursing home next week, yet she is worn out from years of home care.

10:55 A.M. Call from colleague who has a battered woman in his office needing safe house; tell him who to call.

11 A.M. Patient—young wife of addicted Vietnam vet; trying to decide if she should leave him, but today crying over her sick dog.

12 noon Patient—last session with woman whose husband left her a year ago; custody battle over and readjustment good. Hard to say goodbye.

1:00 P.M. Patient canceled. Grab crackers and peanut butter. Contact answering service. Two more calls. Make all my calls: New referral—needs to be seen right away; call a colleague to see him. Regular patient—male executive: What to do? Had to call police last night as wife got drunk and tried to stab him. Patient from night before—feeling better but wants Saturday A.M. appointment. Lawyer—wants to know if I can evaluate an accident victim within next two weeks. Regular patient—wants medications adjusted. Husband—doesn't know if can get me to the airport tonite; will check back later.

2:00 P.M. Patient—40 year-old depressed male school teacher; today he is frightened that he is going to voyeur again. Feeling suicidal.

3:00 P.M. Give secretary itinerary for tonite and tomorrow. Sign correspondence and checks.

3:45 P.M. Arrive home. Pack up things for Durango. Sit down and have a drink. Husband home early at 4:30—is upset about a course he is taking and me. Talk with him a while; he'll take me to airport. Phone rings—secretary saying patient who canceled wants to talk to me right away. Call him. Two other calls to make later. Have to leave for airport at 5:30. Call airport—flight on time.

6:00 P.M. At airport: Plane delayed half-hour. Make rest of calls.

6:45 P.M. Am stuck on the plane right now—another delay—weather problems.

8:15 P.M. Over Pueblo, the stews are finally able to serve drinks. No food service tonight—will grab something in Durango. Flight is bad.

9:15 P.M. Into Durango—message left for me to take cab. Cab comes at ten to ten.

10:20 P.M. Arrive at motel. Told that dining room closed at 10 tonight. Only restaurant two miles down the road. Go to room and wash my hair. Have soft drink from the machine. Watch T.V. Review records for A.M. Asleep by midnight.

Friday

6:00 A.M. Call room service for breakfast. Can't bring it as two employees late. I insist and finally get it at 6:45. Eggs are cold and flat. Caked pack of salt unglues me.

8:00 A.M. At Clinic, etc., etc.

The remainder of this woman's day was deemed satisfying to her with respect to her clinical consultation. However, she did not finally return home until after midnight, encountering similar air-traffic delays, including sitting in the Durango airport for three hours until her flight took off. On her return home, her husband confronted her with his being "fed up" and she could not understand his exasperation with their life-style. During her next therapy session, she attempted to rationalize that he should be able to accept that "that's the way it is being married to a doctor." Only in using her own diary notes with her was it possible to begin to help her get a more objective grasp on a life-style that disallowed her husband to express appropriate concern for her or the relationship. Her notes were also useful in helping to point out how isolated she had become in private practice and how little she reached out and utilized her peers for support, relief, and entertainment.

It was difficult for her to acknowledge her profound underlying exhaustion and the fact that the quality of her work with patients had been slipping. Conscientious, bright, and capable, this young woman had become "lost in her professionalism" and, had she not sought help when she did, a full plunge into the exhaustion stage of burnout might well have permanently disabled her marriage, a successful practice, or even the will to live.[6]

Overall, while burnout may be a general concept to which we may all relate with a sense of commonality, the identification and remediation of the stress reaction must be conducted on the basis of individual "diagnosis," and plans to treat burnout must be tailored to each individual. In this kind of individualized assessment, as was illustrated above, it is important to evaluate three interactive factors that affect the person's life: (1) factors in the health-care setting in which the person functions; (2) factors concerning the selfhood and intimate life of the person; and (3) factors within the patient population, student group, or other clientele the person may be serving.

In the above case in point, a number of changes in life-style were immediately suggested and accepted by this young doctor. She already had a heavy case load of individual therapy clients; she agreed to take no new referrals for a month. In addition, she agreed that, for one year, she would not accept referrals for patients experiencing serious psychotic or borderline disorders. She was excellent in her work with these people, but she was depleted by the demands of those already in her practice, since the open-ended commitment they required had caused her twice in the past year to cancel vacation plans. She wanted to continue her air-flight commuting to Durango for consultation, as she enjoyed the work and the opportunity to get away for a change of scene and pace. This arrangement was considered reasonable insofar as she also agreed not to see patients past noon of the evening she left and not to schedule Saturday morning patients on the day following her return. Her husband was delighted, as this change was linked to her commitment to spend weekends with him. Within the office setting, she increased the amount of secretarial service. She had worked her way through medical school as a secretary and needed to be reminded that she should leave that old role behind and hire a full-time office support system for herself. After a month of the new schedule and weekends spent exclusively with her husband, she and her husband began to entertain friends within their home, a function they had discarded gradually in the previous year.

Interest in how their home looked and felt to them, as well as a shared interest in gourmet cooking and taking classes together triggered new enthusiasm for being at home for them both. Agreed-upon time for each to share what was going on in their professional spheres changed the character of their discussions. Her husband had been eager simply to exchange ideas with her since he was a fourth-year medical student and she more advanced. She, on the other hand, had always wanted to share some of her "victories" as well as defeats with her husband but had feared she would appear to be either bragging or complaining. This "successful" young doctor did more than simply help herself in life-enhancing ways by actively taking charge of her environment and herself; it was learned later that her changes gave her husband renewed hope in continuing his medical education, as he was beginning to feel that, if that kind of life lay ahead for him as an uncontrolled given, he wanted to quit school. The mutual sexual withdrawal they were experiencing when she first sought help required no direct intervention and took care of itself as other aspects of their lives improved.

Collective Burnout Considerations

Individual burnout situations will inevitably occur in any health-care setting regardless of the nature of the setting and the preventive efforts of those responsible for the milieu. However, one often observes a collective burnout syndrome in health-care settings in which few, if any, mental-health, stress-reducing principles are employed within the system. The classic symptoms in such a setting are low worker morale, high rates of absenteeism, high rates of staff turnover, and disregard for subtle to obvious evidences of dehumanizing communications with patients. For those settings that already find themselves in such disarray, or for those who desire to institute built-in principles for preventive purposes, the following recommendations should be considered:

1. Institute regular staff meetings that have the expressed purpose of developing creative ideas for stress reduction for staff and patients. Be willing to bend some of the old rules and experiment. This approach gives a staff the feeling of having more control of what is happening to them; self-esteem grows if employees believe that supervisors are willing to listen to their ideas and try them. If an idea does not work, the group can either go back to the old routine or think of something even more innovative.
2. To the degree possible, allow staff to choose which shifts and days off fit best with their perceived biorhythms and personal responsibilities. When staff talk about requests and trade-offs in an open group discussion, rather than exclusively with the supervisor, there is a higher probability of everyone's getting more of what they want. Even if everyone's needs cannot be met, the staff will have a greater understanding of why certain limitations are necessary.
3. Avoid assignment of difficult situations to newly employed health-care advocates, beginners in the field, or helpers whom you know to be experiencing personal crises at home.
4. Develop planned rotation for staff who are competent to work with difficult, complex patients to less stressful duties as a "break" from the intensity.
5. Sanction relief periods during shifts so that staff members may comfortably remove themselves from direct patient care; let staff know that they will be confronted if they are chronically observed not to take breaks, even when it seems too busy to step away for a while. Encourage staff to listen to their own mind and body messages about relief needs before they become overstressed. With staff who are observed to be chronically avoiding patient contact, discuss where the difficulty lies.
6. Sanction the use of periodic "mental-health days" in lieu of "sick days." Allow employees to be forthright about their use of mental-health days and do not force them into calling in sick. Years of accumulated unused sick days are no longer considered a medal of honor. Neither do employees fully relax and use mental-health days for maximum benefit if they believe they have to lie to get the necessary relief time.

7. Encourage and allow individual staff members to express pent-up feelings. When staff know they can safely express themselves with their supervisor and other staff members, individually or in group meetings, there are fewer withdrawn, resentful staff members and less group tension. The staff's knowing that "talking it out" is a sanctioned avenue of psychological relief lessens the personal, attacking nature of communication that so many supervisors fear. Sharing feelings and exploring strategies in coping helps to reduce the sense of isolation between staff and reinforces an atmosphere of common humanity.

8. To avoid the dead-end syndrome, schedule periodic merit pay raises to which staff can look forward. Learn which of the staff prefer their present level of work with merit raises in contrast to those who prefer promotionary mobility in addition to merit raises. Be willing to mentor staff, teaching and sharing supervisory responsibilities so that, when a promotionary position becomes available, the person can assume it with competent experience and not on the basis of "potential" alone. Supervisors who "share the load" in this manner avoid administrative burnout.

9. Develop or send staff members to training programs to increase competencies in working with complex, frustrating patient problems. Bringing outsiders with expertise into staff meetings is often overlooked as an inexpensive way to increase competencies while solidifying group change in ways of relating to patients.

10. Finally, but not the least important, it is essential that all staff—the newly employed and senior members—know that the setting is dedicated to humanistic health care for patients and that, to accomplish that goal, the staff must strive to be healthy and stay healthy. By explaining that philosophy openly and making opportunities for the staff to accomplish that goal for themselves and others, no supervisor need fear confrontation by any staff member who refuses to learn, grow, or treat patients with the dignity and respect they deserve when they come under their care.

Conclusion

Dedicated, altruistic helpers have been around for centuries. It has seemed that they somehow "belonged to the world," having their intrapersonal matters all in place and functioning well. There is something admirable and refreshing about that traditional mystique about helpers, particularly on the heels of a "me-first" 1970s culture. But the statistics of helper casualties have been mounting, particularly among the dedicated, conscientious ones, and we doubt that these statistics are an artifact of better reporting and documentation. Times have changed in the arena of helping. Pressured by society to save everybody from despair, disease, and inevitable death, it is difficult for helpers to give priority to their personal well-being. But that is where helpers must start in finding a realistic path through the complex field of health care.

Avoiding being a burnout casualty by becoming an unfeeling, robotized human seems a poor trade-off for the helper and a hopeless situation for those who seek to offer humane, cooperative help. Thus, the increased attention given to the human condition of the health-care worker is reassuring, even though it is unfortunate that casualties were so high before appropriate public attention was directed to what people within the health-care system have known for so long. Loath to reinforce the development of technocratic, clone-like helpers or over-responsible rescuers who ultimately burn out, we have presented the advocacy model of helping as a path that, through practiced application, can assist helpers to bridge the large chasm between technical science and humaneness. To the degree that our experience shows that the advocacy model works to preserve the "selfness" of both helper and patient, we believe the model to be a contribution to the prevention of both existential and job-related burnout.

REFERENCE NOTES

1. Jerry Edelwich and Archie Brodsky, *Stages of Disillusionment in the Helping Professions* (New York: Human Sciences Press, 1980). These authors relabel Selye's stages as (1) enthusiasm (alarm/mobilization), (2) stagnation (resistance), and (3) apathy (exhaustion).
2. Michael R. Daley, " 'Burnout': Smoldering Problem in Protective Services," *Social Work* 24, no. 5 (September 1979), p. 376.
3. James M. Mannon, *Emergency Encounters: A Study of an Urban Ambulance Service* (Port Washington, N.Y.: Kennikat Press, 1981), p. 169.
4. Paul Chance, "That Drained-Out, Used-Up Feeling," *Psychology Today* 15, no. 1 (January 1980): 89.
5. Martin Heidegger, *Being and Time*, trans. John Macquarrie and Edward Robinson (New York: Harper & Row, 1962).
6. An article carried by the *APA Monitor 5* (July 1974) carries a report that women psychologists commit suicide at a rate nearly three times that of women in the general population, as do women physicians. The rate for men physicians is one and one-half that of men in general. Interestingly, the rate of suicide among men psychologists is lower than that for men in general. The two researchers, Robert Steppacher and Judith Mausner, also studied the high rate of women who commit suicide in other professions—chemistry and, to some extent, nursing. A more recent article in *Time* concerning M.D. suicides (16 February 1981, p. 57) indicates that physicians commit suicide at a number at least three times the rate for the population at large. Because of these alarming statistics, the American Medical Association and the American Psychiatric Association have initiated a study of such suicides. Other professionals who have high suicide rates are dentists, lawyers, and police.

OTHER SUGGESTED REFERENCES

Herbert J. Freudenberger, "Burnout: The Organizational Menace," *Training and Development Journal* 31 (July 1977): 26–27.

Herbert Freudenberger and Geraldine Richelson, *The High Cost of High Achievement* (New York: Anchor Press/Doubleday, 1980).

H. Steven Moffic and Efrain A. Gomez, "Stress of Working with Mental Health Problems," in *A Clinician's Manual on Mental Health Care: A Multidisciplinary Approach*, ed. H. Steven Moffic and George L. Adams (Menlo Park, Calif.: Addison-Wesley, 1982), chap. 28, pp. 280–300.

Ayala Pines and Elliot Aronson, *Burnout: From Tedium to Personal Growth* (New York: Free Press, 1981).

Chapter 12

What Helpers Are Saying:
Clues to Burnout Prevention

A curiosity bordering on fascination concerning the interaction of the person of the helper and the person of the patient has been with us for many years. It has been particularly evident in our thinking as we have attempted to develop relevant educational experiences for students and as we ourselves have struggled to become presumably adult and helpers of others. Increasingly, as one becomes older, patients and helpers seem to be more alike in their basic humanity, and one ponders on the fine line that sometimes separates the two. At other times it requires deep personal introspection to try to understand the strong barriers that seem to get in the way. A similar interaction occurs between the person of the student helper and that of educators. As one becomes involved in teaching over a number of years, younger helpers seem to sound more and more as one "used to." At other times, there are barriers to understanding each other, and the full gut-level meaning of the term *generation gap* has a powerful impact. However, just as it is important for patient and helper each to come to know the person of the other in the helping process, so also is it important in the student/teacher dyad if positive, meaningful learning is to occur.

Even though there are vast benefits to staying contemporary through "continuing education," chronology does not allow one the privilege of becoming a young student again to refresh old insights. Thus, educators must listen carefully to those who look to them for learning—ferreting out what indeed is the history of growth and development repeating itself and what is significantly different in any particular era.

In this chapter, we summarize what we have heard as students from various disciplines have shared their perceptions, feelings, and wants. In comparing some student expressions with those of older seasoned professionals, it becomes apparent that many feelings of students reflect the age-old struggle to become an adult, but we are impressed with what the youth of today have to cope in the growth process to feel that they have personal meaning. Biased as we are in emphasizing the importance of the uniqueness of each human's personal frame of reference, we also believe that viewing helpers as a group highlights some common themes that are valuable to explore.

In reviewing the statements we have derived from the opinions of beginning helpers, keep in mind that these opinions were part of their essential need system when they chose or entered the field. To the degree that these needs are not met or worked through to self-satisfying resolution, the resultant frustration stressors can become chronic and lay the groundwork for future professional burnout.

Beginning Helpers Care About Others

Beginning health-care workers hold a strong value concerning care as it might be applied to their fellow human beings.[1] Not only does this value hold constant over many years, but helping persons appear to have held some notion about wanting to care or share something with another human for a substantial time prior to taking on a public helping role. When we asked multidisciplinary student interviewees what they had wanted to be "when they grew up," the overwhelming majority included some kind of interpersonal helping role model with whom they identified: teacher, nurse, doctor, or mother. Preadolescent fantasies of a more autonomous nature, such as being an equestrian, mountain climber, or ballet dancer, and the like were reported by less than 1 percent.

Exploring the motivations for helpers to seek a particular professional discipline gives a slightly different emphasis. Within this area, we are impressed with more intellectualized and pragmatic responses for how helpers came to make a particular choice—for example, "Being a teacher didn't pay me enough money"; "I couldn't see myself cooped up with the same kids every day for a year"; "I thought that, as long as it took so many years to be the kind of nurse I wanted to be, I might as well be a doctor"; "It took so many years to be a doctor that I decided I could help sooner in the ways I wanted to by going into social work." Such reasons for becoming one professional or another as being in medicine for the money or going into nursing to marry a physician simply have not held up as motives in our experience. Although we have had helpers tell us that they have entertained such notions as side benefits, they have acknowledged that for those reasons alone "it would not be worth it." Persons who pursue helping only for the gold ring or the wedding ring are likely to exist only in the romantic or sour-grapes fantasies of the onlooker.

In general, beneath the various life circumstances or attitudes that come into play in influencing the choice of one disciplinary orientation over another, the desire to care for or help another is a consistently articulated value held by the majority of health-care workers. Further understanding of what the effects of this choice may be seems to emerge as beginners later appreciate (1) the expectations that patients hold when they seek help, (2) the value-laden philosophies of instructors or employers, and (3) the deeper belief systems within caregivers themselves that they had not previously realized.

CASE IN POINT

Linda, looking back over her beginning years in social work, could not specifically recall why she didn't choose nursing or medicine. "Something stuck in my mind about giving food baskets to the poor and needing to respond to my middle-class guilt; but I got into the field, and, my God, I was surrounded by a philosophy of psychodynamics. Not only that, I got my first job through my uncle, who was a precinct boss. I thought he thought I was caring for people; at next election, I found out I was a political appointee. All I could feel was, holy _____, I'm not a helper; I'm supposed to make people vote Republican. I had to get out and find a job in which I fit better with what people said they wanted."

Beginning Helpers Tend To Be Concerned About Themselves First

Many of our own early student experiences are little different from the experiences related to us by beginning health-care workers in recent years. Content analyses of our recorded early experiences with patients and our conferences with beginning students reveal the material filled with uncertainties about abilities and ambivalence as to who should be up front in the helping dyad. Internal conflict concerning meeting patients' needs and leaving room for oneself are prominent, as exemplified in one of our own journal entries:[2]

CASE IN POINT

January, 1954
Pediatric Nursing Service

Another situation arose shortly that sort of took the starch out of me. A new admission had had emergency surgery for repair of a diaphragmatic hernia that involved abdominal contents in the left side of the chest and a severely displaced heart. Because his postoperative course wasn't satisfactory, I was asked to special him. I went into the room and found him with blood bubbling out of his nose and mouth and suffering from acute dyspnea. Well, two doctors came in, and the three of us worked with suction and endotracheal tubes, trying to get the chest machine to work and in other ways attempting to help him breathe. Because of the shortage of ward help, I volunteered to stay overtime and watch him until his situation was more stable, but I could tell that he wouldn't last through the night. I commented to the doctors that I had been working in these kinds of situations for a number of months and I was getting that old lump in my throat again. "Just stick with where the kid's needs are, and you'll be okay," Dr. _____ said. Tonight I have been sitting here trying to study for a psychology quiz tomorrow, but I keep thinking about that kid and the lump in my throat. I *think* I did all that I could. Is it immature to feel like this? I don't ever want to be a stony-hearted nurse, but, on the other hand, I shouldn't let these things bother me as much as they do.

In several university settings, we carried out a rudimentary survey of beginning health-care workers with whom we had had no previous experience. Two of the questions asked were "When you are approaching a patient for the first itme, what is the first thing that comes to your mind?" and, conversely, "What is the first thing that comes to the patient's mind?" Responses to both questions were rated with respect to who was the initial focus of concern. Helper responses to both questions consistently show a predominant preoccupation with themselves. This self-preoccupation was far stronger for those helpers having less clinical experience than for those who had spent more time with patients. The majority of these imagined response reactions tended to be stated in question form by the early beginner. For example, to the question "What is the first thing that comes into your mind?" common responses were "What will I say?" "Will they have confidence in me?" and "Will I know how to do the right thing?" In contrast, a more experienced beginner's response typically was less questioning, less personalized, and suggestive of more capacity to see another's viewpoint; for example, "how they (the patient) presently view their situation," and "what understanding they have about how a nurse may help them."

To the question as to what is uppermost in the patient's mind, early beginners imagined that the patient also was concerned with specifically who they the helpers were and how competent they would be. Common responses were "Will this person be able to help me?" "Will I like this person?" "Does this person know what to do?" Again, as helpers experienced more contact with patients, they tended to articulate a range of possible initial concerns of the patient that were less personally focused on the characteristics of the helper.

Does this mean that beginners in the helping professions are egocentric in an unfeeling way and desire to come out on top at all costs? We think not when we carefully examine the responses. More in-depth analysis shows that the ultimate concern is the patient and that, as a result of their efforts, students are concerned that patients will get what is believed to be needed. In general, that beginning clinicians want to feel secure in being liked and respected reflects a healthy growth goal in the developmental phase of adulthood.[3] Specifically, survey responses reflect a subtle recognition that, unless helpers are respected, patients may not trust them. Students therefore sense that something has to occur first within themselves if they are to help another. This recognition is most apparent in the many responses expressing the desire to be comfortable with a repertoire of technological and interpersonal abilities. Comparison of responses between least experienced and more experienced beginners also dramatizes another growth adage: as experience and confidence in one's abilities increase, projecting one's own self-doubt onto others decreases.

As with our own early experience, parenthetical comments made by the survey group and interviewees suggest that beginning helpers want some internal peace regarding whether they "ought" to feel insecure and preoccupied with how they appear to their patients. We respond to this ambivalence positively. It is a basic process that goes on in self-evaluation as people learn to know who they are as autonomous beings, what the limits of their human abilities are, and how they are going to "fit" or challenge the view of others. If the conflict is too intense or the students are attempting to work on these struggles in an environment that holds an external offer of values that they cannot refuse, or both, such conflict can be resolved simply by rigid conformity. However, the majority of our interview and written reactions indicate that beginning health-care workers have a high degree of willingness to keep struggling so that some resolution fits what they can live with. They want to talk it out, but they express considerable uncertainty about how they can meet that personal need in their educational environment.

CASE IN POINT

A medical intern was interviewed concerning his personal feelings about his patients. When asked what he did if he felt in conflict and needed to talk to the teaching staff, he replied, "I think there is an underlying feeling that wanting to talk out feelings about patients is 'too personal.' The staff man on my service would probably think I was a kook if I wanted to rap with him about the my needs/patient needs kind of things, or he'd just say, 'Yeah, you got to be careful, or they'll run all over you.' "

Lest it appear that only the external environment disallows internal feelings or pressures one to conform, it is important to point out that human beings carry inner "shoulds" and "oughts" that they bring with them into health-care studies. Our experience in settings within which there are high degrees of freedom to explore oneself without outside dictates has found many students to have "always" believed that to care for someone includes thinking about another with no consideration of oneself.

CASE IN POINT

Tracy, a senior student nurse, was interviewed about her greatest source of difficulty in learning to help patients. She described the clash that she felt between her long-held notions of caring for someone and the new insights that she was experiencing, "I'm just beginning to let myself face up to a kind of missionary attitude that I believe I have. I feel sorry for everybody and want to do everything for them. I was brought up that way—always to think of others first. Now I'm having to face that, if I do this all the time with all my patients, I'm really insisting that they respond 'my way.' One of my instructors is helping me to understand how this can put my patients in a situation of having to do nothing or thinking that they can never do anything back for me. I never thought about its being important for them to give me anything back. That's hard for me to admit, and it's going to take me a while to change. I had a boyfriend tell me that one time also, but I just thought that he was unappreciative."

"Older" student helpers, as inferred from survey responses, seemed in far less conflict about whether they were capable, safe, or "ought" to feel a certain way. Their general responses indicate far less concern about what patients think of them than do those of their less experienced peers. However, one wonders whether they have not learned to "write a good line," since our experience in talking with them behind the scenes has also been that they still have similar, albeit not so intense, feelings. As might be expected, when their educational experience nears an end, the personalized struggles of the older students become suddenly transformed into questioning their competency to find a job of their liking. That job seeking becomes a personal crisis time for both students and faculty is expressed by a faculty member who compared part of her function to that of an employment bureau.

CASE IN POINT

Every year about May or June I want to leave town. Trying to get the students to focus on their patients is almost impossible. They want to talk about how good this or that job might be, whom I know there, and other such information—in general, what to do with the rest of their lives. One fellow had applied to 15 different places and wanted me to write 15 different letters of recommendation for each one, so he wouldn't "feel like a form letter." Impossible!

In reviewing the developmental progress of the clinical student, one notes two points at which focus on the needs of oneself seem to be highly prominent: at the onset of clinical experience and nearing the end of student status. At the onset of working directly with patients, the student focus includes a high degree of concern as to how to "make it" with patients; later, the concern appears to be directed more at how they will make it in the outside job world. To initiate emphasis on humanistic values and behaviors with students late in their careers is better than nothing, but our experience suggests that prime readiness for the most meaningful impact is far earlier.

Older, practiced professionals seem to be in less open conflict than is seen with younger helpers. They have weathered the initial crises of competency and job seeking. For the most part—for better or worse—personal resolutions seem to have been made. Appearing unruffled with what they are doing or believing that they are doing right by themselves and others, most seem to have found personally unique mechanisms for satisfaction and/or coping with stress.

CASES IN POINT

Dr. _____ was interviewed at the point at which he had just celebrated 20 years of an apparently successful career of medical practice and teaching. He was asked how he felt his original desire to help had turned out for him.

"Well, you know how it is. You learn some things over life. I grew up on the streets of Scranton and early had some notion that I could make things better for everybody. In medicine, I had to realize that I was not God and that if you followed your patients long enough they all died if you didn't beat them to it. I had a chief of staff tell me that one night at the right time; he was kind about it and let me damn mortality. I've had to learn to do the best that I can and try to help the patients put themselves forward the best that they can and struggle it out in the here and now. Sure I'm future oriented, but who knows about tomorrow?"

Anna agreed to talk about her helping experiences and wanted to meet in a cocktail lounge to "get away from things for a while." I knew that she was reputed to be an excellent nurse and that her students thought that she "shared"; yet she found difficulty in talking of her ten years of experience and comparing philosophies. She wanted to know everything about my field of endeavor and coquettishly discouraged inquiries about herself. When I told her of my interest concerning humanism in health care, she immediately commented, "That is too heavy when you are caring for patients." She turned away from me to the bartender to order another drink. She said that she did not want to talk about it anymore.

Dr. _____, 40 years old and a prominent transplant surgeon, was asked about how he integrated his personal life with his heavy professional demands.

"When I was younger, I used to get into conflict about 'doing medicine' versus doing other things, but I've learned to put things together so it isn't an either/or kind of thing. Some people may see me as too involved in my practice, but it's inconceivable to me not to check on my surgery patients no matter what time it is. I learn something afterward from how they're doing, and I think that they need me around. It may be old-fashioned, but as a physician I believe that I'm a servant of the people, and it is them I must serve. It doesn't hurt."

Judy, age 32, seemed a relaxed, effective nursing supervisor. It was known that she had recently married a social worker who was beginning private practice and that they were attempting to integrate their four children by previous marriages into a new family "system." When asked how she was able to do all of this and yet project such a "together" aura, she replied: "If I thought I had to cope with it just every once in a while, it would feel like madness, I'm sure. I know I have to deal with it all, all of the time. I also know it's *what* I want and I am not ambivalent about it. Neither is my husband. We don't sit around and stew about whether we should have tried it or not, even when it's tough. I think our commitment to it is our glue."

In spite of what superficially appears to be a settling in, as we have previously reviewed, older helpers do have existential crises over the course of their lives. As full members of humanity, professionals have to cope with problems like anyone else—for example, shaky marriages, raising the children "right," getting along on the job, making ends meet, and alterations in physical health. Some miss such problems and others grind through them, but most older professionals appear to experience a third acute phase of focusing on themselves first and foremost. This phase correlates with a well-documented developmental phase of adulthood[4] in the "average" population: that point somewhere in the middle years of one's life when a global existential question, "What am I doing with my life?" reappears. As one of our colleagues related, "You won't believe this, but it's just like in the books. Just at the time when you seem to have your life most in place—with a good job and the kids raised—you feel as though you just walked out of a bomb shelter and got the full impact of the realization that, my Lord, you are not immortal and the question arises whether you have time to carry out all your plans." Recognition of this phase is sometimes less clearly delineated but is reflected in such career concerns as "What am I doing in administration when I should be teaching or practicing with patients?" or "I don't feel that I have the time to spend with the students and patients anymore, and I feel that I need to focus just on my research."

Since health-care workers are faced with existential issues of life and death earlier and with more intensity than most, one might assume that they have come to terms with the impact of mortality in smoother ways than has the general population. Of course, many persons in the health-care professions have used their experiences to examine and reexamine their own life philosophies broadly; these are emotionally rich people and steady, growth-enhancing humans to be around. As a part of maturing, one observes such professionals to have developed the capacity to put outer events more to the test of inner values instead of being manipulated by external factors;[5] but shifts occur for them also. Following are our recorded reflections on one of the most productive persons we have known.

CASE IN POINT

He probably is the most humanistic physician we know. Courageous in staying practical with what patients wanted, in spite of all the automatic practices and newfangled treatments, he would always start with basics: physical comforts, emotional warmth, and the understanding arm to lean on. What a capacity to listen! He had been through more than one war right at the front lines. He saw death again and again; he also knew that people could die emotionally and that they have the capacity to kill each other that way also. We often talked of a kind of grasp of something about life that he seemed to act on again and again: "I know that I'm a mortal being and have only so much time." We always presumed that that was where much of his energy came from. We had not seen him for years, and in talking with us the other night he shared his recent realization that he was not going to live forever; a radical surgery of his own had caused that to happen. He wanted to talk about where he was going. When we knew him before, he always seemed to know.

In summary, our personal and interviewing experience suggests that even those who have spent a lifetime helping others grapple with issues of "Why me?" and "Where am I going?" stand unprepared when there seem to be no more challenges or when there appears to be only a limited time left to grapple with those still on the horizon. Although we emphasize the importance of assisting beginning clinicians to struggle with their developmental crises early in their education, we also suggest a closer look at what older professionals have available when in later life they, too, have need to focus once again on themselves.

Helpers Want and Learn by Interpersonal Experience

Most professional curricula designed to educate health-care workers require a number of years of preclinical course work before students are allowed to apply their knowledge interpersonally with real human beings. The higher the educational degree to be earned, the longer is the period of time before patients are encountered. This preclinical educational practice symbolizes in part the recent emphasis on the mechanical use of technology. Realistically, time is required to master the understanding and safe use of the principles of technical procedures, but this time lag between theory and real practice also conveys an attitude that certain knowledge is more important than the intrinsic values and feelings of human beings—two powerful forces that ultimately decide whether technological knowledge will help others.

The preclinical delay also overlooks what happens to the students who are to become professional helpers. Students, wanting to help and struggling with personal dilemmas concerning the meaning of adult life and the results of their occupational choice, are put on existential hold until some later time.[6] It is a wonder that, when clinical experience does occur, students still want to help others or that they still have the capacity to appreciate the frame of reference of the human beings whom they are now supposed to help. As a faculty member bemoaned at a recent medical school admissions committee meeting, "After those years, we then expect clinical applicants to be an amalgam of self-confidence, security, and humility."

We find students to be more aware than we were in our early experience that something has to shift in the preclinical years of helping education. They seem to have a keener sense of the impact of our mechanistic era. This sense is derived not only from their social experience but also from the greater amount of technology that they have to incorporate immediately. To obtain the humanistic experience that they do not see forthcoming in their preclinical years, many students seek it on their own outside the educational system. To obtain human contact and expression of their need to help, many work as aides in hospitals or nursing homes or volunteer in street clinics serving young people like themselves.

CASES IN POINT

Jason, a second-year medical student, was asked why he had worked for three years in the downtown street clinic.

"I needed extra money, but that wasn't the whole story. I wanted to do something that helped others, and I knew it would be a long time before I'd ever see a patient. I also needed something to keep me from going mad in that competitive intellectual jungle—grade points, talking nice to certain profs, and beating the other guy out. Just call it *survival till you get there;* there's nothing you can do about it with the faculty."

Bill was a top-grade senior undergraduate in psychology; he probably knew more psychological theory already than a lot of Ph.D. candidates. However, he did not know what to do with it. He wandered into my office wanting to get some experience for a self-study course. All that he wanted to do was to spend some time with patients, just talking, listening, and watching others do the same thing. Six months later, I wondered if he had ever decided to go into graduate school. I checked up on him and found him working in a child-care center, trying to "get it together" before he went on to graduate school. He wanted to know if his dropping out for a while would hinder his being accepted into a program the following year. I had to say that that would probably make it tougher. He is still looking for a place that will accept him. I am afraid that he will be lost to the field. I would hire him tomorrow if he had the credentials.

However, students do not seem entirely alone in wanting a fuller humanistic education.[7] Signs that something is happening within faculty ranks are increasing—many of their feelings are not so different from those of the students. Following are the comments of an anonymous physician, as recorded in the minutes of a medical school faculty meeting at the University of Colorado.

CASES IN POINT

It appears that the students whom we receive are good at the craft of going to school and that education is obtained only as an incidental by-product. . . . Perhaps the primary use of the grade-point average as a criterion for the selection of future physicians is an absurd cultural custom, as is the use of biological age as a criterion to determine the level of material to which a child in school is to be exposed.

An older nursing instructor, interviewed about developments in nursing education, expressed frustrations repeatedly heard from students as well.

"By the time the students have put in two years of academic studies and finally get to try themselves out in nursing, they seem either to wake up and find that they don't want to do this after all or they feel that they've lost confidence in their basic human abilities; then I find myself teaching them 'interpersonal dynamics,' as if they were from another planet. It's unfair to everybody."

On this same theme, Steven Muller, president of Johns Hopkins University, publicly voiced his concern about the failure to expose students to human values in higher education:

The failure to rally around a set of values means that universities are turning out potentially highly skilled barbarians: People who are very expert in the laboratory or at the computer or in surgery or in the law courts but who have no real understanding of their own society. We are not turning out very self-confident people, and in a democracy that is a potentially catastrophic problem because our society depends on people who are not passive, but active, who are prepared to make choices and take responsibility. That requires individuals who have self-confidence—and to have that confidence requires a value structure.[8]

Glick, who believes as we do that there need not be something inherently contradictory between science and humanity or between technology and compassion, echoed Muller's concern:

> The crisis of humane medicine is the result of the failure of secular democratic societies to inculcate moral and ethical values into their educational systems.[9]

There are many reasons why faculty and students need to see eye to eye and to increase the mutual capacity to listen. The tragic college upheavals of the 1960s and early 1970s point to the urgency of generations' understanding each other if we are to deal productively with our rapid transitions, to say nothing of survival as a human culture. For students preparing for health-care professions, it seems even more critical. If it is essential for health-care workers to learn to appreciate the frame of reference and values of others, the preclinical years can no longer be ignored for the interpersonal distance they encourage, not only with patients but between student and teacher as well. Relegation of each other to stereotypes is no model for the helping process that the student is hoped to be learning. A shift must occur away from faculty's being seen as sitting around for hours devising Skinner-box objectives, curricula, and learning laboratories and from students' being perceived as learning to beat the system.[10]

Student frustration about delayed personal contact with teachers and patients in the preclinical years carries over into the beginning clinical years. Our survey data show that clinical students not only wanted more interpersonal experience "back then" but also right now. When clinical students were asked what kinds of things would be helpful to them in coming to grips with the interpersonal skills that they desired, two prominent themes emerged: *trust* and *reality.* Most want practice, practice, and more practice with real live people in situations that are not contrived and the opportunity to check themselves out with professionals who foster mutual respect in the student/ teacher dyad.

Few beginning health-care workers from a variety of disciplines desire more course work in assisting them to gain competence or reality in interpersonal process skills. Many are critical of the lecture-theory courses in basic psychology, sociology, or human development. Such courses seem to the student so far back in their curriculum as to be presently useless or to have material included that they did not perceive as appropriate to themsleves or helpful in getting along with others.

CASE IN POINT

A premedical student was asked how useful his required psychology course was to him. He thought that it was a drag, explaining, "By the time that we got through cats, dogs, pigeons, and monkeys and got to human beings, it was the end of the quarter. Then we got into some abnormal stuff about humans, and it kind of freaked me out because I saw a lot of myself in the material. Like I read something about paranoid persons and that there is generally a kernel of truth in what they are uptight about. For a long time I kind of worried if I were paranoid in the way that the book was talking about until one of my frat brothers told me, 'You're damn right, you should be paranoid; if you don't make it through that course with an

A from that ____, you're not going to get admitted.' So I forgot it; but I'm wondering about running into my first paranoid what-have-you; maybe I'll be just like him except for the white coat."

Wanting to learn about people and to practice helping abilities in a real way is a part of the counterculture values of students today. Students want more experiential happenings. The desires also reflect a need for a sense of belonging to a group to which students aspire to gain rank. Apparently, trying out certain skills in laboratory situations beyond a certain point strikes the beginning health-care worker as not being trusted, and they feel increased insecurity, rather than less. This feeling of not being capable is further perceived when patient contacts appear to be so contrived by instructors that the student feels protected from the mainstream of what the patient or other staff members or both have to cope with. Many say not only that they feel left out of the mainstream because of what they are allowed to do within the setting but also that often their period of time within a setting is so short that they never encounter the "difficult" patient or "their" patient's full gamut of difficulties.

CASES IN POINT

Mary, a senior baccalaureate nursing student, sought consultation because her first patient died and she needed to "put it together" for herself. She expressed open grief at the loss. She was also resentful of what she saw as the unreality of her student status.

"Here I am 23 years old; I have two kids and went through a messy divorce along the way. Maybe I'm just eager to feel competent in something and want to do more before I'm ready, or maybe I want to finish something with somebody. I felt so cut off when I came in for my few hours with my patient and found that he had died in the night. I thought that someone should have called me or something; yet I'm *only* a student, and I suppose that they thought, 'What could she do?' See, I don't know what I could have done, but I think that now I'll never know."

Clare, a social-work student in the final quarter of her graduate work, expressed concern at not having enough "real experience" to fall back on when she took a full-time job.

"My practicum involves being here only two half days a week. It's hard to feel a part of things. Everybody is running their buns off on the in-between days; sometimes I wonder if it's going to be like that for me some day. Right now I think maybe I'm getting just the simple cases because I'm not very sharp; but I'm going to be out in the slave market, looking for a full-time job in three months."

Themes of reality and trust are most prominent in students' expression of their most frequently stated need—*feedback from others*. For any individual striving to gain full membership in a designated group, including the human race, it is important that an aspirant receive (1) clear guidelines as to expected behaviors and (2) some form of open disclosure as to whether one is "making it" with the group. Unless this information becomes known, one cannot fully evaluate whether one's own values and abilities fit with the superordinate goal[11] and with the expectations of those already in the group. Questions of concern include "Are the actions of the group in keeping with what they say we are to be?" "Can I do what is expected?" "Do I want to do what the group formally expects?" "Will this group allow any of my input?"

In some occupations, feedback about one's performance can be given in the form of quantifiable measures; for example, production workers in a technological laboratory might be satisfied with their standing on the basis of written feedback about their accomplishments. This is not so with beginning health-care workers. They seem to be clearly aware that much of their sense of productivity and personal identity is rooted in interpersonal-process variables. They want feedback experience to occur within an interpersonal process. Particularly do younger beginning students want closeness and feedback from those whom they perceive as models of their particular profession. Older students, still wanting close contact with their mentors, seem more open to feedback from those in other disciplines—particularly those disciplines concerned with the understanding of human behavior.

As shall be seen, even when the faculty participate actively, students are frequently displeased and uncomfortable with how these fully professional models participate with them in a supervisory capacity. Often highly critical of how they are responded to, beginning helpers seem to be saying two things at once: "Please tell me what to do" and "Don't keep telling me what I am; I want to find out for myself." On the face of it, one might think that some students are merely demanding for demanding's sake and that one cannot win for losing. This view might be justified if it were a rare phenomenon. To the contrary, these behaviors—uncertainty, feelings of momentary chaos, and simultaneously wanting and disavowing structure—are all a part of an experience of growth, change, and learning to adapt to life's evaluative realities. In testing both the limits of autonomy and the strictures of a particular discipline, students are what they are for good reasons. It is a "critical period"[12] of potential for growth; lifetime decisions are at stake. Particularly with assertive, individualistic students, these conflicts are most intense and misunderstood, since both students and faculty frequently overlook the fact that the health-care disciplines (and interdisciplinary efforts) require a capacity to embrace a group or team allegiance as well as a capacity to be competent in one-to-one interchanges.

In attempting to resolve both professional and personal identity issues, just as in earlier developmental phases, students are naturally concerned with a highly personalized feedback system. They want feedback to be ongoing and spontaneously available. They want it transmitted through live human beings in the form of professionals from their discipline with whom they can verbally share and whom they can observe functioning competently in their own right as practitioners of what they are teaching.

Hungry to model after someone "in the know," some students grow angry at the lack of models or when their models do not live up to their expectations. One student from a large school of nursing stated: "We need more interaction by way of participation from the faculty. They act as though they don't care, even when they say that they do." Even the distance placed between student and teacher when written "interpersonal" exercises are requested is perceived as contributing to unreality; for example, written analysis of the interpersonal record of what went on between patient and self leaves many students unimpressed. Some find such a procedure better than nothing, but the general opinion holds that it primarily forces one to be a certain way on paper with no opportunity to hash out the process realistically. Many of the students frankly relate that they fudge on who said what to whom.

CASES IN POINT

Ron, a newly graduated social worker, was still vehement about what he referred to as the instructors' "ineffectual, idiotic written exercises."

"The emphasis is still on how you say something in *their* terms, and you never see them do what they say that you should have done. I had such contempt for writing those things. Every day we had to turn in something in format form. One day I was called in and told, 'You are in serious trouble' because there weren't two pages, but I knew that they were bullshit!"

Cathy reflected what many nursing students expressed—the fear of being herself with patients and submitting that experience in a form that did not seem to aid in learning what she desired.

"I think that the IPRs (interpersonal records) were important in reverse maybe. I learned to listen carefully but only so that I could remember what to write down. That makes you forget your own natural responsiveness. It tied me up with what I was going to say that would sound okay on paper. I learned that wasn't the way for *me* to improve. I got to the point that I turned stuff in to the instructor and behind the scenes talked to patients in the way that I wanted to."

Students are also aware that when they have close interpersonal contact with the faculty, the probability of their being "listened to" is heightened. Unlike cricital periods of growth in early childhood, later developmental levels find persons having considerable capacity to verbally articulate their internal reactions, their opinions of external influences, and what they perceive to be helpful to them in integrating new and old experiences. Simply having the faculty accessible is not enough. Having someone appreciate their verbal capacity to contribute to their own growth process is what students also say they want. Several criteria in evaluating whether an instructor is useful emerge from student commentary: Will that person allow, encourage, and respect my unique needs for feedback at a particular time in my struggle to be competent?

Some students state that someone's indiscriminately "watching over your shoulder" and "making irrelevant comments afterward" is sheer terror if that is not what they, the students, perceive as helpful at the time. These same students are, however, able to delineate specific situations in which direct observation of their work is perceived as necessary or what they would rather have had the instructor require or request.

CASE IN POINT

Maggie, an assertive, self-reflective student nurse, sought consultation because she was furious with one of her instructors. She wanted to work out ways to confront her with what she wanted in supervision without "blowing up."

"I was humiliated with Jonesy standing over me while I was trying to help the doctor start the IV. So I never did the real procedure before with a patient and a doctor; but we practiced in lab and I had a good picture in my mind of it. Besides the doctor had done it before, and he would have been willing to help me. If it had gone well, it would have been kind of neat to tell Jonesy about it; maybe she didn't trust me to tell her if it didn't, but I would have. When I did my first catheterization of Mrs. ____, I wanted her there. I know that it sounds funny, but I was scared that I wouldn't recognize the urethra if it was staring me in the face."

Interrelated with wanting a visible faculty who allow personal expression of what would be the most helpful method of external evaluation, students want to trust that the feedback obtained as a result of observation or self-report will be focused on the specific issue about which they are the most concerned. "Other things" that their instructors pick up on are viewed as observations that need to be made. However, these other observations can be perceived by students as irrelevant or picky if the student's primary concern is not given major focus. Students are also quick to clarify that they need as much help defining their strengths as they do those areas in which they feel weak.

CASE IN POINT

Jo-Ellen was ecstatic about what she thought to be a top-notch feedback conference after what she considered a tough, observed patient interview.

"What a kick to have someone tell you that responding in such and such a way was excellent. So much of what I hear back is 'You should have done this and that.' I have had some instructors act as if teaching is totally telling you how you could improve. I think that I have arrived at confidently doing a number of things. It makes my day when someone else thinks so too. Now when someone points out something that I did well that I didn't have the slightest idea that I was good at, it makes my whole week."

Less easily articulated is student sensitivity to (1) the degree of confidence they have in feedback from certain faculty and (2) the general spirit with which any feedback is given. Apparently, their mentors can do all the right things mechanistically with both students or patients but can leave students feeling as though they "put people down." One student remarked, "I want my supervisors to know that I won't always like what I hear. Somewhere in between my coming off like a dumb bunnie and a snot, I have a *me* inside that I'm trying to hang onto and give a boost: *that's* what I want respected when someone tells me how I need to shape up. Why does anyone have to be condescending about it?" Those instructors that seem to embody most of the student's positive appraisal and with whom they feel most comfortable are those who

(1) are open to both observation and feedback about their own functioning and (2) convey an attitude that they themselves are continuous learners, needing the students to enhance their own learning/helping process.[13]

The bird's-eye view of student desires for feedback in their learning to carry out a helping process is impressive in its similarity to what patient wants and desires seem to be: like all human beings, beginning helpers want to be individualized, neither over-estimated nor underestimated; they want someone they respect to guide their work and be available for direct and indirect feedback that is "right on." They want to be able to trust that realistic feedback will be given in ways that leave them with a sense of integrity and dignity. Highly uncomfortable and uncertain but having substantial notions of what would feel helpful, students want to be listened to. They want educators who are able to understand their frame of reference.

Obviously the student/teacher dyad is an analogous microcosm of the process variables important in any helping process. Without the students' having the opportunity to contribute their input to the teacher/learner helping process, the teacher runs a high risk of missing the students' frame of reference and losing their respect. It seems an incredible task for student or teacher or both to attempt to apply humanistic helping principles with patients if they have been violated in the learning process. Related to wanting a professional feedback person with whom to learn experientially is the desire of beginning helpers for opportunities to find out more about the personal characteristics of the group to which they aspire. They want to know if their mentors are role playing or "for real." Many young health-care workers (as well as older professionals) are unconvinced that one has to be one way at work and another at home. Most are seeking to learn just how congruent or real one can be across all spheres of social interchange. Beginners' questions about older professionals seem to be "What are they 'really' like?" "How can I be like that person if I like what I see?" and "How can I avoid becoming like that if I am repelled by what I see?"

CASE IN POINT

John, a psychology student, was hanging around outside the faculty office rather sheepishly. I wondered what he was about, since he always was forthright about what was on his mind. Perhaps he wanted to talk about a couple of jobs that he was applying for. He had been a little down because no one was putting out the red carpet for anyone any more, much less new graduates. Imagine my surprise when he wanted to talk about *me* and the observations he had made about me as a person. He was apologetic, and I was uncomfortable as he struggled to explain that he had always observed me to take a briefcase home, that I seemed bushed lately, and that he had heard by the grapevine that my marriage was rocky. Newly married, he wondered if that was something that he could prevent from happening to him. Initially I recoiled inside, wondering if it were any of his business. "I don't need your concern; I'll tell you when I do," I thought to myself; but he wasn't trying to help *me,* I realized. He was trying to help himself, and to do this he had to check out my reality—something I had always stressed with the students, and he was doing it! I laughed inside at that simple insight. Jestingly I told him that, if I ever saw him carry a briefcase home at night, I would flunk him. He was not sure exactly what I meant, and we talked a long time about being a "human professional."

As in the other preceding examples, John was struggling with his occupational group membership *and* his entire sense of personal identity. This is all part of the normal phase of early adulthood. It happens to patients and to helpers; but the struggle seemed formidable to John at this point in his educational path, when there seemed to be a more serious crossroad of personal and professional values. John's lengthy conversation revealed that he considered it critical to obtain some answers firsthand from someone whom he identified with professionally but had reservations about as a personal model. He needed to sort out some personal questions: "Am I to infer that I must carry work home every night? May I not have as much time to spend with my wife as I should like? Do I *have* to do these things along with all the other shifts that I have willingly made to become a competent, respected member of this profession?"

Jesting with John about flunking him if he carried home a briefcase was more than flippant. It was a serious commentary to sensitize John to the fact that he did not have to do anything. He could decide if he wanted to take work home at night. If he decided to do so, it should represent something other than a burden over which he felt no control. He was essentially on his own at that point, having passed all the external hurdles and being about to obtain the official credentials of his profession. Anxiety provoking as it might be, he had a responsibility to pursue what his self-system told him and, in the process, to set aside his imitation of others and his reliance on the power that he had attributed to his "gods." Unless students experience the realness of their mentors, imperfect as they may be, a critical aspect of what is to be learned about the helping process is unfulfilled: there is no mechanical way to be like another. We are all ultimately ourselves.

Beginning Helpers Tend To Devaluate Critical Thinking

It is no surprise and quite normal that, irrespective of professional discipline, beginning helpers experience phases of being more outer-directed—that is, reliant on external feedback during critical periods in their aspiration to become one of their professional group. As we have seen, these periods are marked by a high degree of personalization about their own functioning and a strong need for others to be skilled in humanistically evaluating them. However, beginning helpers do not simultaneously perceive themselves as having or needing analytic evaluative process abilities as critical elements of their own repertoire of helping skills. They tend to deemphasize or overlook them completely.

This blind spot is dramatically exemplified in recorded survey contacts with multidisciplinary groups asked to explain their role in the total schema of patient care. As if tightly holding to the desire to help in some diffuse way, beginning health-care workers more frequently than not were caught up in abstract verbiage about what they did. They described what they saw themselves responsible for in ways that did not discriminate one profession's role from that of another. This might be a heartening theme if one were looking for signs of potential for interdisciplinary effort, but that was not the significance of these responses.

Most significant were the responses that they did not give. In the content analysis of expressed role functions, less than 10 percent of the students—beginners and advanced—utilized descriptive terms that even vaguely approximated the concept of evaluation (for example, assessment, appraisal, analysis, diagnosis, problem solving, and planning). Even beginners in the medical profession—historically geared toward a diagnostic/evaluative model—rarely mentioned evaluation of patient, family, milieu, or team functioning as a part of their role. In general, the content of student perception of their role suggested (1) absence of positive value ascribed to evaluative functions (internal or external) and (2) that, in spite of their more outer-directed efforts, students are somehow not receiving or hearing feedback from others in the form of defined operations that guide them to act in a comfortably autonomous or interdependent team fashion.

The following examples of role-function concepts are from a random sample[14] of responses given by both male and female students of nursing, medicine, physical therapy, and social work who had had a minimum of one year's clinical work with patients. To emphasize the overlapping responses, they are deliberately not labeled as to what profession each represents.

Q: *What is your role in the total schema of patient care?*
A: To be aware of everything.
    Medical treatment—sometimes emotional support.
    My role is to be close to patients and listen to their needs as well as to facilitate helping action.
    Doing the most that I can for the individual patient within my limits.
    Doing what the physician orders.
    Delineating the role of disease and coordinating referral for help.
    To be aware of all the surroundings that affect the patient directly and indirectly.
    I am a necessary part of patient care, both psychologically and physically. Priority should be given to medical care, then nursing care, then to my role.
    Part of the team to improve the patient's health.
    Assessment and treatment of individual and/or family functioning and coordination of resource systems.
    Treating the patient in modes that I am capable of, including listening and explaining what I am doing and answering other questions when I can and may.
    Total patient care!
    To get the patient back home in as normal a condition as possible.
    Firsthand care—responsibility, respect for individual feelings, kindness, teaching, interpersonal communication, sincerity, helping, and caring.
    To facilitate understanding and treatment of patients and their families who need my service.

Ferreting out reasons why something does *not* seem to be occurring is often more difficult than comprehending why something is happening. That students overlook their own evaluative capacities or cannot translate them into action terms or both is complex to understand. In spite of their heightened awareness of what is going on around them and their ability to say what they want, they seem unaware of these underdeveloped human potentials. That these evaluative functions are deliberately negated or not seen as necessary by educational instructors is too simplistic an explanation and, in reality, does not seem to be the case. Older professionals working directly with students perceive themselves as more than adequately emphasizing the evaluative mode in their teaching and are mystified as to why their emphasis does not "take."

CASE IN POINT

One faculty member from a large baccalaureate school of nursing was given general feedback as to the content analysis of her group's responses to the question: "What is your role in the total schema of patient care?" She was shocked that only 5 of the 38 students expressed role behaviors that even remotely correlated with the concept of evaluative function.

"I think that all we have talked about the past year is assessment, determining goals, problem solving, and other evaluative functions. It's almost unbelievable. After all that, it's discouraging."

Although by no means presuming to understand fully how young students perceive the concept of evaluation, we will explore some of the factors that may be influencing deemphasis of an evaluative posture. As an initial basis for understanding, the recent sociocultural transformations and their influence on behavior seem most apparent. Even though beginning students are maturing adults at the time that they enter their clinical years, they are recently children of our culture and deserve evaluation within that context.

As much as there is in common between the old and the young, our impression is that, regardless of sex and professional discipline, beginning students are found to "think differently" from older health-care workers. We think that that impression makes developmental sense for some obvious reasons. For example, in reflecting on the fact that a person early develops internalized evaluative skills, we have to acknowledge that these abilities, if they are to be fully actualized, depend highly on the context in which they are experienced—that is, actualization of evaluative skills depends on how much they are needed and valued and how one is responded to when utilizing them. Cultural transitions of the past 20 to 30 years have devalued critical thinking processes. This kind of atmosphere denies young persons valuable skills applicable in all problem situations. As a result, every new situation can come to be viewed as a completely new phenomenon, requiring solutions to be found in tools or guides external to oneself.

Through a host of interacting variables in contemporary life, children in increasing numbers are observed to gradually relinquish their own creative appraisal and reliance on their own growing judgment. Consider (1) the increasing number of parents whose life circumstances preclude them from working through this exciting, though time-consuming, growth process of their children or those parents who simply say that they do not know how;[15] (2) massive television input that can quickly substitute for individual evaluation and challenging, problem-solving thought; (3) educational settings at all levels in which is presented "the" only way to think, feel, and behave and in which knowledge is offered in such a way as to leave the learner with the impression that everything has already been discovered;[16] and (4) the significant advance of group peer pressures to be "in" at all costs.

A further aspect of our times that affects old and young alike is the ease with which certain problems have been solved as a result of technological advances, leading to the myth that solutions can be brought to bear on all problems instantly;[17] for example, living in a "penicillin culture," wherein drugs are seen to quickly take care of historical scourges of humankind, has one kind of implication for what comes to supplant the critical ingredients of many helping encounters. Just as importantly, such advances have to be viewed as to their impact on critical thinking processes in general, specifically as to how much effort people are willing to make in deriving alternative solutions to problems that "take time."

Beginning health-care workers in the 1970s and 1980s whose development has been influenced by the aforementioned factors have a high chance of evolving with a different sense of the meaning of *problem,* how they feel about identified problems, and what should be done about them.

CASES IN POINT

A junior baccalaureate nursing student was asked to describe some of her most difficult times in "getting with" patients.

"One of the hardest things for me, when I first started, was to realize that people aren't always willing to talk openly about themselves. It's not like the TV med shows. Some of those shows are pretty real, but you get the whole deal in an hour—a big messy problem and a happy or sad ending all in one swoop. Real-real is someone's just not talking or being delirious and your not being able to make rhyme or reason out of it. At that point I want to give up. It just blows my mind when somebody can't get where I'm at."

A first-year social-work student was discussing why he went into a helping field. His manner was forceful and tinged with anger.

"I want sheer power to try to beat down the system. I want my people to get a fair shake!"

When asked about which specific aspect of the system he was going to take on, he said that he was not sure. Primarily he emphasized "for openers, letting more of us into the field." When further asked what his people were telling him they wanted him to help them do, he began to quote what some of the leaders of his ethnic group were saying. I asked him how he was getting along in being helped to evaluate what his clients were saying they wanted. He initially was angry at the question but he thoughtfully responded, "That's a big problem so far. Some of my own people don't want what they should. My instructors don't seem to dig that."

In our discussions with well-functioning older professionals, it is apparent that they have come to value their own evaluative abilities highly. Many are keenly aware that beginners need these well-honed skills to carry with them as a valuable tool in defining and evaluating health-care problems; yet, they too seem to have a blind spot. This is particularly evident in their verbal expression and the educational programs for which they are responsible that fail to acknowledge that young persons of the past two decades have had to struggle to hang onto evaluative abilities or simply give up early to let someone or something else come up with the answers.

To have to think on one's feet and depend on one's own resources in an earlier era when not so many external supports were available contributed much to the positive value placed on self-reliance. Developmentally, self-reliance happened earlier in the lives of those who are now older professionals. It allowed self-reliant evaluative skills to become incorporated into one's frame of reference about oneself and others. However, experiencing forces that contribute to a more passive-recipient, conforming set of behaviors when one is 25 or 50 years of age is a different developmental story from experiencing these forces when one is 5 or 15. Factors in recent history that older professionals could integrate with their already developed evaluative abilities seem to have influenced the younger generation differently. How difficult it is to appreciate the frame of reference of a younger group within a field in which there is so much vital commonality of motive, but it is a group that has come to think in significantly different ways.

Some Implications for Educators

We hold that, early in the educational experience of beginning health-care workers, both students and educators need to be highly sensitive to a phenomenon wherein feelings, ideas, and internal evaluative, critical thinking abilities lie dormant as a result of being culturally underfed or underappreciated, or both. We also propose that, unless specific humanistically oriented educational experiences occur within which students can come to value and trust the potential of their own internal capacities, these will not be perceived as valuable clinical judgment skills that helpers must carry with them as they increase distance from the externally provided input of instructors and supervisors.

We have observed that those helpers who do not trust or value their own internal evaluative abilities have a difficult time trusting patients to use their strengths of self-reliance and responsibility. For beginning health-care workers to become humanistic helpers working from an advocacy base, we believe that educators must become models of advocacy for their own students. We believe that educators must do mutual goal setting with groups of students and individual students. We know that this practice will alter many traditional educational programs as new values and new ways of approaching problems come to the fore. To embark on such an endeavor, older professionals must make a vigorous commitment to get close to students personally, sharing their own evaluative abilities and creative experiences in order to turn students on to their own possibilities.

In this process of understanding students' frame of reference, we suggest that health-care workers of all age groups remain sensitized to the following factors:

1. Because beginning students have grown up within the context of self-diminishing sociocultural factors, taking a chance on one's own feelings, ideas, and internal evaluative skills may be one of the *least practiced* behaviors that a student brings into the field.[18]

   For some students, the educational experience must heighten awareness of dormant skills and their critical value in providing safe, effective humanistic help. For others, experiences may have to be specifically devised within which students can take the first steps in developing a more trusting, self-reliant mode of thinking through new and complex situations. Students who already have reflective, self-evaluative abilities available to them require experiences to enhance further growth.

2. Having long experienced personal evaluation within educational settings as "something that happens at the end of the quarter" that judges one by another's standards, students tend to attach highly ambivalent feelings to any concept implying evaluation, assessment, analysis, or any other judgmental processes. This ambivalence can result in a backlash when students are expected to value the evaluative process and utilize it with others.

   When students express conflict about whether it is appropriate to make value judgments or state that evaluation of a patient is picking someone apart and somehow unfair, it is often a reflection of their own uncomfortable history of perceiving the process to be a negative experience. Students are also aware that much, if not most, of the evaluation carried out about them has been derived from examination results, attendance records, and other nonpersonal, paper-and-pencil products. These methods provide little modeling experience in being evaluated as a total person within an interpersonal process. Students simply may not know where to start formally evaluating another in the humanistic way that they believe is deserved.[19]

3. Aspects of preclinical and clinical education do teach methodical, analytical problem-solving skills. However, for students who are concerned with humanistic values and know that they need to understand human experience, many contemporary evaluative methods miss the boat. Within this mode, methods of assessment are (a) generally defined as needing to "meet the rigors of science" and (b) stressed within the context of experimental design as emphasized in the "hard sciences" (for example, mathematics, chemistry, and physics). Assessment skills taught only via an experimental laboratory model can confuse health-care students who know that they do not have the option to control whom they will care for, as do laboratory scientists who control the material with which they work.[20] At the same time that a health-care student is experiencing hard-science course work, subjective feelings, clinical

evaluation, and human-oriented judgments are often downgraded as involving a fuzzy art or are referred to as *soft science.* In combination, these factors can result in students' perceiving an analytical, evaluative process as a mechanical, add-on splinter skill that is not comprehensively sound to use with human beings; or students may come to perceive that a process of analysis applies only to certain materials, to the exclusion of others.

Overall, educational programming for health-care workers requires a high degree of scrutiny as to the potential for eroding the value placed on evaluative methods. Educators who sniff at soft science and retreat from the need to teach a critical thinking process to be applied to humanistic problems might better stay within an area of functioning in which devaluation of the student's primary task is not visible to new learners. At the same time, health educators who claim to teach from humanistic objectives have to be careful that they are neither so vague as to provide the student with no structure nor so structured as to develop sterile, meaningless objectives.[21]

4. Historically, in attempting to integrate behavioral science into clinical education, health-care faculties initially relied on Freudian theoretical formulations. Characterized primarily by hindsight evaluation of limited aspects of a person's life, Freudian approaches provide students with little skill in coping with right-now problems. The Freudian framework also strongly emphasizes a disease model and subtly nurtures an evaluative attitude of looking for pathology. To the degree that clinical evaluation stresses only pathological behaviors, students will tend to focus on what they do not yet know or think that they should know. If an evaluation process that focuses on the total person, including strengths and potentials, is highly valued and taught, students tend to feel more comfortable. This approach allows them to appraise health—a concept with which students are initially more familiar.[22]

5. Finally, if educators are to become more sensitive to the needs of "student society" and devise humanistic experiences accordingly, they simultaneously must be selective in choosing applicants for their programs. Student applicants are young adults with most of their character traits already established. Some already have a rigid, narcissistic value set so that no amount of humanistic higher education will essentially alter their view of life or how they will continue to relate to other human beings. Educators must be prepared, therefore, to define the "kind of person" they believe will develop into an intelligently safe and humanistic health-care professional and seek only such candidates in the admission process. Students in general do not like to face such an evaluation hurdle, which clearly reflects that "many are called, but few are chosen." However, most experienced educators in any of the professions hear the well-known reality in Glick's comments regarding higher education in health care:

> Unfortunately, medical training can disillusion and render cynical even some quite decent students, but rarely can it convert a basically self-centered and egotistic person into a humanitarian. Such a goal would strain almost any educational system.[23]

Summary

Health-care workers from a variety of disciplines have the tenacious value of wanting to help others. Throughout the course of their growth and development as adults, there appear to be three critical periods of uncertainty and internal change about what holding to this value means. These periods seem to be marked in part by a high degree of self-focus, even though the ultimate direction of concern is that of patient care. Roughly, these periods seem to be (1) when beginning students are struggling to perceive themselves as competent and are concerned that they will be seen as such by patients and discriminating professionals; (2) when older students wonder whether, as members of the profession, they can find a position that satisfies both personal and professional values; and (3) when middle life brings personalized recognition of mortality, which heightens the seasoned professional's sensitivity to whether enough time is left to be everything that one had hoped.

Health-care workers seem to have more awareness at a young age that something about the nature of intrapersonal and interpersonal experience is critical for becoming an effective person and professional. Although both beginning and older professionals agree that one learns by experience, the younger generation seems more keenly aware and more verbal about the need to alter their educational experiences in order to legitimatize the interpersonal experience that they desire. They do not want to develop desirable abilities on the side. They also want the mystery taken out of understanding and meeting patients at their own level.

Highly critical and often harsh and demanding behind the scenes, beginning and older students alike tend to be superficially conforming. As they come closer to the end of their educational experience, one sees more of this. As a group, professional students are hardly revolutionary in pressing their ideas about what they want for themselves and their patients—a characteristic that may be unfortunate in view of the humanistic values at stake. That they are not more individually or collectively assertive is understandable, however. Students easily recognize that they have limitations to their power within the educational system similar to those of patients within the vast health-care system. Keenly discriminating about whom they can be open with and trust not to label them in negative ways, students are aware of needing to play both sides against the middle to stay within the ranks of their respective disciplines. Lest students continue to take enforced roles similar to that of patients, or simply burn out, health-care education faculty need to take the first major step in freeing up the rich resources that students can bring to bear on humanizing health care. That innumerable older professionals recognize and advocate for student concerns in activizing ways is an encouraging trend.

Several other messages are clear, particularly with respect to the potential for learning an interpersonal helping process. If beginning health-care workers of any discipline are to regard others positively, be congruent, and develop capacities for empathic evaluation, (1) these qualities must be highly regarded in selecting applicants to health-care programs in addition to grade-point considerations and (2) preclinical and beginning clinical students must see humanistic values operative in their educational life space. Aspirants to the helping professions must be able to experience these behaviors with others besides patients. They must be able to experience humanistic interaction with those with whom they initially identify and seek to emulate.

We believe that, alongside our marvelous technology, time and space exist in all health-care settings for caring what happens to people, respecting and accepting their feelings, and helping all participants in the culture to grow. We believe that this kind of humanism is possible regardless of the rank or experience of the persons who come together in the name of health. However, this humanism will not happen by osmosis or by relying on theory alone. This humanism of which we speak is not a wishy-washy feeling state or limited to platitudes in books. It is action, motivated by deep respect for one's own and another's full range of feelings and the meaning about life that is being communicated to one another. Making this kind of humanism visible takes hard work—work in the form of an internal, intrapersonal evaluation process and in the form of willingness to take interpersonal risks.

This kind of advocacy-oriented humanism in behalf of oneself and others will not emerge by consumers' waiting for health-care personnel to act or by students' waiting for educators to offer it, or by staff helpers' waiting for administrative mandates. Whoever is concerned has the right to speak out and demand a humanistic existence in the health-care field. Where are any of us going if we do not?[24]

REFERENCE NOTES

1. Mayeroff states, "To care for another person, in the most significant sense, is to help him grow and actualize himself" (p. 1). "In caring as helping the other grow, I experience what I care for (a person, an ideal, an idea) as an extension of myself and at the same time as something separate from me that I respect in its own right" (p. 5). See Milton Mayeroff, *On Caring* (New York: Harper & Row, 1971). We like Mayeroff's book and recommend it. However, we did not think that the term *caring* would be as useful to carry through the text as the term *helping*.

2. In response to a request to the pediatric nursing instructor for feedback about this episode, she wrote on the margin of the journal entry: "This is not an immature feeling that you describe. It is feeling as humans must feel for other humans if we really believe the things that we say we believe. As we get more experience, we may have more perspective or be able to use our inner resources more advantageously to help us through these situations without developing an external sadness; but we can't stop feeling."

3. Arthur W. Chickering, *Education and Identity* (San Francisco: Jossey-Bass, 1969). Particularly helpful is part I, in which Chickering discusses the young adult's struggles with achieving competence, managing emotions, becoming autonomous, establishing identity, clarifying purpose, and developing integrity. See also John Janeway Conger, "A World They Never Knew: The Family and Social Change," *Daedalus* 100 (1971): 1105–38. This article is concerned with contemporary family/adolescent struggles in the process of becoming adult.

4. Kenn Rogers, "The Mid-Career Crisis," *Saturday Review,* Feburary 1973, pp. 37–38. An excellent article for review is Roger L. Gould, "The Phases of Adult Life: A Study in Developmental Psychology," *American Journal of Psychiatry* 129 (November 1972): 33–43. Gould's study speaks of the ages of 16 to 18 years signaling to young people the motto "We have to get away from our parents"; a shift occurs between the ages of 22 to 28 years, at which time individuals believe that what they are doing is the true course to follow in life. A further shift is observed between the ages of 29 to 34 years, when people feel weary of devoting themselves to the task of being what they are supposed to be and want to be what they are. A middle-aged phenomenon was noted in ages 35 to

43, when existential questioning about self, values, and life continued but with a tone of "quiet desperation and an increasing awareness of a time squeeze" (see pp. 37–38). Gould's work for the public market is excellent and useful for patients to read as well: *Transformations: Growth and Change in Adult Life* (New York: Simon & Schuster, 1978).

5. A particularly well-written and dramatic portrayal of a man's experience in becoming a professional can be found in David S. Viscott, *The Making of a Psychiatrist* (New York: Fawcett Books, 1973).

6. Chickering, *Education and Identity*, pp. 320–45.

7. Organized nursing has formally taken the lead in integrating psychiatric and behavioral-science concepts throughout the clinical aspects of nursing education curricula. That nursing educators were serious about integrating humanistic approaches into the curricula is evidenced by the federally supported grants that developed in the late 1950s and early 1960s to support curriculum study and implementation. However, private correspondence with several project directors of such integration studies suggests that variable resistance to full faculty acceptance of integrated behavioral science material beyond lip service was encountered. The medical profession continues to struggle with the status of behavioral science in their curricula. See George L. Engel, "The Best and the Brightest: The Missing Dimension in Medical Education," *The Pharos* (October 1973): 129–33. It is interesting to note that nursing faculty early moved ahead in espousing interdisciplinary education. See Madeleine Leininger, "Interdisciplinary Health Education for the Future," *Nursing Outlook* 19 (1971): 787–91.

8. Steven Muller, "Universities Are Turning Out Highly Skilled Barbarians," *U.S. News and World Report*, 10 November 1980, pp. 58–59.

9. Seymour M. Glick, "Sounding Board: Humanistic Medicine in a Modern Age," *New England Journal of Medicine* 34, no. 17 (23 April 1981): 1038.

10. Student-centered teaching is by no means a new concept; the materials are all available for its inception. As an example, see Samuel Tenebaum, "Student-Centered Teaching as Experienced by a Participant," in *On Becoming a Person*, ed. Carl R. Rogers (Boston: Houghton Mifflin, 1961), pp. 297–313. See also Sidney Jourard, "Fascination and Learning-for-Oneself," in *Disclosing Man to Himself* (New York: Van Nostrand Reinhold, 1968), chap. 10. The University of Wisconsin began experimenting with an independent study program in the medical school in 1974.

11. *Superordinate goal* is a term coined by Sherif and Sherif in the mid-1950s. It has the unique quality of being a commonly desired goal that cannot be ignored by group members and that cannot be attained by the resources and efforts of one subgroup alone. See Muzafer Sherif and Carolyn W. Sherif, *Outline of Social Psychology* (New York: Harper & Bros., 1956), p. 330.

12. The "critical period" hypothesis has been around for some time in the field of developmental psychology. During critical periods, behavioral processes of a particular nature seem to proceed most rapidly; that is, there are optimal times for the formation of primary social attachments or for certain kinds of learning. Erik Erikson uses a critical period model in his theory of human personality development. See Erik H. Erikson, *Childhood and Society* (New York: Norton, 1950). For an excellent by-line on Erikson, see Erik Erikson, "The Quest for Identity," *Newsweek*, 21 December 1970, pp. 84–89.

13. Hildebrand studied the opinions of both faculty and students at the University of California concerning effective professors. Items most often checked regarding good teachers included "invites criticism of his own ideas," "contrasts the implications of various theories," and "is valued for advice not directly related to the course." For a summary, see "Grading the Profs," *Human Behavior*, November 1973, p. 33; or Milton Hildebrand, "The Character and Skills of the Effective Professor," *Journal of Higher Education* 44, no. 1 (1973): 41–50. See also Maxine Greene's *Teacher as Stranger* (Belmont, Calif.: Wadsworth, 1972).

14. Random sampling refers to a procedure in selecting subjects (or, in this case, responses) that allows chance alone to determine which subjects or responses from the whole population are to be selected. This procedure is used so as not to allow the bias of the experimenter (or writer) to influence which subjects or responses to use.

15. In our experience with individual parents and groups of parents who have sought assistance in "managing" their children, the prevailing difficulty, as acknowledged by the parents themselves, is their lack of self-confidence in knowing the "right" thing to do and acting on their own best judgment. In further exploring what they would like to do, we find that most parents are not really off base; they seem not to know what they know or find it difficult to take risks with their own ideas or both.

16. Any of John Holt's writings speak to this situation repeatedly. See John Holt, *Escape from Childhood* (New York: Dutton, 1974).

17. See Alvin Toffler, *Future Shock* (New York: Random House, 1970). Required reading for any student or faculty member.

18. Dressel's research on critical thinking abilities of college students was distressing in the late 1950s and still is. See Paul L. Dressel, "On Critical Thinking," in *Evaluation in the Basic College at Michigan State University*, ed. P. L. Dressel (New York: Harper & Bros., 1958).

19. Arthur W. Chickering, *Education and Identity* (San Francisco: Jossey-Bass, 1969). See particularly chapter 10, "Curriculum, Teaching, and Evaluation," pp. 196–219.

20. A. R. Feinstein, "What Kind of Basic Science for Clinical Medicine?" *New England Journal of Medicine* 283 (1970): 847–52.

21. Instructors of any of the health-care disciplines are referred to Arthur J. Combs, "Educational Accountability from a Humanistic Perspective," *Educational Review* (September 1973): 19–21.

22. Freud has advanced the most comprehensive and profoundly influential theory of human behavior. Everyone who works in a person-oriented field utilizes varying degrees of insights from his massive work, sometimes without realizing it. It is not a matter of being pro-Freudian or anti-Freudian; the task is to appreciate what his formulations have to offer and some of his pitfalls in appreciating the total human. Freud based his theories on his work with mental patients. He focused primarily on historical, recalled early experience information about his patients. He was a "reductionist" in the sense of hoping to find that human behavior could be reduced to chemical and physical dimensions. Social implications of his theories (generally ignored by Freud himself) evolved later by those called neo-Freudians (for example, Harry Stack Sullivan). There are formulations concerning human behavior other than Freud's. For an excellent resource by which to evaluate the philosophical underpinnings of the integrated behavioral-science concepts in any health-care curriculum, see Frank Goble, *The Third Force: The Psychology of Abraham Maslow* (New York: Pocket Books, 1971). Of particular interest are chapters 1 (concerning historical perspectives) and 14 (regarding mental health).

23. See Glick, "Sounding Board," p. 1038.

24. An excellent companion piece to *Future Shock* is a very salient book by Alan Gartner and Frank Reissman, *The Service Society and the Consumer Vanguard* (New York: Harper & Row, 1974). The single most useful book to tie together the vast social changes and obtain a picture of the impact on all aspects of life—particularly health—is Marilyn Ferguson's *The Aquarian Conspiracy: Personal and Social Transformation in the 1980s* (Los Angeles: Tarcher, 1980).

Annotated Glossary

The following glossary defines terms that have been used throughout the text. As is apparent, certain concepts lend themselves better to succinct definition than do others. Complete texts have been written concerning the nature of some. To assist students wishing to pursue the meaning of the terms further, additional references are included.

ACTUALIZATION A term suggested for greater realization of the potentials of human existence than is usual (Bugental). Maslow explains that all definitions of actualization accept or imply (1) acceptance and expression of the inner core, or self—that is, realization of these latent capacities and potentialities, "full functioning," and availability of the human and personal essence and (2) minimal presence of ill health, neurosis, psychosis, or loss or diminution of the basic and personal capacities.

    J. F. T. BUGENTAL *The Search for Authenticity* (New York: Holt, Rinehart & Winston, 1965), p. 263.

    ABRAHAM H. MASLOW *Toward a Psychology of Being*, 2d ed. (Princeton, N.J.: Van Nostrand, 1968), p. 184.

ANXIETY A variable pattern of interacting fundamental emotions. Anxiety is a natural phenomenon that a person experiences in the face of threat to values essential to existence, sense of being, and identity. Izard hypothesizes that anxiety includes fear and two or more of the fundamental emotions of distress—for example, anger, shame (including shyness and guilt)—and the positive emotion of interest/excitement. Clinical anxiety may be expressed by many observable behaviors; yet, each person has a characteristic way of feeling anxious. A person may variably express a feeling of vague uneasiness, apprehension, or impending doom, as if disintegrating, or "falling to pieces." Somatic behaviors involve increased tension of skeletal muscles or changes in the cardiovascular and gastrointestinal systems. Not all anxiety indicators are felt or consciously experienced.

> CARROLL E. IZARD   *Patterns of Emotions: A New Analysis of Anxiety and Depression* (New York: Academic Press, 1972), p. 47.

> ISIDORE PORTNOY   "The Anxiety States," in *American Handbook of Psychiatry*, ed. Silvano Arieti (New York: Basic Books, 1959), vol. 1, pp. 307–23.

ATTITUDE   A relatively enduring organization of interrelated beliefs held by persons that describe, evaluate, and advocate options with respect to an object or situation. Attitudes show variation between individuals and cultures. Although attitudes can be changed, they are relatively resistant to alteration. They cannot be directly observed but must be inferred from motoric expressions, verbal statements of opinion, or physiological changes because of exposure to the object of the attitude.

> MILTON ROKEACH   *The Nature of Human Value* (New York: Free Press, 1973), pp. 17–19.

> G. D. WILSON   "Attitude," in *Encyclopedia of Psychology*, ed. H. J. Eysenck (New York: Herder & Herder, 1972), vol. 1, p. 95.

AUTONOMY   In the general sense, the term refers to the maintenance of the integrity of the subjective experience of the self—for example, to resist certain external pressures, to make decisions based on internalized standards, and to persist in certain behaviors that have helped over time in coping with life's difficulties (Bonner). It is a complicated term, since "too much" autonomy—behavior completely unregulated by external influences or behavior overdetermined by highly unique internal values—is often seen in psychotic episodes or acts of crime. "Too little" autonomy can lead to overreliance on the willfulness of others and confusion about one's sense of individuality (Jahoda). It is a highly personalized experience, yet intricately involved with prevailing social values.

> HUBERT BONNER   "Autonomy," in *A Dictionary of the Social Sciences*, ed. Julius Gould and William L. Kolb, compiled under the auspices of UNESCO (New York: Free Press, 1964), p. 46.

> MARIE JAHODA   "Mental Health," in *The Encyclopedia of Mental Health*, ed. Albert Deutsch and Helen Fishman (New York: Watts, 1963), vol. 3, p. 1070.

BELIEF   Rokeach defines belief as "any simple proposition, conscious or unconscious, inferred from what a person says or does, capable of being preceded by the phrase 'I believe that . . . .' " The content of a belief may *describe* an object or situation as true or false, *evaluate* it as good or bad, or *advocate* a certain course of action as desirable or undesirable. Beliefs are central to the concepts of attitude and value. They are considered intellectual operations that predispose one to visible action.

> MILTON ROKEACH   "The Nature of Attitudes," in *International Encyclopedia of the Social Sciences*, ed. David L. Sills (New York: Macmillan, 1968), vol. 1, p. 450.

COPING   Lazarus defines two classes of coping: (1) action tendencies aimed at eliminating or mitigating the anticipated harmful confrontation that defines a threat and (2) purely cognitive maneuvers through which appraisal is altered without action directed at changing the objective situation (for example, defense mechanisms). Allport describes the purposes of coping as the following: to fulfill needs and to find safety, love, self-respect, freedom from worry, opportunities for growth, and ultimately a satisfying meaning of existence.

GORDON W. ALLPORT   *Pattern and Growth in Personality* (New York: Holt, Rinehart & Winston, 1961), p. 262.

RICHARD S. LAZARUS   *Psychological Stress and the Coping Process* (New York: McGraw-Hill, 1966), pp. 258–59.

CULTURE   The traditional, or learned, ways of behaving that become established in an on-going social group (Spencer). In addition to the socially standardized behavior—actions, facts, feelings—of some enduring group, culture also involves the material products of, or aids to, the behavior of that group (Honignann).

JOHN J. HONIGNANN   *Culture and Personality* (New York: Harper & Bros., 1954), p. 22.

KATHRYN SPENCER   "Introduction," in *Socio-Cultural Elements in Casework* (New York: Council on Social Work Education, 1969), p. 5.

DEFENSE   A mental operation that functions unconsciously and has as its goal the reduction of threat to self-esteem and the resulting felt anxiety. Defenses reduce threat by denying its existence, altering its meaning, or diverting its emotional impact (Korchin). Defenses take a number of forms in guarding against self-blame and unpleasant or disagreeable memories or in concealing unacceptable impulses, desires, or beliefs. Examples of defenses are repression, rationalization, denial, projection, displacement, reaction formation, sublimation, dissociation, and conversion.

SHELDON J. KORCHIN   "Stress," in *Encyclopedia of Mental Health*, ed. Albert Deutsch and Helen Fishman (New York: Watts, 1963), vol. 6, pp. 1977–78.

PHILIP POLATIN   "Mental Mechanisms," in *Encyclopedia of Mental Health*, vol. 4, pp. 1156–59.

DEVIANT   Generally, behavior or a condition (physical or psychological) that falls beyond the bounds of what is expected. Since society and subcultures within society frequently vary from one to another and further change over time, the definition of behavioral deviance is tentative, culture bound, and time bound.

RUTH BENNETT AND ELIZABETH SANCHEZ   "Psychopathology or Deviance, Treatment or Intervention?" in *Psychopathology*, ed. Muriel Hammer et al. (New York: Wiley, 1973), pp. 77–78.

LEONARD P. ULLMAN AND LEONARD KRASNER   *A Psychological Approach to Abnormal Behavior* (Englewood Cliffs, N.J.: Prentice-Hall, 1969), p. 6.

ECLECTIC   A term derived from the Greek *eklektikos,* meaning "selective." Eclecticism refers to the practice of choosing ideas, suggestions, and therapeutic procedures from different systems of fact without necessarily accepting the whole system from which certain parts are drawn. In everyday practice, it refers to a commitment to being guided by what is the most effective help for patients, in contrast to devotion to any particular theoretical doctrine.

JOEL FISCHER   "An Eclectic Approach to Therapeutic Casework," in *Interpersonal Helping*, ed. Joel Fischer (Springfield, Ill.: Charles C. Thomas, 1973), pp. 321–22.

EMOTION   A complex set of behaviors that may be experienced in various combinations: (1) as felt experience that is private to the individual, is experienced in a characteristically distinct way, so that the individual can verbally label and recognize it but that is difficult to communicate verbally, as one can communicate thought; (2) as a visceral response that involves smooth muscles and the autonomic nervous system, sometimes felt and describable and sometimes not consciously experienced; and (3) as an overt motoric response, involving large skeletal muscles or facial, postural, and gestural reactions (Peters). Izard states that the fundamental emotions are interest, joy, surprise, distress, anger, disgust, contempt, shame (shyness and guilt), and fear. Others acknowledge love as a basic emotion. Combinations of emotions can result in other sets of complex behavior (for example, anxiety and depression). No one seems to speak about what sexual feelings are. In attempts to describe the subjective experience of emotions, people often use group or highly individualistic slang terms that convey greater meaning than those used in textbooks.

CARROLL E. IZARD   *Patterns of Emotions: A New Analysis of Anxiety and Depression* (New York: Academic Press, 1972), p. 2.

HENRY N. PETERS   "Affect and Emotion," in *Theories in Contemporary Psychology*, ed. Melvin H. Marx (New York: Macmillan, 1963), pp. 435–46.

ETHICS   A branch of philosophy concerned with moral rights and obligations and the nature of commendable behavior or character. Ethical theory systematically explores the characteristics of beliefs, value judgments, and the general principles that justify their application. Ethical values and behaviors differ from one culture to another and from one historical period to another. Individually, ethics may vary with age, maturation, and the degree to which a person is controlled by, or free from, conflict.

MAURICE LEVINE   *Psychiatry and Ethics* (New York: Braziller, 1972), pp. 46–47.

M. REINHARDT   "Ethics," in *Encyclopedia of Psychology*, ed. H. J. Eysenck (New York: Herder & Herder, 1972), vol. 1, p. 336.

EUSTRESS   A term coined by Selye to describe positive stress. In deriving this word, Selye employed the Greek prefix *eu*, meaning "good," as is in *euphoria*.

HANS SELYE, INTERVIEWED BY LAURENCE CHERRY   "On the Real Benefits of Eustress," *Psychology Today* 11, no. 10 (March 1978): 63.

EXISTENTIALISM   The doctrine that states that existence precedes essence. Sartre describes this as meaning that people first of all exist, encounter themselves, and surge up in the world, defining themselves afterward. It emphasizes the capacity to become aware of one's existence, which distinguishes human beings from the rest of nature; and it implies that one can respond to the fact of one's own existence and thus exercise some responsibility for it (May and Basecu).

ROLLO MAY AND SOBERT BASECU   "Existential Psychology," in *International Encyclopedia of the Social Sciences*, ed. David L. Sills (New York: Macmillan, 1968), vol. 13, p. 76.

JEAN-PAUL SARTRE   "Existentialism," in *Existentialism from Dostoevsky to Sartre*, ed. Walter Kaiymann (New York: Meridian Books, 1956), pp. 288–91.

GESTALT   Gestalt is a German word that refers to a pattern or to the particular form of organization of the parts that go into a configuration. Gestalt psychology maintains that human nature is organized into patterns or wholes, that it is experienced by the individual in these terms, and that it can be understood only as a function of the patterns, or wholes, of which it is made. The gestalt view is that the whole is different from the sum of its parts and can never be understood from the study of its parts alone. Gestaltists maintain that the parts can never be thoroughly understood until after the meaning of the whole has been discovered.

FRANZ ALEXANDER AND GLENN W. FLAGG   "The Psychosomatic Approach," in *Handbook of Clinical Psychology*, ed. Benjamin B. Wolman (New York: McGraw-Hill, 1965), p. 858.

FRITZ PERLS   *The Gestalt Approach and Eye-Witness to Therapy* (Palo Alto, Calif.: Science & Behavior Books, 1973), pp. 3–4.

HEALTH   A long-established definition of *health* is that of the World Health Organization: "Health is a state of complete physical, mental, and social well-being and not merely the absence of disease or infirmity." Objectively, this definition fits well the meaning intended in this text. In practice, how one determines when someone is in a complete state of physical, mental, and social well-being raises problems. There may be wide discrepancies between the objective and subjective views of this state of being. A more sociological definition of *health* is the state of optimum capacity of individuals for the effective performance of the roles and tasks for which they have been socialized (Parsons).

TALCOTT PARSONS "Definitions of Health and Illness in the Light of American Values and Social Structures," in *Patients, Physicians, and Illness,* ed. E. Gartly Jaco (New York: Free Press, 1958).

WORLD HEALTH ORGANIZATION *Constitution of the WHO* (Geneva: The World Health Organization, 1946).

HEALTH CARE Organized health care as perceived by professionals consists of four major components: (1) maintenance and promotion of health, (2) prevention of disease, (3) cure of disease, and (4) rehabilitation to social usefulness. Health care as perceived by consumers is what they do to take care of themselves. This is influenced by such characteristics as lifestyle, beliefs, attitudes, personal health habits, and willingness and ability to use formal health-care services.

JOHN D. GRANT *Health Care for the Community* (Baltimore: Johns Hopkins University Press, 1963), p. 48.

MONROE LEARNER "Health as a Social Problem," in *Handbook on the Study of Social Problems,* ed. Erwin O. Smigel (Chicago: Rand McNally, 1971), pp. 299–300.

HEALTH DELIVERY SYSTEM A system organized and designed to make health-care services directly available to individual persons. Achieving these ends entails a massive supportive organization and structure that includes persons engaged in hundreds of occupations, both professional and nonprofessional.

ARNOLD REISMAN AND MARYLOU KILEY, EDS. *Health Care Delivery Planning* (New York: Gordon & Breach, 1973), p. 28.

RUSSELL G. MAWBY "Innovation: Key to Better Health," *Hospitals* 47, no. 1 (1973): 32–34.

HELPING (INTERPERSONAL) Interpersonal helping can be described as informed, purposeful intervention either directly with, or on behalf of, a given person or persons (clients). The goal of such intervention is to bring about positive changes either directly in the clients' functioning or in environmental factors immediately impinging on the functioning. These interventions are intended to enhance aspects of the clients' feelings, attitudes, or behaviors, or all three, in such a way that their personal and social functioning will be more satisfying and beneficial to them (Fischer).

JOEL FISCHER "Introduction," in *Interpersonal Helping,* ed. Joel Fischer (Springfield, Ill.: Charles C. Thomas, 1973), p. xvii.

HUMANISM The view of human beings that insists that they are best seen as they normally see themselves. The individual is seen as a conscious agent with a sense of willfulness who functions as an integrated whole. Humanism starts with the assumption that people have dignity simply because of their existence and that to strip them of that dignity is to degrade them so outrageously that we call that degradation inhumane.

IRVIN L. CHILD *Humanistic Psychology and the Research Tradition: Their Several Virtues* (New York: Wiley, 1973), pp. 13, 15–16.

ALBERT ELLIS *Humanistic Psychotherapy* (New York: Julian Press, 1973), pp. 1–2.

HOWARD MUMFORD JONES *American Humanism: Its Meaning for World Survival* (Westport, Conn.: Greenwood Press, 1957), pp. 101, 103.

INTELLIGENCE A controversial concept about which there are many definitions. Generally, intelligence is described as a collection of cognitive abilities—for example, (1) the ability to reason or to think abstractly, (2) the ability to learn or to profit from experience, (3) the capacity to adapt, and (4) the capacity to solve problems (Wechsler). Intelligent behavior is thought to require all these abilities. In addition, it is dependent on such ingredients as drive, persistence, motivation, and goal awareness. An even broader definition of intelligent behavior would include acknowledgment of its relationship to the individual's capacity to perceive and respond to moral, aesthetic, and social values.

J. MCV. HUNT *Intelligence and Experience* (New York: Ronald Press, 1961), p. 362.

PHILIP E. VERNON "Ability Factors and Environmental Influences," in *The Causes of Behavior*, 2d ed., ed. Judy F. Rosenblith and Wesley Allinsmith (Boston: Allyn & Bacon, 1966), p. 386.

DAVID WECHSLER "Intelligence: Definition, Theory, and the I.Q.," in *Intelligence: Genetic and Environmental Influences*, ed. Robert Cancro (New York: Grune & Stratton, 1971), pp. 50–55.

INTERVIEW A planned verbal transaction between two or more persons. The purpose of an interview is to give and get information about a specific topic in a way that furthers understanding through obtained facts and perceptual interpretation (that is, the view of each about the topic at hand). Effective interviews involve openly spelled out transactions: the motives of both parties in undertaking the interview and stipulations about the consequences of the interview for each. Interchange within the process of the interview per se is dependent on the situation in which an interview is taking place, subject matter discussed, the ability of each to appreciate the frame of reference of the other, and the ability of both parties to put facts and feelings into communicative actions that are clearly understood by the other.

LOUIS BERNSTEIN AND RICHARD H. DANA *Interviewing and the Health Professions* (New York: Appleton-Century-Crofts, 1970).

ROBERT L. KAHN AND CHARLES F. CANNELL "Interviewing," in *International Encyclopedia of the Social Sciences*, ed. David L. Sills (New York: Macmillan, 1968), vol. 8, p. 149.

INTROSPECTION The observation and analysis of one's own mental state and activities, or asking another to use these methods to get an idea of conscious experience. Thus, people's reports of their own feelings, thoughts, decisions, and fears involve introspective data.

BENJAMIN B. WOLMAN "Clinical Psychology and the Philosophy of Science," in *Handbook of Clinical Psychology*, ed. Benjamin B. Wolman (New York: McGraw-Hill, 1965), pp. 12–13.

MOTIVATION A process of arousing and sustaining action in dynamic interaction with the process of regulation and direction of behavior; for example, energy transformation from bodily structures interacts with goals, attitudes, interests, and aims to mobilize activity that is in some sense selective. Since the process of motivation is difficult to see in a concrete sense, one determines its presence by the goals toward which behavior seems to be directed and the quality of the action taken to achieve those goals.

ABRAHAM H. MASLOW *Motivation and Personality*, 2d ed. (New York: Harper & Row, 1970).

NEUROSIS A clinical diagnostic term utilized to describe a defensive life-style designed to exclude from consciousness certain classes of subjective experience and mental content. The goal of this behavior is to reduce experienced tension and anxiety. Various forms, or styles, of such behavior are described—for example, obsessive/compulsive, paranoid, hysterical, and impulsive styles (Shapiro). Neurotic behaviors may be present in varying degrees; in general, they retard full development of intellectual abilities, affect, and involvement in new experiences.

SILVANO ARIETI, ED.   *American Handbook of Psychiatry*, vol. 1, part II, "The Psycho-
neuroses and Allied Conditions" (New York: Basic Books, 1959), pp. 235–417.

DAVID SHAPIRO   *Neurotic Styles* (New York: Basic Books, 1965), pp. 196–98.

NORMAL   Technically, a statistical concept meaning that a given human trait, such as physiological or psychological patterns of one kind or another, falls within some accepted range
of variability. The measures to obtain a profile of "normal" may be from random or selected
samples of the general population. When an individual's characteristics are compared with
those estimated to be true of the general population, "normality" means some approxima-
tion to what seems to be true of the total population. The term also has connotations of a
state of being relatively free of psychological and physical difficulties; that is, some persons
referred to as *healthy* are called *normal.*

PERSONALITY   Little agreement is found on the definition of *personality.* In 1937, Allport
listed some 50 definitions. More recent surveys describe at least 15 approaches. One way of
looking at personality is that it is the dynamic organization within individuals of those interrelating systems that determine their characteristic or distinctive thought and behavior (Allport). *Systems* here is meant to signify a person's biological drives, cognitive and physical
attributes, values, sentiments, interests, and other traits as they operate consciously and unconsciously. Personality is thought of as evolving during the process of development and
maturation (Sullivan).

GORDON W. ALLPORT   *Pattern and Growth in Personality* (New York: Holt, Rinehart &
Winston, 1961), p. 28.

HARRY STACK SULLIVAN   *Personal Psychopathology* (New York: Norton, 1972), pp. 47–48.

PHENOMENOLOGY   The descriptive science of pure experience without intended theoretical or
practical applications (Beloff). The phenomenological approach is to examine an object or
situation as it appears to the senses, as it is experienced, or as it is symbolized. It is the study
of what a person experiences or perceives about something else; such study does not demand
that pure experience fit any known law or "truth."

JOHN BELOFF   *Psychological Sciences: A Review of Modern Psychology* (London: Crosby
Lockwood Staples, 1973), p. 63.

PHILOSOPHY   The formal study of knowledge, particularly general principles that furnish the
rational explanation of anything. Out of philosophy, formalized bodies of knowledge (for
example, the sciences) have emerged. Philosophy, like science, is neither pure speculation
nor pure logical analysis. Both activities go on. Philosophers, as differentiated from sages,
submit their speculations to the discipline of critical thinking.

JEAN PIAGET   *Insights and Illusions of Philosophy* (New York: World, 1971).

PSYCHOSIS   A clinical diagnostic term used to describe complex behavior characterized by
thought disorder and actions deemed inappropriate to a norm of social reality. As a behavioral complex (syndrome), it can be temporary or relatively enduring. Many psychotic syndromes are classified as *functional,* referring to a status of no known causes originating
within the nervous system. Psychotic behavioral manifestations may also accompany inter-
ference with brain function and may be observed secondary to infection, trauma, senility
changes, and alcohol or drug intoxication (or sensitivity). Clinically, the traditional criteria
for diagnosing psychosis involve the presence of the following characteristics:

1. Difficulty with orientation as to identity, time, and place
2. Expression of emotions that do not coincide with the reality of the context as perceived by
   others

3. Expression of thought that is not immediately intelligible as expressed verbally, not relevant to ongoing events, and not connected in terms of the sequence of the conversation
4. Faulty memory function for recent or past events or both
5. General behavior in relation to people and things in the environment seemingly determined by overpersonalized reference points exclusively within oneself and not easily correctable by outside input to the contrary; often, but not always, expressed in delusions, hallucinations, or misinterpretation of reality as others experience it
6. More or less pervasive substitution of behavior from earlier levels of development

SILVANO ARIETI, ED.   *American Handbook of Psychiatry*, vol. 1, part III, "The Functional Psychoses," pp. 419–563, and vol. 2, part VIII, "Organic Conditions," pp. 1003–1316 (New York: Basic Books, 1959).

PSYCHOTHERAPY   The literal translation is treatment of the mind. More broadly, psychotherapy refers to a systematic learning process with individuals (or groups) in which the concern is for learning new aspects of oneself, new ways of relating to others, and new ways of behaving (Rogers). Measures are psychotherapeutic if they are achieved through their relationship with, or behavioral impact on, another, as contrasted with physiological measures (for example, drugs and mechanical treatments).

CARL R. ROGERS   "Some Directions and End-Points in Therapy," in *Psychotherapy: Theory and Research*, ed. O. Hobart Mowrer et al. (New York: Ronald Press, 1953), p. 66.

JOHN G. WATKINS   "Psycho-therapeutic Methods," in *Handbook of Clinical Psychology*, ed. Benjamin B. Wolman (New York: McGraw-Hill, 1965), pp. 1143–44.

RAPPORT   The feeling of confidence, trust, and harmony that is established between two or more persons in an interpersonal relationship—a feeling of which both parties are aware.

BARRY M. BROWN   "The Multiple Techniques of Broad Spectrum Psychotherapy," in *Clinical Behavior Therapy*, ed. Arnold A. Lazarus (New York: Brunner/Mazel, 1972), p. 175.

JAMES C. COLEMAN   *Abnormal Psychology and Modern Life*, 3d ed. (Glenview, Ill.: Scott, Foresman, 1964), p. 565.

ROLE   In general, a role represents the behavior expected of the person who occupies a given position or status in society (Sarbin). It is a concept basic to understanding the social systems of groups and an individual's psychosocial development. Developmentally, adequate role learning involves generally knowing how one is expected to act by others and having considerable awareness of how others are going to behave in complementary situations. Role behavior is often consciously expressed. At times, but not always, it is consciously felt. Certain role behaviors may not always feel congruent with one's inner sense of identity. One may "play" a role to cope with a difficult situation temporarily, is in contrast to "taking" a role.

THEODORE R. SARBIN   "Role: Psychological Aspects," in *International Encyclopedia of the Social Sciences*, ed. David L. Sills (New York: Macmillan, 1968), p. 546.

EDWARD STAINBROOK   "Society and Individual Behavior," in *Handbook of Clinical Psychology*, ed. Benjamin B. Wolman (New York: McGraw-Hill, 1965), p. 219.

STRESS   A variably used term denoting anything from an engineering-science phenomenon to its colloquial use in describing "nervous strain." It is not nervous strain. Selye defines *stress* as the nonspecific response of the body to any demand placed on it both internally and externally. Stress-producing factors are technically called *stressors*. Stressors are not necessarily causative of damage (see *eustress*). Whether the agent is pleasant or unpleasant is immaterial; the effects of stressors highly depend on the intensity and duration of the adaptive demand placed on the body, as well as one's perceptions of any given situation.

RICHARD S. LAZARUS   *Psychological Stress and the Coping Process* (New York: McGraw-Hill, 1966).

HANS SELYE   *The Stress of Life* (New York: McGraw-Hill, 1956).

HANS SELYE   "The Evolution of the Stress Concept," *American Scientist* 61 (1973): 692–93.

SYSTEM   A complex unity formed of many, often diverse, parts subject to a common plan or serving a common purpose; a set of units combined by nature or art to form an integrated, organic, or organized whole—an orderly working totality; or a group of bodies moving together in an interrelated pattern or under the influence of related forces or attractions (Iberall). A systems view of reality is described by von Bertalanffy as a perspective philosophy. He states that science is one perspective of reality in retracing some of its formal aspects; others are derived from art, music, religion, and other fields. Von Bertalanffy views the systems approach as giving some answers to the question of meaning, "which is nothing else than connections within a whole or system."

ARTHUR S. IBERALL   *Toward a General Science of Viable Systems* (New York: McGraw-Hill, 1972), p. 7.

LUDWIG VON BERTALANFFY   "System, Symbol and the Image of Man," in *The Interface Between Psychiatry and Anthropology*, ed. Galdston Iago (New York: Brunner/Mazel, 1971), p. 117.

STYLE   A form, or mode, of functioning—the way, or manner, of a given area of behavior—that is identifiable in an individual through a range of specific acts (Shapiro). There are body movement styles that come to be identified with a particular person; the ways in which one thinks or perceives may also be of a particular form, or style.

DAVID SHAPIRO   *Neurotic Styles* (New York: Basic Books, 1965), p. 1.

THERAPEUTIC   The prevention or treatment of disease by techniques (for example, drugs, mechanical devices, and vaccines) or the influences of a person or both. Inherent in this definition is the notion that what is therapeutic makes an obvious difference, or change. Even when specific disease is not involved, measures are said to be psychotherapeutic if they are achieved through an interpersonal relationship or behavioral impact on the one being "treated," as contrasted with physiological measures.

VALUE   A value is a special form of belief within one's total belief system about (1) how one ought to behave or (2) the end state of existence, which is or is not worth attaining (Rokeach). Values can also be defined as things or acts that are chosen by and desirable to an individual or society within a certain frame of reference (von Bertalanffy). Values cannot be seen but are inferred from people's behavior—what they attach value to, what they say that they believe in, and the choices that they make under varying conditions. Values may be consciously felt and capable of being articulated or may be unconsciously held. Psychologically, values serve to clarify the purpose and meaning of life, setting standards of culturally acceptable behavior. Given a variety of opportunities on which to act, values can be viewed as guideposts against which one evaluates directionality and risk taking (Menninger).

KARL A. MENNINGER WITH PAUL W. PRUYSER   "Morals, Values, and Mental Health," in *Encyclopedia of Mental Health*, ed. Albert Deutsch and Helen Fishman (New York: Watts, 1963), vol. 4, pp. 1244–45.

MILTON ROKEACH   "The Nature of Attitudes," in *International Encyclopedia of the Social Sciences*, ed. David L. Sills (New York: Macmillan, 1968), vol. 1, p. 554.

LUDWIG VON BERTALANFFY   "The World of Science in the World of Value," in *Challenges of Humanistic Psychology*, ed. James F. Bugental (New York: McGraw-Hill, 1967), p. 336.

Appendix A

Interdisciplinary Questionnaire

INTERDISCIPLINARY QUESTIONNAIRE

The purpose of this open-ended questionnaire is to assist in exploring how students in the "helping professions" perceive the process of help.

Your responses will not be shared with instructors; compiled data will become the basis for a written overview of where students in various disciplines "are at" when they are beginning to work directly with patients in clinical settings.

Thank you.
Jane Chapman, Ph.D.

1. Area (check one): nursing _____ medicine _____ physical therapy _____
   social work _____ other _____

2. Level of education thus far: _____

3. Have you started to work with patients yet? Yes _____ No _____
   a. If yes, how long have you been working with patients? _____

   b. If no, when will you begin clinical practice? _____

4. Age: _____ Sex: male _____ female _____

5. When you were a child, what did you want to be when you grew up?

   _____

INTERDISCIPLINARY QUESTIONNAIRE (*Cont'd.*)

6. When you are thinking of approaching a patient to offer some kind of help, what is your first thought?

7. According to your educational experience what could happen to help you learn or handle your interactions with patients most effectively?

8. How much right do you think that patients have to direct what will be part of their treatment?

9. When patients learn that they are going to be hospitalized, what do you think is uppermost in their minds?

10. When patients learn that they are to be recipients of your professional services, what do you think is uppermost in their minds?

11. Please list the four most important factors that you believe influence hospitalized patients.

    a. _____

    b. _____

    c. _____

    d. _____

12. If you wanted to get to know a patient, where or from whom would you get the information?

13. In the schema of total patient care what is your role?

14. Which of the preceding role functions do you believe is the most important aspect of your intervention with a patient?

15. Do you prefer an inpatient or outpatient setting in which to practice? (check one)

    a. Inpatient _____ Why? _____

    _____

    b. Outpatient _____ Why? _____

    _____

16. Have you ever been hospitalized? Yes _____ No _____

    a. If yes, for what? _____

    b. For how long? _____

INTERDISCIPLINARY QUESTIONNAIRE (*Cont'd.*)

17. Have you ever had a serious illness for which you were not hospitalized?
    Yes ____ No ____

    a. If yes, describe: _____

18. With whom of the following do you prefer to work now (or eventually) (check one):

    a. Adults ____ Why? _____

    b. Children ____ Why? _____

    c. Undecided ____

Appendix **B**

Letter of Resignation

Dr. Blank
Director, Psychiatric Division
XYZ Hospitals

Dear Dr. Blank:

I hereby submit my resignation from the psychiatric division of the XYZ Hospitals to be effective at the earliest possible date.

This I do because of my conviction that the administrative system within the psychiatric division, since it acquired such large powers in early 1971, has set out on a disastrously regressive course of medical authoritarianism. I believe that this system is entirely against the best recent developments in American mental-health science and that it has impaired and will more impair staff morale and training as well as interagency coordination and cooperation. Also I believe that the system has already had a substantially bad effect on the quality of patient care and will have an even worse effect as time passes. Accordingly, I wish to separate myself from such a system as quickly as I can.

In the hopes of being taken more seriously and at the risk of being misunderstood, I believe that I had better do something that I have never considered doing before. This is to make some point of my professional position. I believe that I speak as the senior clinician of the division, not only in terms of variety of experience and of postgraduate training, but also in terms of number and significance of contributions to knowledge within the field. I speak also as one who has never sought power save that of one voice in a cooperating group and as one who has had a major academic career, which I forsook because of my conviction that the most important future developments would come in the community sector. When I made this decision, I chose to work in the XYZ system because my analysis indicated that it represented the most advanced model in the field. I still believe that the future of American mental-health science lies in the community area, and I believe that XYZ Hospitals with its neighborhood health centers does have the most advanced delivery system in the field. However, I have lost all confidence in the quality of care that, hindered and injured by an outdated administrative structure, can be developed in the XYZ system. What is the system that has come to disappoint me so?

Let us look first at what are the most significant recent developments in the field and then review the present administrative practices in that light. As I see it, after the psychotropic drug developments of the late 1950s, the most significant progress in the past ten years has been in three main areas:

1. Chiefly through the efforts of psychologists focused on learning theory, there has been a great simplification and clarification of the previously dominant Freudian theory. The pruning away of the dense and obscure overgrowth of Freudian theory has resulted in a much more lucid and easily grasped group of concepts, the essence of which is that mental maladjustments and the bad feelings that are their by-products are produced by faulty attitudes consequent to unfortunate experience. The field then shifted to its present focus of developing better techniques for more speedily, accurately, and powerfully changing these attitudes. Action techniques, revitalized psychodrama, and fearlessly experimental confrontations that use the clinician as a totally open humanist are some of the great improvements to which the field has come; and many subdisciplines (nursing, occupational rehabilitation, recreational therapy, and others along with psychology and psychiatry) have had large and, I judge, about equal parts in developing this new technology.*

2. These technical advances have been accompanied by, and have really initiated, crucial changes in organizational structures within the mental-health field. Psychotherapeutic techniques became no longer the particular province of the psychiatrist but were shared at least equally by many other subdisciplines. Thus came about an equalization of disciplines, with each having its particular expertise and its general contribution. The psychiatrists, with their medical background, have the particular competence of drugs and somatic treatments. The

*The physician who authored this letter uses the term *technology* in a different sense than that utilized in this text. *Technology* as we have used it involves those material products of science in health-care practice in the form of equipment, chemicals, and mechanistic procedures.

psychologists have the particular strengths of projective testing, advanced theory, and research know-how. All the other subdisciplines, such as nursing, recreational therapy, social work, and vocational counseling, have their particular subspecialty strengths; and all these subdisciplines have in equal strength the general contribution of the new psychotherapeutics. This new reality resulted inevitably in a sharing of power, an interdependent cooperativeness. Any decision regarding a patient's care became not the final province of the traditional authority, the psychiatrist, but rather a composite, reflecting the contributions of all the many, now coequal, subdisciplines that have been developed and found necessary for the speedy and effective resolution of problems as complex as mental difficulties. This process of subdiscipline equalization led, in other words, to a great democratization of organizational process within the mental-health field. In this development, the field was greatly guided by Lewin's work and its subsequent development at the Harvard Business School, the National Training Laboratory, and the Organization and Communication Center of the Massachusetts Institute of Technology. This work demonstrated that only for the most static and simple problems does the traditional authoritarian model furnish the best mechanism for problem resolution. The more complex the problem and the more subsystems that need to be involved in its resolution, the greater the need for a non-authoritarian, democratic, or consensus-seeking process. This latter model has come to be seen as particularly appropriate in mental health, in which field, as was the theme of a recent University of Wisconsin conference on the new hospital psychiatry, "medicus rex" is dead. However, I understand that this new development has also come to be increasingly accepted and practiced in the more complex and advanced sectors of the business community.

3. Of course, the most important consequence of these developments for the mental-health field has been improved ways of helping people. This is what it is all about. Here the shift, as would be expected, has been to group action that involves patients as greatly responsible and empowered members of a therapeutic community. Patients have come to be distinguished only as having less training in the resolution of psychic problems, for which resolution they need to be speedily and accurately schooled. This schooling is done by the cooperation and egalitarian group interaction of patients and representatives of all the mental-health subdisciplines. This is best done in a climate of fearless sharing in which professionals reveal themselves as human above all else and in which they are, if you will, basically patients with more advanced training, who become most effective when they can share their personal, as well as professional, experiences with the resolution of psychological problems; and the process depends a great deal on the identified patients' getting a variety of much repeated feedback from various experience levels and in a variety of styles and phrasings about their behavior (attitudes really) as they reveal themselves in such groups. These groups, then, are characterized by openness and by the fearless authenticity of individuals working to create a composite and rich mix of subdiscipline know-how and personal experience.

Now how has the psychiatric division's system related itself to these developments? Before its acquiring the vastly extended powers that it got in January of 1971, the present system, although evidencing little, if any, effective awareness of these newer developments, nevertheless tolerated their existence and their application in many sectors of the division. Perhaps it did this because it needed the strength of their representatives for the great struggle in which it was so long engaged with the central administrative organization of the XYZ Hospitals. In any event, since that struggle was resolved and motivated by I know not what fears, it has moved rapidly in a most unhealthy direction. It has flagrantly asserted the traditional "superiority" of the psychiatrists and has moved to place members of this subdiscipline in positions of increased authority whenever possible. It has come to the open undoing of policy previously established by cooperating groups and to the archaic practice of government by the arbitrary dictum of titular authority. It has positioned itself against such concepts as openness and spontaneity in groups involving the training of professionals. In short it has embarked on an invidious reinforcement of an antiquated status quo that flies in the face of the best recent learning, that impairs interdisciplinary cooperation, and that guarantees an inferior product in terms of patient care. Indeed, I believe that the present system actually contributes to the worst psychic disease of our time, the alienation of human beings one from another because of a deadly cycle of pride, force, fear, and pride.

All this is serious enough, but I must go further. To paraphrase that old maxim of Lord Acton's, it seems that the more inappropriate the power, the speedier the corruption; and already disturbing signs of corruption within the present system are appearing. Not only is there such a climate of fear that even the leaders of the most established and successful elements are feeling a deep sense of disquiet and disappointment, but also there are more gross matters, such as the suppression of appropriate group communications, cruel and unusual punishment for dissent (for example, by abrupt and isolating transfers and by the use of ridicule and coercion), and even such matters as the apparent rewriting of performance evaluations.

Such considerations as these have greatly hastened my departure from this regressive system. I believe that they explain why the overall rate of resignations within the division has stepped up so substantially. Others, as I know, are not in a position that would permit them to go with the appropriate protest that they would like to make. Fortunately I am in such a position. This increases my responsibility to them and to the clients, who are the main sufferers from an inferior system that is going backward.

I must, therefore, protest as strongly as I can at the same time that I depart with all reasonable dispatch.

Very truly,
John Doe, M.D.

Appendix **C**

Understanding Narcissism: A Key to Coping with a Complex Behavior

Some behaviors encountered by helpers do not fit into the usual diagnostic categories or models of personality theory. In part, this is because our contemporary culture has contributed to the development of new forms of character disorders, and our experience with these syndromes precedes documentation. For example, some writers have termed the 1960s and 1970s the "me" culture, leading to the development of what is called the "new narcissism."

In working with a disordered patient population characterized by social deviance and substance abuse, the most difficult personality disorder to work with successfully is the narcissistic character disorder. To understand and effectively intervene in the behavior of these persons, one must understand the roots of narcissism and child-development theory. Following are a few developmental concepts about narcissism. These concepts are important to understand in working with adults who remain narcissistic in their basic orientation:

1. All human beings are born with a primary narcissistic orientation. At birth, infants are thoroughly egocentric (self-centered), overwhelmed by physiological and emotional needs that can be met only by the adults in their life space. There is no way

for infants to act in their own behalf except to cry (or scream) in response to felt discomfort (hunger, pain, being cold).

2. Narcissistic infants begin to comprehend that others exist in their life space as they gradually differentiate between external and internal experience. The process of differentiating that there is a "you" and a "me" shows outward evidence at approximately two to two and one-half years of age when the child begins to actively rebel against parent guidance and wishes and when language expands to include such words as "me do," "you do," and "I do."

3. During the critical period from birth to three years of age, if the child is parented poorly (neglected and/or abused or extremely indulged), the primary narcissistic position can solidify and prevent the appropriate gradual growth and development into secondary narcissism.

4. Primary narcissism is a normal, valuable characteristic of the young infant and child. It is survival in the earliest development of a "self" and aids in the task of differentiating oneself from others. It is an insistent drive and expresses itself powerfully as "me, me, me" at a time when the helplessness of the vulnerable child requires defense in coping with an immense and ambiguous universe.

5. How adults respond to the egocentric "me, me" messages of the young child is critical.

   a. If the child's messages are not heard by parents, the child may turn in to the self and conceptualize that "there is no one to rely on but myself," thus developing an alienated, detached style (as seen in neglected children).

   b. If the child's messages are punished severely by parents, the child may struggle to keep trying but conclude that the self is bad or that negative attention is better than none and thus continue to seek attention at all cost (as seen in abused children).

   c. If the child's messages are too quickly rewarded and all narcissistic demands met, the child may develop a "power trip" of demanding, never able to perceive a reciprocity with others, insisting on receiving, no matter what the circumstances (as seen in the overindulged immature child with whom parents are fearful to draw lines and face the narcissistic wrath when the child is disallowed anything).

6. Shifting to a secondary narcissistic process is essential to healthy older childhood and adult development. Characteristics of secondary narcissism are:

   a. Appropriate retention of concern for self and having confidence that certain self-directed behaviors will fulfill one's needs without total reliance on others—that is, *learning to do for oneself.*

   b. Knowing that one can ask others (without insistent demanding) to help one out once in a while and that help will be received—that is, *learning to ask.*

   c. Appreciating that giving to others is the other side of the coin in learning to survive well in the world if equity and reciprocity in relationships are to be accomplished—that is, *learning to share.*

Telltale signs of developmental retardation at primary narcissistic levels in adult behavior are:

a. Extreme emphasis on self as the center of the universe with little to no concern for others.

b. Extreme anger or withdrawal when things don't go according to their plan.

c. Vague to definitive notions that the reason for lack of success is the world's fault.

d. Resistance to comprehending that rules applying to society in general have relevance to themselves.

e. A poverty of close, intimate relationships and the inability to stay with any one partner for a sustained period of time.

Therapeutic Structures in Outpatient and Group Living Programs for Clients with Narcissistic Personality Disorders

1. People with narcissistic disorders have a self-styled view of the world in which few, if any, traditional ground rules are seen as applying to them. Therefore, expect some form of rebellion or defense against *any* rules (with passive aggression or active aggression).

2. Spell out what is expected clearly—verbally and in writing; keep all ground rules logical, reasonable, and tied to reality.

3. There is a difference between being authoritarian and oppressive in implementing ground rules versus being firm and matter-of-fact. Even if you are appropriately firm and matter-of-fact, you will be accused of being unfair and authoritarian by these clients. Few people have been straight and confrontive with these people in their life without engendering their wrath. Ride with it. Stand your ground with calm confidence. Firmness is not easy in any case, and it becomes particularly difficult if there is not staff solidarity and support in standing behind each other.

4. To help these clients get over the hump and struggle with the immaturity of primary narcissism, they need to be helped through the battle of wills that their parents were unable to healthily engage at earlier developmental levels.

5. Keep in mind that persons engulfed in primary narcissism have developed their total personality around their egocentric view; to see your point of view feels to them as if they are selling their souls or going to die if things don't go their way.

6. An eternal message to these clients must be that life is a series of options and choices, that nobody (even the helper) can have it both ways, and that nobody will drop dead for anybody in life just because they demand it. This is a tough lesson learned by healthy people beginning at age two and gradually learned through childhood. These clients have a lot of catching up to do.

7. These clients must have the opportunity to learn that there can be positive payoffs for giving up the primary narcissistic grip on their approach to problems. A good program for these clients spells out "what can happen if" and spells it out in small achievable goals leading to larger ones. The primary narcissist wants it all in one leap with no effort. Therefore, much support to "hang in there" and "keep trucking" must be given along the way. Many will rationalize that there is "big

money" or "big time" if they keep doing what they were doing. They need reminding that, if such were the case, they would not be where they are, and that most people keep a clear head so they avoid chronic social disasters.

8. Keep in mind that narcissistic clients have few friends and that their families have probably wearied of them because of their chronic inability to give and take or be concerned about the effect of their behavior on others. Program efforts should be made to foster new sharing and beginning friendship experiences—for example, group socialization, group therapy, competitive sports, group home responsibilities done on the buddy/mutual dependency system, volunteer work in the community.

9. After the rebellion stage (if effectively worked through with the client), expect moderate to deep depression. It is not easy to gain insight into what one has been doing and to give up old behavior, even if it was negative and ineffective. Frequently, there is intense guilt felt when these clients realize how much they have hurt or disregarded others and themselves during their unconscious primary narcissistic state. At this time, they need concrete suggestions and structures to help them "make up for the past" and get back with themselves and others who are still significant—for example, helping them rehearse "scripts," as they have impoverished verbal language skills in how to apologize, lend support to others, or ask directly without strong defenses or demands.

10. Help them learn new, more mature defenses—for example, sublimation or modeling healthy, successful people. They must hear the message that to be more mature does not mean being a patsy or pushover and that there are more self-productive ways to "get yours" in life than what they have been doing.

11. They need to learn that there is a fine, but important, line between assertively standing up for oneself and the insistent self-servicing that primary narcissistic people demand. One critical difference lies in the explanations clients give for themselves in evaluating situations and their feelings—for example, a client can be given support for anger and dealing directly with the boss when the boss adds tasks to a job that were not agreed on mutually. However, if a client simply "does not feel like" doing what was agreed on and becomes angry, this reaction cannot be supported.

12. Expect progress to take time.

Index